SHORT-TERM PLAY THERAPY FOR CHILDREN

Short-Term Play Therapy for Children
Second Edition

Edited by

Heidi Gerard Kaduson
Charles E. Schaefer

THE GUILFORD PRESS
New York   London

Library of Congress Cataloging-in-Publication Data

Short-term play therapy for children / edited by Heidi Gerard Kaduson,
Charles E. Schaefer. — 2nd ed.
     p. ; cm.
   Includes bibliographical references and index.
   ISBN-13: 978-1-59385-330-3
   ISBN-10: 1-59385-330-0
   1. Play therapy. 2. Children—Counseling of. 3. Family psychotherapy.
4. Child psychotherapy. I. Kaduson, Heidi. II. Schaefer, Charles E.
[DNLM: 1. Play Therapy—methods. 2. Child. 3. Psychotherapy, Brief.
WS 350.2 S5587 2006]
RJ505.P6S53 2006
618.92'891653—dc22   2006011630

*To those play therapists who continue
to strive for the psychological health of our children*

About the Editors

Heidi Gerard Kaduson, PhD, RPT-S, specializes in evaluation and intervention services for children with a variety of behavioral, emotional, and learning problems. She is past president of the Association for Play Therapy and codirector of the Play Therapy Training Institute in Hightstown, New Jersey. She has lectured internationally on play therapy, attention-deficit/hyperactivity disorder, and learning disabilities. Dr. Kaduson's publications include *The Playing Cure* and *101 Favorite Play Therapy Techniques* (Volumes I, II, and III). Dr. Kaduson maintains a private practice in child psychotherapy in Monroe Township, New Jersey.

Charles E. Schaefer, PhD, RPT-S, is Professor of Psychology at Fairleigh Dickinson University in Teaneck, New Jersey. He is cofounder and director emeritus of the Association for Play Therapy, and founder and codirector of the Play Therapy Training Institute in Hightstown, New Jersey. He has written or edited more than 50 books on parenting, child psychology, and play therapy, including *The Therapeutic Use of Child's Play, Foundations of Play Therapy, Handbook of Play Therapy, Play Therapy with Adolescents,* and *Empirically Based Play Interventions for Children.* Most recently, he is coeditor (with Heidi Gerard Kaduson) of *Contemporary Play Therapy: Theory, Research, and Practice.* Dr. Schaefer maintains a private practice in child psychotherapy in Hackensack, New Jersey.

Contributors

Alisa B. Bahl, PhD, private practice, Santa Cruz, California

Julie A. Blundon, MA, Department of Psychology, Fairleigh Dickinson University, Teaneck, New Jersey

Lois Carey, LCSW, Center for Sandplay Studies, Nyack, New York

Meena Dasari, PhD, Department of Psychology, New York University School of Medicine, New York, New York

Loretta Gallo-Lopez, MA, private practice, Tampa, Florida

Amy D. Herschell, PhD, Child and Adolescent Psychiatry, Western Psychiatric Institute and Clinic, University of Pittsburgh School of Medicine, Pittsburgh, Pennsylvania

Linda B. Hunter, PhD, LCSW, Behavioral Communications Institute, Palm Beach, Florida

Heidi Gerard Kaduson, PhD, Play Therapy Training Institute, Hightstown, New Jersey; private practice, Monroe Township, New Jersey

Susan M. Knell, PhD, Spectrum Psychological Associates, Cleveland, Ohio

Wendy Ludlow, LCSW, private practice, Bronx, New York

Sandy Magnuson, EdD, Department of Applied Psychology and Counselor Education, University of North Colorado, Greeley, Colorado

Cheryl B. McNeil, PhD, Department of Psychology, West Virginia University, Morgantown, West Virginia

Erik Newman, MA, Department of Psychology, Fairleigh Dickinson University, Teaneck, New Jersey

Scott Riviere, MSW, KIDZ, Inc., Lake Charles, Louisiana

Charles E. Schaefer, PhD, Department of Psychology and Center for Psychological Services, Fairleigh Dickinson University, Teaneck, New Jersey; Play Therapy Training Institute, Hightstown, New Jersey; private practice, Hackensack, New Jersey.

Holly E. Shaw, PhD, private practice, Austin, Texas

Risë VanFleet, PhD, Family Enhancement and Play Therapy Center, Boiling Springs, Pennsylvania

Mary K. Williams, MSW, private practice, Fayetteville, Arkansas

Preface

As managed care continues to curtail the length of treatment for children who have psychological difficulties, the importance of short-term play therapy remains paramount. Therapists are challenged by the additional stress that children encounter in a more demanding, competitive, and critical world. We have an obligation to find ways to help these children heal.

This volume is an up-to-date presentation of how to do short-term play therapy with children who have psychological problems of varying degrees. The second edition includes revised and updated revisions of some of the same chapters (children with attention-deficit/hyperactivity disorder, involving and empowering parents of disruptive children, play therapy groups for sexually abused children, and the use of play group therapy for children with social skills deficits), incorporating new treatments and techniques that have had clinical significance. Five entirely new chapters have been added detailing the use of short-term play therapy for different disorders and/or treatment pro-tocols (short-term play therapy for bipolar children, cognitive-behavioral play therapy for children with anxiety, family sandplay therapy, a behavioral/solution-focused model for enhancing play therapy with parent training, and group sandtray play therapy). Furthermore, this book also now includes different play therapy approaches to similar problems or disorders that were discussed in the first edition (release play therapy for posttraumatic stress disorder, short-term play therapy with disruptive children, short-term play therapy for families of adoptive children, and short-term play therapy groups for children of divorce).

With the increasingly large numbers of children being diagnosed with bipolar disorder, posttraumatic stress disorder, anxiety, and disruptive disorders, this second edition of *Short-Term Play Therapy for Children* was put together to enhance the therapist's abilities to treat these disorders within the continuing managed care format.

Many professionals in the mental health field find that they do not have the resources to help them work with children with severe difficulties. This book covers play therapy for individuals, families, and groups. Chapters in each of these sections provide an introduction to the specific play therapy approach, a description of the differences and difficulties found in treating the particular population, and detailed, step-by-step methods that are used to help children manage. Each of the chapters explains the protocol for the approach and includes case studies to illustrate the success of the treatment.

When doing short-term play therapy, it is beneficial to structure the treatment carefully. The prescriptive approach to treatment followed in the book allows the therapist to be able to assist the child in the healing process even though the time allotted is limited. This book provides creative and effective techniques to help play and other child therapists become more adept in brief play therapy and offer the safety, security, and enjoyment needed for children to work through their difficulties in a playful, therapeutic format with long-lasting results.

Contents

PART I

INDIVIDUAL PLAY THERAPY

CHAPTER 1

Release Play Therapy for Children with Posttraumatic Stress Disorder

HEIDI GERARD KADUSON

In order to have the proper perspective on how posttraumatic stress disorder (PTSD) affects children, one must first understand what a trauma is. A psychic trauma is an emotional shock or wound that has long lasting effects. It results when an individual is exposed to an overwhelming event and is rendered temporarily helpless and unable to use ordinary coping and defensive operations of the ego in the face of intolerable danger, anxiety, or instinctual arousal (Eth & Pynoos, 1995).

PTSD is a psychiatric disorder that can occur following the experience or witnessing of life-threatening events such as military combat, natural disasters, terrorist incidents, serious accidents, or violent personal assaults like rape. Adults who suffer from PTSD often relive the experience through nightmares and flashbacks, have difficulty sleeping, and feel detached or estranged, and these symptoms can be severe enough and last long enough to significantly impair a person's daily life.

Contemporary research on the biology of PTSD has confirmed that there are profound and persistent alterations in physiological reactivity and stress hormone secretion in people with PTSD. The brain is an analyzing and amplifying device for maintaining a person's internal and external environment (MacLean, 1988), and if emotional arousal is intense and persists, as has often been experienced by trauma survivors, the person may develop conditioned emotional and biological responses with long-term effects. High levels of emotional arousal are likely responsible for the observation that traumatic experiences initially are imprinted as sensations or states of physiological arousal that often cannot be transcribed into personal narratives (van der Kolk & Fisler, 1995).

PTSD is not a new disorder. There are written accounts of similar symptoms that go back to ancient times. Careful research and documentation of PTSD began in earnest after the Vietnam War. The National Vietnam Veterans Readjustment Study estimated in 1988 that the prevalence of PTSD in the group studied was 15.2% at that time and that 30% had experienced the disorder at some point since returning from Vietnam (Zatzick et al., 1997).

PTSD has subsequently been observed in all veteran populations that have been studied, including World War II, Korean conflict, and Persian Gulf populations, and in United Nations peacekeeping forces deployed to other war zones around the world. There are remarkably similar findings of PTSD in military veterans in other countries. For example, Australian Vietnam veterans experience many of the same symptoms that American Vietnam veterans experience (Creamer & Forbes, 2004).

PTSD is not only a problem for veterans, however. Although there are unique culture- and gender-based aspects of the disorder, it occurs in men and women, adults and children, Western and non-Western cultural groups, and all socioeconomic strata. A national study of American civilians conducted in 1995 estimated that the lifetime prevalence of PTSD was 5% in men and 10% in women (Kessler, Sonnega, Bromet, Hughes, & Nelson, 1995).

PTSD was formally recognized as a psychiatric diagnosis in the *Diagnostic and Statistical Manual of Mental Disorders*, third edition (DSM-III; American Psychiatric Association, 1980). At that time (1980), little was known about what PTSD looked like in children and adolescents. Today we know children and adolescents are susceptible to developing PTSD, and we know that PTSD has different age-specific features. Although a diagnosis of PTSD required the patient to have the symptoms for over a month's duration, a diagnosis of acute stress disorder, in DSM-IV (American Psychiatric Association, 1994), covers those children who have symptoms like PTSD, but for a duration of at least 2 days and less than 1 month.

A diagnosis of PTSD means that an individual has experienced an event that involved a threat to his or her own or another's life or physical integrity and that this person responded with intense fear, helplessness, or horror. There are a number of traumatic events that have been shown to cause PTSD in children and adolescents. Children and adolescents may be diagnosed with PTSD if they have survived natural or human-made disasters—floods; violent crimes such as kidnapping, rape, murder, or suicide of a parent, sniper fire, and school shootings; motor vehicle accidents such as automobile and plane crashes; severe burns; exposure to community violence; war; peer suicide; and sexual and physical abuse.

A few studies of the general population have examined rates of exposure and PTSD in children and adolescents. Results of these studies indicate that 15–43% of girls and 14–43% of boys have experienced at least one traumatic event in their lifetimes. Of those children and adolescents who have experienced a trauma, 3–15% of girls and 1–6% of boys could be diagnosed with PTSD (Giaconia et al., 1995; Cuffe et al., 1998).

Rates of PTSD are much higher in children and adolescents recruited from at-risk populations. The rates of PTSD in these at-risk children and adolescents vary from 3 to 100%. For example, studies have shown that as many as 100% of children who witness a homicide of a parent or sexual assault develop PTSD (Kilpatrick & Williams, 1997). Similarly, 90% of sexually abused children (Hamblen, 2004), 77% of children exposed to a school shooting (Ackerman, Newton, McPherson, Jones, & Dykman, 1998), and 35% of urban youth exposed to community violence develop PTSD (Margolis & Gordis, 2000).

Certainly not all children develop PTSD. There are, however, many factors that have been shown to increase the likelihood that children will develop PTSD:

- Quality of pretrauma attachment relationships and overall adjustment
- Amount of social support (the more, the better)
- Type of disaster (human-made disaster leads to more PTSD than natural disaster)
- Human aggression (abuse, etc., leads to more severe symptoms of PTSD)
- Degree to which trauma is life-threatening (the less, the better)
- Parents' reactions (the less distressed, the better)
- Degree to which primary attachment figures are available and supportive
- Communication (the more open, the better)
- Cumulative stressors (the fewer, the better)
- Degree of exposure (the more direct the exposure, the more likely PTSD)

In general, children and adolescents who report experiencing the most severe traumas also report the highest levels of PTSD symptoms. Family support and parental coping have also been shown to affect PTSD symptoms in children. Studies show that children and adolescents with greater family support and less parental distress have lower levels of PTSD symptoms. Finally, children and adolescents who are farther away from the traumatic event report less distress (Pynoos et al., 1987).

In terms of gender, several studies suggest that girls are more likely than boys to develop PTSD (Pfefferbaum et al., 1999, 2000). A few studies have examined the connection between ethnicity and PTSD. Although some studies find that minorities report higher levels of PTSD symptoms, researchers have shown that this is due to other factors such as differences in levels of exposure. It is not clear how a child's age at the time of exposure to a traumatic event impacts the occurrence or severity of PTSD. Some studies find a relationship; others do not. Differences that do occur may be due to differences in the way PTSD is expressed in children and adolescents of different ages or developmental levels (Vernberg & Varela, 2001; Shelby, 1997).

Researchers and clinicians are beginning to recognize that PTSD may not present itself in children the same way it does in adults. Criteria for PTSD now include age-specific features for some symptoms (DeWolfe, 2001; Pynoos & Nader, 1993):

Infancy through preschool
1. Helplessness and passivity; lack of usual responsiveness
2. Generalized fear
3. Heightened arousal and confusion
4. Cognitive confusion
5. Difficulty in talking about event; lack of verbalization
6. Difficulty in identifying feelings
7. Sleep disturbances, nightmares
8. Separation fears and clinging to caregivers
9. Regressive symptoms (e.g., bed wetting, loss of acquired speech and motor skills)
10. Inability to understand death as permanent
11. Anxieties about death
12. Grief related to abandonment by caregiver
13. Somatic symptoms (e.g., stomachaches, headaches)
14. Startle response to loud/unusual noises
15. "Freezing" (sudden immobility of body)
16. Fussiness, uncharacteristic crying, and neediness
17. Avoidance of or alarm responses to specific trauma-related reminders involving sights and physical sensations

School-age children (6–11 years old)
1. Responsibility and guilt
2. Repetitious traumatic play and retelling
3. Reminders triggering disturbing feelings
4. Sleep disturbances, nightmares
5. Safety concerns, preoccupation with danger
6. Aggressive behavior, angry outbursts
7. Fear of feelings and trauma reactions
8. Close attention to parents' anxieties
9. School avoidance
10. Worry and concern for others
11. Changes in behavior, mood, and personality
12. Somatic symptoms (complaints about bodily aches, pains)
13. Obvious anxiety and fearfulness

14. Withdrawal and quieting
15. Specific, trauma-related fears; general fearfulness
16. Regression to behavior of younger child
17. Separation anxiety with relation to primary caretakers
18. Loss of interest in activities
19. Confusion and inadequate understanding of traumatic events most evident in play rather than in discussion
20. Unclear understanding of death and the causes of "bad" events
21. Magical explanations to fill in gaps in understanding
22. Loss of ability to concentrate and attend at school, with lowering of performance
23. "Spacey" or distractible behavior

Preadolescents and adolescents (12–18 years old)
1. Self-consciousness
2. Life-threatening reenactment
3. Rebellion at home or school
4. Abrupt shift in relationships
5. Depression, social withdrawal
6. Decline in school performance
7. Trauma-driven acting-out behavior: sexual acting out or reckless, risk-taking behavior
8. Effort to distance from feelings of shame, guilt, and humiliation
9. Flight into driven activity and involvement with others or retreat from others in order to manage inner turmoil
10. Accident proneness
11. Wish for revenge and action-oriented responses to trauma
12. Increased self-focusing and withdrawal
13. Sleep and eating disturbances; nightmares

Very young children may exhibit few PTSD symptoms. This may be because eight of the PTSD symptoms require a verbal description of one's feelings and experiences. Instead, young children may report more generalized fears such as stranger or separation anxiety, avoidance of situations that may or may not be related to the trauma, sleep disturbances, and a preoccupation with words or symbols that may or may not be related to the trauma. These children may also display posttraumatic play in which they repeat themes of the trauma. In addition, children may lose an acquired developmental skill (such as toilet training) as a result of experiencing a traumatic event.

Clinical reports suggest that elementary school-age children may not experience visual flashbacks or amnesia for aspects of the trauma. However, they do experience "time skew" and "omen formation," which are not typically seen in adults. Time skew refers to a child's missequencing trauma-related events when recalling the memory. Omen formation is a belief that there were warning signs that predicted the trauma. As a result, children often believe that if they are alert enough, they will recognize warning signs and avoid future traumas. School-age children also reportedly exhibit posttraumatic play or reenactment of the trauma in play, drawings, or verbalizations. Posttraumatic play is different from reenactment in that posttraumatic play is a literal representation of the trauma, involves compulsively repeating some aspect of the trauma, and does not tend to relieve anxiety but to actually increase it (Terr, 1991). An example of posttraumatic play is an increase in shooting games after exposure to a school shooting. Posttraumatic reenactment, on the other hand, is more flexible and involves behaviorally recreating aspects of the trauma (e.g., carrying a weapon after exposure to violence).

PTSD in adolescents may begin to more closely resemble PTSD in adults. However, there are a few features that have been shown to differ. As discussed earlier, children may engage in traumatic play following a trauma. Adolescents are more likely to engage in traumatic reenactment, in which they incorporate aspects of the trauma into their daily lives. In addition, adolescents are more likely than younger children or adults to exhibit impulsive and aggressive behaviors.

Besides PTSD, children and adolescents who have experienced traumatic events often exhibit other types of problems. Perhaps the best information available on the effects of traumas on children comes from a review of the literature on the effects of child sexual abuse. In this review, it was shown that sexually abused children often have problems with fear, anxiety, depression, anger and hostility, aggression, sexually inappropriate behavior, self-destructive behavior, feelings of isolation and stigma, poor self-esteem, difficulty in trusting others, and substance abuse. These problems are often seen in children and adolescents who have experienced other types of traumas as well. Children who have experienced traumas also often have relationship problems with peers and family members, problems with acting out, and problems with school performance.

Along with associated symptoms, there are a number of psychiatric disorders that are commonly found in children and adolescents who have been traumatized. A commonly co-occurring disorder is major depression. Other disorders include substance abuse; other anxiety disorders such as separation anxiety, panic disorder, and generalized anxiety disorder; and externalizing disorders such as attention-deficit/hyperactivity disorder, oppositional defiant disorder, and conduct disorder.

TREATMENT INTERVENTIONS FOR PTSD

Although some children show a natural remission of PTSD symptoms over a period of a few months, a significant number of children continue to exhibit symptoms for years if untreated. Few studies have PTSD treatments to determine which are most effective for children and adolescents. A review of the studies of PTSD treatments for adults shows that cognitive-behavioral therapy (CBT) is an effective approach. CBT for children generally blends both cognitive and behavioral interventions, including having the child directly discuss the traumatic event (exposure), anxiety management techniques such as relaxation and assertiveness training, and correction of inaccurate or distorted trauma-related thoughts (Berliner & Saunders, 1996; Foa & Rothman, 1998). Although there is some controversy regarding exposing children to the events that scare them, exposure-based treatments seem to be most relevant when memories or reminders of the trauma distress a child. Children can be exposed gradually and taught relaxation so that they can learn to relax while recalling their experiences. Through this procedure, they learn that they do not have to be afraid of their memories. CBT also involves challenging children's false beliefs, such as "the world is totally unsafe." The majority of studies have found that it is safe and effective to use CBT for children with PTSD (Mannarino, Cohen, & Berman, 1994; Mannarino & Cohen, 1996; March & Mulle, 1998).

CBT is often accompanied by psychoeducation and parental involvement. Psychoeducation in this case is education about PTSD symptoms and their effects. It is as important for parents and caregivers to understand the effects of PTSD as it is for children. Research shows that the better parents cope with the trauma, and the more they support their children, the better their children will function. Therefore, it is important for parents to seek treatment for themselves in order to develop the necessary coping skills that will help their children.

Psychological first aid has been prescribed for children exposed to community violence and can be used in schools and traditional settings. Psychological first aid involves clarifying trauma-related facts, normalizing the children's PTSD reactions, encouraging the expression of feelings, teaching problem-solving skills, and referring the most symptomatic children for additional treatment (Pynoos & Nader, 1988).

Eye movement desensitization and reprocessing (EMDR) combines cognitive therapy with directed eye movements (Shapiro, 1998). Although EMDR has been shown to be effective in treating both children and adults with PTSD, studies indicate that it is the cognitive intervention rather than the eye movements that accounts for the change. Medications have also been prescribed for some children with PTSD. However, due to the lack of research in this area, it is too early to evaluate the effectiveness of medication therapy.

But what about the child who cannot "talk" about it? Such children are considered to be fine because they are not showing the symptoms in a verbal sense. Children will tend to play out traumas on their own if they can. It may be that no adult will ever see the play. However, if the support system is weak for these children (parent pathology), or if the trauma was too intense and too frequent, then they may not even attempt to play out the trauma on their own. Children do heal themselves through their play if they can. But if conditions prevent such play, then that is when release play therapy shows the most promise and positive clinical results (Kaduson, 1997).

There has been great interest and activity over the years devoted to the study of the child's play as a basis for psychotherapy. Treating children's problems by exploiting their own methods of treating themselves has a sound basis, analogous to a study of the cure of disease by determining the organism's own methods of protection (Kaduson, 1997). Because many of the symptoms that children have are seen in their play, it is the natural course of intervention.

THERAPEUTIC POWERS OF PLAY

One of the most important aspects of play therapy is the actual therapeutic powers of play (Schaefer, 1993). Certainly, when we are talking about PTSD, there are clear indications that the following therapeutic powers are at work in helping children assimilate a trauma and gain mastery over the event through their own means of communication, namely, play.

Communication is one of the most important powers of play. Play is to the child what verbalization is to the adult—the most natural medium of self-expression. Because play is the language of the child, it allows the child to "speak" to us without words. There are two types of communication: unconscious and conscious. Children play out unconscious material without direct awareness at first. They reveal thoughts, feelings, and conflicts that they are totally unaware of. Children project their feelings onto miniature figures or puppets, thereby allowing their unconscious thoughts to rise to consciousness. Play provides a window into the otherwise invisible inner world of children. The play is "as if" it were real, so children are protected from flooding of the event when they are not ready for it. Conscious material is also communicated through play because children use their natural expression (play) to communicate events, traumas, and so forth, without using words. Play allows children to enact those thoughts and feelings of which they are aware but cannot express in words. This helps them to report their traumas in a nonthreatening way.

Abreaction is the reliving of past stressful events and the emotions associated with those events, even if a child could not express those emotions at the actual time of the trauma. Children use abreactive play to work through their traumas and assimilate the material a piece at a time. This concept was used by Sigmund Freud (1920/1955) to help explain how trauma victims resolve their experiences. Repressed memories are brought to consciousness and relived with the appropriate release of affect. Freud applied the concept to children, and he noted (1920/1955) that play offers young children a unique opportunity to accomplish this mental work. According to Freud, the post-traumatic anxiety can be resolved only if the therapist is able to get the child to relive the trauma with appropriate release of affect. This assimilation model fits well with the work of Piaget (1950), in that the traumatic experience is gradually assimilated into a schema (frame of reference) that is developed by the therapist–client interaction (Schaefer, 1993).

In abreaction, children have to do the opposite of what they want to do. They want to avoid processing the trauma. This can be done by (1) avoidance of knowledge of the event (amnesia), (2) avoidance of affect (numbing), (3) avoidance of behavior (phobic responses), and/or (4) avoidance of any communication about the event (Schaefer, 1997). Of course, the problem with such avoidance is that one cannot process the traumatic experience unless one relives it. The best way to expose young children to traumatic memories is through structured play.

Abreaction is enhanced through the act of repetition. Freud (1914/1958) maintained that children unconsciously recreate, in their play, situations related to the original traumatic event, and the frequency of the play is related to the intensity of the trauma. Therefore, every new repetition of play weakens the negative response associated with the trauma and seems to strengthen the child's sense of mastery of the event.

By means of the brief intervention of release play therapy, the play therapist can, in the playroom, present the child with miniature play objects representing the trauma scene and can encourage the child to play out the trauma. In this way the children can reexperience an event or a relationship in a different way, and with a more positive outcome than that of the original event. For children to benefit from play reenactment of past traumas, a number of therapeutic processes must be present (Ekstein, 1966):

1. Miniaturization of experiences by use of the small play objects.
2. Active control and domination of events that are possible in play.
3. Piecemeal assimilation of a traumatic event by repetitiously playing out that event.

As children play in later sessions with the play therapist, different distressing details of the trauma are likely to be emphasized until, piecemeal, the event is brought into complete awareness and the reality of it accepted and integrated into the psyche.

Mastery is another therapeutic power of play that impels children to play out their traumas. Because play is a self-motivated activity, it tends to satisfy children's innate need to explore and master the environment (Berlyne, 1960). When children have experienced a traumatic event, their sense of efficacy is diminished. Yet through the play in release play therapy, children become competent and feel satisfied by the sense of efficacy.

Also at work with mastery is systematic desensitization (Wolpe, 1958). Children's play can reduce anxiety through the process of exposing them to a fearful situation while they are relaxed in play. The pleasure of play can counteract and neutralize the fearfulness, so that the children can perform the desired behavior of working through the event. The repetition of play allows for the desensitization of the traumatic experience, so that the child gains a sense of power and mastery at the same time.

Catharsis is the release of tension and affect. It also refers to the arousal and discharge of strong emotions (positive and negative) for therapeutic relief (Schaefer, 1993). In release play therapy, children can release the intense feelings of anger, grief, or anxiety that have been difficult or impossible to express before, either due to the intensity of the trauma or because of the lack of a support system that would allow such expression. This discharge results in a sense of relief.

Fantasy compensation also allows children to create their own realities. In the world of imagination, children do not have to be satisfied with current realities or their own limitations. In release play therapy, children can have the power through their fantasy to compensate for their real-life weaknesses, hurts, losses, or fears and satisfy unmet needs while playing out the traumatic situation repetitively and safely in the playroom.

Pretending gives children power over the world, even when they do not have much control in real-life situations (Schaefer, 1993). It is the one area in which children can make reality conform to their wishes. Therefore, when they revisit a traumatic event through play, they can modify the circumstances to fill their own needs, place a support system around themselves even if it didn't exist during the trauma, and make the ending turn out better than they experienced in the first place.

With the therapeutic powers in play, release play therapy can give children a chance to assimilate a traumatic situation slowly and with enjoyment as they face the frightening event through their play.

ORIGINS OF RELEASE PLAY THERAPY

David Levy (1932) originated release therapy during a time when he was observing many children experiencing the same responses to night terrors or nightmares. It was already known that children handle their own emotional difficulties through their imaginative play. When they play, they get rid of tensions arising out of anxiety. Presumably, if children's behaviors were appropriate during the event that caused the anxiety, no tension residuals would have remained (Levy, 1932). When a child's method of dealing with the anxiety is unsuccessful, symptoms of the presence of the anxiety are still at hand.

During this research, Levy found that the reasons that the children did not naturally abreact certain situations had do with a number of factors: (1) the strength of the stimulus (because fears are of varying intensity and duration); (2) the summation of events (several traumas may occur simultaneously or in close time relation; (3) the children's sensitivity to the stimulus (at different ages, different effects may occur with certain situations); (4) children may have been sensitized through a specific past experience that intensifies the response; and (5) whether any children who experienced a traumatic situation had any psychological problems prior to the event.

TYPICAL RESPONSES TO A TRAUMATIC SITUATION

Based on the foregoing discussion, an example is used to illustrate how children naturally abreact. Although many children go through daily difficulties, it is their play and the conditions of the situation that allow them to "work it through" in their play. The following example illustrates this procedure.

A 5-year-old girl, Julie, was playing with her friend (also 5 years old) in the ocean close to shore. They were both jumping in the waves and screaming with delight. Julie's mom wanted to take a picture of the two children, so she walked toward the water and called for Julie and her friend to get close together for the picture. Mom was directing Julie to move a bit farther out in the ocean so that she could frame the shot better. Without Mom's knowledge, and in a split second, Julie fell into a sinkhole in the ocean and went underwater. People around her saw this and began grabbing for her in the water. The ocean's water was not clear, so it was difficult for them to see her. Mom's immediate response was to move the camera, thinking that Julie was fooling around. In a few seconds, it was clear to Julie's mom that something had happened. She started screaming for help, and the lifeguard came quickly. He took Julie out of the water, and she immediately vomited the salt water onto the beach. Mom held her while they both cried, and then they went back to their blanket. At this point, Julie's friend was just watching from her own blanket about 5 feet away. Mom sat on the blanket, holding Julie; then, without notice, Julie pulled away and started digging furiously in the sand to make a hole big enough to put her doll in. After she covered the doll with sand, she pulled it out again, and repeated the same action again and again while her mother watched. After about five repetitions, Julie asked her mother to get her some water. Mom just took a bucket and ran to the water's edge to scoop up the water. She filled the bucket and returned to the blanket. Julie then dug another hole, put water in the hole, and then the doll. She covered the doll completely with water and repeated this action several times. She then wanted more water, so Mom went to the ocean again and filled the bucket. During this short time, Julie's friend asked her innocently if she wanted to go back into the ocean. Julie said, "Not yet." When Mom returned again with the water, Julie took her doll, put the doll in the bucket of water, and then pulled her out quickly and made her "vomit" onto the sand. Julie repeated this three times. Then she threw her doll in the air and grabbed her friend's hand, and they both returned to the water, playing as if nothing had ever happened.

Julie was able to naturally abreact because she had all of the conditions that made it easy for her to repetitively revisit her scary situation without feeling out of control. The trauma was of short duration and intensity (although she had swallowed some water, she was never unconscious), her support system was strong (people helping immediately, as well as her mother's being right there and holding her), and this had never happened to Julie before. She was able to play it out right away without someone stopping her, perhaps by saying, "Don't worry honey, it's OK now. You don't need to do that." Whenever these words are spoken, it stops a child from doing what is naturally helpful to work through a fearful situation.

RELEASE PLAY THERAPY FOR CHILDREN WITH PTSD

In order to work with a child who is diagnosed with PTSD, it is very important for the therapist to get enough information from the intake with the parents, caretakers, or whoever was present so that the therapist can help the child play through the event, rather than avoid the thoughts and feelings associated with it. Although the intake information may not be totally accurate, if the therapist can replicate the situation closely enough, children can play through the event slowly so that they can assimilate the feelings at a pace that they can tolerate. This is always a short-term approach. If the conditions are right, a child might be able to play it out in one to ten sessions. The therapist will be very directive, while following the lead of the child. As illustrated shortly, a child may play "around" the event or withdraw from the actual play when his or her anxiety becomes too great. It is the therapist's responsibility to help the child get closer to the event, and to keep in the event, by using humor or other creative means to join the child in the experience. This can give the child more ego strength and allow for a greater feeling of safety and an opportunity to revisit something that was very scary the first time around.

It is important in release play therapy to remain playful and lighthearted even if the situation was so frightening that the child may have dissociated or stopped playing at all. If that happens, the child is in a severe state of PTSD. Because during the event the child felt hopeless and helpless, his or her only protection was to dissociate. This does not mean that the child cannot play about it at some time, but it does mean that at the time of the trauma, the child was frozen and experienced so much fright that he or she removed the ability to feel at all. When this reaction is followed by play disruption—the child stops playing altogether—then the introduction of play must be done at a slower pace, through less threatening media. This approach is illustrated in detail in the following case study of Ronald.

CASE ILLUSTRATION

Ronald was a 4-year-old boy who was no longer able to play anything following a traumatic event when his best friend, Adam, was mauled by Ronald's dog, Angel. This event happened by accident, as follows: Ronald and Adam were playing army in the living room of Ronald's house. Angel, his dog, was asleep in the living room close to the boys. When Adam got up to back up his army men during the play, he stepped on Angel's paw. Angel was a male dog, and Adam had a male dog as well. These dogs did not like each other and could not be in the same backyard together. Therefore, when Adam stepped on Angel, Angel must have smelled the scent of Adam's dog, and from a deep sleep he jumped onto Adam and bit him on his head, ear, and neck. All of this happened in front of Ronald, and it took only a couple of minutes before Ronald's parents were right there, pulling Angel off Adam. In order for the family to feel safe again, Ronald's parents decided to have Angel "put to sleep." They were afraid that this could happen again.

Prior to this event, Ronald would engage in imaginary or symbolic play every day after preschool. His parents did not necessarily attend to this play, but they knew he was fully involved in it because when it was dinnertime, they had to wait until he "finished" his play. After Adam was attacked by Angel, Ronald stopped playing altogether. He became withdrawn, aggressive toward his parents, and did not want to see his best friend, Adam, again. Interestingly, Adam showed no signs of PTSD at all due to the events that immediately followed the attack.

After the intake with his parents, Ronald was brought to the therapist's playroom for his intake. Because he was not able to play out what happened, the therapist began the play session by asking Ronald draw a picture of anything. His response to this was, "I can write—do you want me to write?" The therapist had asked for a picture, but it was clear that Ronald could not even do that at this stage in his PTSD. Therefore, the therapist said yes to his request, and Ronald wrote, "I am mad because Angel bit my friend." His affect was totally flat during this writing. Because he was only 4 years old, he clearly was intellectually advanced, but his play was gone.

Color Your Heart Technique

After Ronald wrote his sentence, the therapist told him to come to the floor, and she took a piece of paper and drew a heart on it. She asked Ronald to pick colored markers to represent the following feelings: love, sad, mad and missing. He picked pink for love, blue for sad, purple for mad, and green for missing. The therapist then drew a heart and told Ronald to color in the heart, showing how much of each feeling he had toward Angel, his dog. Although this color your Heart technique is usually done with the four basic feelings (happy, sad, scared, and mad), the therapist changed the feelings so that Ronald could slowly get to those typical feelings after expressing his feelings about the loss of his dog. The aim was to go slowly to the trauma.

Each week when Ronald came to therapy, he filled out the heart again, and this became an assessment tool to see how he was processing the loss of his dog. At first, the artwork was all about being mad, with little other expression of feeling. Over several weeks, it eventually showed more love for the dog, a lot of missing, a large amount of sad, and very little anger.

Brave Bart

After the third week of Color Your Heart, it was clear to the therapist that Ronald was ready to go closer to the trauma. To guide him to do this in a non-threatening way, the therapist read *Brave Bart* (Sheppard, 1998) to Ronald in the session. She did not add anything to the story, because this is by far one of the best ways to introduce a traumatic event to a child. In the story, Bart "has something very bad, sad, and scary happen." The narrative never says what that something was, but it clearly relates what happens to an individual when a traumatic event occurs. Bart is a cat, so this is a nonthreatening story that gives the vocabulary of trauma to the child and introduces the idea of playing again.

Play Begins

Through Ronald's release play therapy sessions, it was seen what he perceived had happened right after Angel was pulled off Adam. Ronald was not able to play it out at first, but he remembered more and more pieces of the event as he was encouraged to "show" what happened. As in many cases of PTSD in children, telling the story does not relieve the child of any anxiety, because that is not the emotional language of a child. It is only when the child plays it out that the relief is felt and the anxiety dissipates.

During the fourth session, the therapist began to take out miniatures to start the play of what had happened. At first Ronald had no interest in the toys presented, except when the therapist went to take out a dog. Ronald said that the dog did not have to look like Angel, and he picked one that looked nothing like his own dog. The therapist began to play out what happened, with the limited information she had received from the parents. With the therapist playing the story, the situation allowed Ronald to get involved as a director at first, correcting errors that the therapist made on purpose. The therapist put affect in the play where it would have been appropriate if Ronald had not dissociated. When the therapist "couldn't get it right," she said to Ronald, "Show me what happened." Ronald began again to "tell the story," and the therapist would repeat, with a bit of laughter, "Show me what that looks like. I don't get it." By the end of the fourth session, Ronald had moved one of the figures in the play about 2 inches toward the scene. The session was over, but all pieces of the abreactive play were kept separate from other figures so that on the next visit, Ronald could get started where he left off.

In the next two sessions, the therapist asked Ronald if he wanted to draw to show what happened, but he declined. She had set up the play as it had been left the week before so that Ronald could just take it from that point or start again. Each week he chose to start again to show what happened, and the play became more detailed, more fantastic, and accompanied with much more affect. Through his play, over the next two sessions, Ronald showed that when Adam was attacked, Ronald felt as though he "just fainted right down on the floor." When the therapist asked where Ronald's parents were, Ronald showed her by bringing both parents figures to take Adam into the kitchen and rinse his wounds. Ronald indicated that Adam was crying the whole time. He did not indicate any emotions of his own. This is true in many cases of PTSD in children; the child with PTSD notices the emotions of others (they were crying, laughing, etc.) and reports no feelings for him- or herself. When the therapist asked Ronald who took care of him when this happened, his response was that there wasn't anyone because they all had to help Adam. Not only Ronald's parents, but also Adam's parents, were all around Adam, taking care of him and then taking him to the hospital. Adam stated in his play that he went to sleep, and then hours later his mother woke him up by "throwing a bucket of water on his face" (his own exaggeration to explain how he returned to a conscious state).

In the next session, the therapist reviewed what Ronald had shown her, by playing it out with him and stating, "Then you fainted to the floor." In this play session, Ronald said, "I mean it was like I went to sleep but my eyes were open. I could see everything but I was stunned and couldn't move, and I was wheezing" (he illustrated the fright that he now recalled and the noise of wheezing because of the fright). This was the turning point of the release play therapy. Ronald had played it out so that pieces of the real event were being assimilated into his schema of the trauma, until he could become comfortable enough to allow the feelings he had not felt at the time of the trauma. In this way, he was able to feel safe in the play and so could experience the fear for the first time.

In the eighth session, Ronald was clearly more playful and showed the therapist what happened from the beginning to the end of the incident. The therapist did not have to add affect anymore, because Ronald was doing that all by himself. When he finished the play scene this time, he asked if he could draw a picture of what had happened. This was the first time he was willing to draw, and he spontaneously suggested it. In this session he drew a picture of himself and Adam in the living room, with his dog, Angel, on the floor, and a lot of blood surrounding Adam. As he drew it, he told the story again but with more detail and affect, showing that he had released all of the anxiety that caused his play disruption.

At the next and final session, Ronald entered the playroom and asked if he could play something else. According to his parents' reports, Ronald had "just started playing again like he had before his dog mauled Adam." He was sleeping better at night, and he was no longer being aggressive with his parents. Once he had assimilated all the pieces of the trauma and managed to feel the anxiety in the safety of the playroom with a trained play therapist, he was able to let it go. He returned to his "playful self." Because this session would be his termination session, the therapist made a chain of construction paper that represented the eight weeks of release play therapy they had shared together. She made a written comment on each link to summarize each week, and she and Ronald connected all the construction paper links together as a final project. Ronald wanted to come back again next week, but he was instead encouraged to stay in touch with the therapist and let her know how he was doing with the start of kindergarten. It was important not to allow dependence on the therapist to develop, when, in effect, Ronald had done all the work himself, and he would once again use his natural play abilities to emotionally deal with his world.

CONCLUSION

Release play therapy has been clinically used successfully with all type I traumas (Terr, 1991). Type I traumas are single, sudden, and unexpected. Therefore, in selecting cases suitable for release play therapy, it is advisable to consider the following criteria (Levy, 1938):

1. The child should be between 2 and 10 years of age (although it can work for older children with some modifications).
2. There should be a definite reactive pattern triggered by a specific stressor (e.g., a frightening experience, divorce of parents, birth of a sibling).
3. The problem should not be long-standing.
4. The traumatic experience should be in the past, not continuing at the time of referral.
5. The child should be from a relatively normal family situation.

With the foregoing criteria met, it has been shown that children do not have to know the nature of their difficulties, or of their relationship to the therapist, in order to improve. The emotional release and positive therapeutic relationship are basic therapeutic elements leading to the resolution of the trauma.

Release play therapy helped dozens of children after the tragic World Trade Center attack on September 11, 2001. These children were able to work through their fears, anxieties, and sadness through playing out their perceptions of what happened that frightening day. Within weeks many children, like Ronald, returned to their carefree childhood experiences, although at some level they had changed for good. The same is likely to happen with the victims of Hurricane Katrina as the children begin to heal.

REFERENCES

Ackerman, P. T., Newton, J. E., McPherson, W. B., Jones, J. G., & Dykman, R. A. (1998). Prevalence of post traumatic stress disorder and other psychiatric diagnoses in three groups of abused children (sexual, physical, and both). *Child Abuse and Neglect, 22*(8), 759–774.

American Psychiatric Association. (1980). *Diagnostic and statistical manual of mental disorders* (3rd ed.). Washington, DC: Author.

American Psychiatric Association. (1994). *Diagnostic and statistical manual of mental disorders* (4th ed.). Washington, DC: Author.

Berliner, L., & Saunders, B. E. (1996). Treating fear and anxiety in sexually abused children: Results of a controlled two-year follow-up study. *Child Maltreatment, 1*(4), 294–309.

Berlyne, D. E. (1960). *Conflict, arousal and curiosity.* New York: McGraw-Hill.

Creamer, M., & Forbes, D. (2004). Treatment of posttraumatic stress disorder in veteran and military populations. *Psychotherapy: Theory, Research, Practice, 41*(4), 388–398.

Cuffe, S. P., Addy, C. L., Garrison, C. Z., Waller, J. L., Jackson, K. L., & McKeown, R. E. (1998). Prevalence of PTSD in a community sample of older adolescents. *Journal of American Academy of Child and Adolescent Psychiatry, 37*, 147–154.

DeWolfe, D. (2001). *Mental health response to mass violence and terrorism: A training manual for mental health workers and human service workers.* Rockland, MD: Center for Mental Health Services.

Ekstein, R. (1966). *Children of time and space, of action and impulse.* New York: Appleton Century Crofts.

Eth, S., & Pynoos, R. S. (1995). Developmental perspective on psychic trauma in childhood. In C. R. Figley (Ed.), *Trauma and its wake: The study of treatment of posttraumatic stress disorder* (pp. 36-52). New York: Brunner/Mazel.

Foa, E. B., & Rothman, B. O. (1998). *Treating the trauma of rape: Cognitive-behavioral therapy for PTSD.* New York: Guilford Press.

Freud, S. (1955). Beyond the pleasure principle. In J. Strachey (Ed. and Trans.), *The standard edition of the complete psychological works of Sigmund Freud* (Vol. 18, pp. 1–64). London: Hogarth Press. (Original work published 1920)

Freud, S. (1958). Remembering, repeating and working-through. In J. Strachey (Ed. and Trans.), *The standard edition of the complete psychological works of Sigmund Freud* (Vol. 12, pp. 145–156). London: Hogarth Press. (Original work published 1914)

Giacona, R. M., Reiknherz, H. Z., Silverman, A. B., Pakiz, B., Frost, A. K., & Cohen, E. (1995). Traumas and PTSD in a community population of older adolescents. *Journal of American Academy of Child and Adolescent Psychiatry, 34*, 1369–1380.

Hamblen, J. (2004). *PTSD in children and adolescents* (National Center for PTSD Fact Sheet). Available at www.ncptsd.va.gov/facts/specific/fs_children.html

Kaduson, H. G. (1997). Release play therapy for the treatment of sibling rivalry. In H. G. Kaduson, D. Cangelosi, & C. Schaefer (Eds.), *The playing cure* (pp. 255–273). Northvale, NJ: Aronson.

Kessler, R. C., Sonnega, A., Bromet, E., Hughes, M., & Nelson, C. B. (1995). Posttraumatic stress disorder in the national comorbidity study. *Archives of General Psychiatry, 52*, 1048–1060.

Kilpatrick, K. L., & Williams, L. M. (1997). Post-traumatic stress disorder in child witnesses to domestic violence. *Journal of Orthopsychiatry, 67*, 639–644.

Levy, D. M. (1932). The use of play technique as experimental procedure. *American Journal of Orthopsychiatry, 3*, 266–275.

Levy, D. M. (1938). Release therapy in young children. *Psychiatry, 1*, 387–390.

MacLean, P. D. (1988). *The triune brain in evolution: Role in paleocerebal functions.* New York: Plenum Press.

Mannarino, A. P., & Cohen, J. A. (1996). Abuse-related attributions and perceptions, general attributions, and locus of control in sexually abused girls. *Journal of Interpersonal Violence, 11*, 162–180.

Mannarino, A. P., Cohen, J. A., & Berman, S. R. (1994). The Children's Attributions and Perceptions Scale: A new measure of sexual abuse-related factors. *Journal of Clinical Child Psychology, 23*, 204–211.

March, J. S. (Ed.). (1995). *Anxiety disorders in children and adolescents.* New York: Guilford Press.

March, J., & Mulle, K. (1998). *OCD in children and adolescents: A cognitive-behavioral treatment manual.* New York: Guilford Press.

Margolis, G., & Gordis, E. B. (2000). The effects of family and community violence on children. *Annual Review of Psychology, 51*, 445–479.

Pfefferbaum, B., Nixon, S., Tucker, P., Tivis, R., Moore, V., Gurwitch, R., et al. (1999). Posttraumatic stress response in bereaved children after Oklahoma City bombing. *Journal of the American Academy of Child and Adolescent Psychiatry, 38*, 1372–1379.

Pfefferbaum, B., Seale, T., McDonald, N., Brandt, E., Rainwater, S., Maynard, B., et al. (2000). Posttraumatic stress two years after the Oklahoma City bombing in youths geographically distant from the explosion. *Psychiatry, 63*, 358–370.

Piaget, J. (1950). *The psychology of intelligence.* London: Routledge & Kegan Paul.

Pynoos, R., & Nader, K. (1988). Children who witness the sexual assaults of their mothers. *Journal of the American Academy of Child and Adolescent Psychiatry, 27*, 567–572.

Pynoos, R., & Nader, K. (1993). Issues in the treatment of posttraumatic stress in children and adolescents. In J. P. Wilson & B. Raphael (Eds.), *International handbook of traumatic stress syndromes* (pp. 535–549). New York: Plenum Press.

Pynoos, R., Frederick, C., Nader, K., Arroyo, W., Steinberg, A., Eth, S., et al. (1987). Life threat and posttraumatic stress in school-age children. *Archives of General Psychiatry, 44,* 1057–1063.

Schaefer, C. E. (1993). What is play and why is it therapeutic? In C. E. Schaefer (Ed.), *The therapeutic powers of play* (pp. 1–5). Northvale, NJ: Aronson.

Schaefer, C. E. (1997). In H. Kaduson, D. Cangelosi, & C. E. Schaefer (Eds.), *The playing cure.* Northvale, NJ: Aronson.

Shapiro, F. (1998). *EMDR: The breakthrough therapy for overcoming anxiety, stress and trauma.* New York: Basic Books.

Shelby, J. S. (1997). Rubble, disruption, and tears: Helping young survivors of natural disaster. In H. Kaduson, D. Cangelosi, & C. E. Schaefer (Eds.), *The playing cure* (pp.143–169). Northvale, NJ: Aronson.

Shelby, J. S. (2000). Brief therapy with traumatized children: A developmental perspective. In H. G. Kaduson & C. E. Schaefer (Eds.), *Short-term play therapy for children* (pp. 69–100). New York: Guilford Press.

Sheppard, C. H. (1998). *Brave Bart: A story for traumatized and grieving children.* Pointe Woods, MI: Institute for Trauma and Loss in Children.

Terr, L. (1991). Childhood traumas: An outline and overview. *American Journal of Psychiatry, 148,* 10–20.

van der Kolk, B. A., & Fisler, R. (1995). Dissociation and the fragmentary nature of traumatic memory: Background and experiential evidence. *Journal of Trauma Stress, 9,* 505–525.

Vernberg, E. M., & Varela, R. E. (2001). Posttraumatic stress disorder: A developmental perspective. In M. W. Vasey & M. R. Dadds (Eds.), *The developmental psychopathology of anxiety* (pp. 386–406). New York: Oxford University Press.

Wolpe, J. (1958). *Psychotherapy by reciprocal inhibition.* Stanford, CA: Stanford University Press.

Zatzick, D. F., Marmar, C. R., Weiss, D. S., Browner, W. S., Metzler, T. J., Golding, J. M., et al. (1997). Posttraumatic stress disorder and functioning and quality of life outcomes in a nationally representative sample of male Vietnam veterans. *American Journal of Psychiatry, 154,* 1690–1695.

CHAPTER 2

Cognitive-Behavioral Play Therapy for Children with Anxiety and Phobias

SUSAN M. KNELL
MEENA DASARI

Anxiety disorders, which include phobias, are among the most prevalent psychiatric disorders in children and adolescents (see references in Albano, Chorpita, & Barlow, 2003). In the past several years, there has been increased interest in these disorders due to their prevalence and responsiveness to psychotherapy. It is estimated that in a class of 30 children, 5 to 6 children will meet criteria for an anxiety disorder. Moreover, unlike treatments for other childhood disorders, cognitive-behavioral therapy has consistently emerged as a highly effective treatment for anxiety and phobias. This chapter (1) discusses assessment and treatment and (2) describes the use of cognitive-behavioral play therapy for anxiety and phobias in young children.

Fears and worries are considered part of normal child development, which makes identification of childhood anxiety disorders more complicated. For some children, specific fears and phobias may mask an emerging or existing anxiety disorder (Muris, Merckelbach, Mayer, & Prins, 2000). In addition, there is little understanding of normal, developmentally appropriate anxiety. Clinicians are often faced with the challenging task of differentiating between fears and worries that may be a normal aspect of development, and those that are more clinically significant and worthy of diagnosis and treatment. Clinical anxiety can be differentiated from normal anxiety by understanding three factors: (1) intensity, (2) impairment in functioning, and (3) flexibility of response (Barrios & Hartman, 1997; Klein & Pine, 2002).

It is also important to make a distinction between fear and anxiety. Fear is a biologically based response that usually occurs in the presence of real danger. For example, when a child is crossing the street and is suddenly faced with an oncoming car, the child's body reacts physiologically (e.g., racing heart) and responds by jumping backward. In contrast, anxiety is a learned response that usually occurs in the absence of real danger or in response to a perceived threat. A concept commonly used to understand anxiety is "false alarm." For example, during a thunderstorm, a child's body may react physiologically (e.g., shaking, nausea), even when no real threat of death or harm exists.

The most widely accepted model for understanding the maintenance of fears and anxiety is the cognitive-behavioral model. The cognitive-behavioral model, which proposes that there is a relationship between situations, thoughts, emotions, and behaviors, is particularly useful in better understanding anxiety. It is based on the assumption that people's emotions and behaviors are determined largely by the way they think about the world, with these thoughts being triggered by situational cues (Beck, 1967, 1972, 1976). It is the perception of events, not the events themselves, that determines how an individual understands life circumstances. Cognitive theory asserts that an individual's thoughts determine (or guide) his or her emotional experiences and subsequent behaviors.

ANXIETY DISORDERS IN CHILDHOOD

Anxiety disorders are highly prevalent in children and adolescents, affecting approximately 12–20% of the general population (Achenbach, Howell, McConaughy, & Stanger, 1995; Gurley, Cohen, Pine, & Brook, 1996; Shaffer et al., 1996). If anxiety disorders in children are untreated, symptoms may persist and worsen into adulthood (Albano et al., 2003). Research has shown that children with untreated anxiety disorders are also at greater risk for developing a depressive disorder. Therefore, early identification and intervention are crucial to prevent poor developmental outcomes.

According to DSM-IV, anxiety disorders are a broad category that includes nine specific disorders related to anxiety (American Psychiatric Association, 1994). Separation anxiety disorder is usually diagnosed in early childhood, and its core symptom is excessive anxiety concerning separation from home or from caregivers. Generalized anxiety disorder, previously known as overanxious disorder, is characterized by excessive and uncontrollable worry about multiple events that is present for at least 6 months. Social phobia is usually diagnosed in adolescents, with a core symptom of marked and persistent anxiety about one or more social or performance situations due to excessive worries about embarrassment or rejection. Obsessive–compulsive disorder is commonly diagnosed between ages 10 and 12 years and involves either recurrent, intrusive obsessions and/or time-consuming compulsions. Posttraumatic Stress Disorder can be diagnosed only if the child experienced or witnessed a traumatic event and is currently reexperiencing the event, avoiding associated stimuli, and hyperaroused. Finally, panic disorder involves a core symptom of unexpected panic attacks and persistent concerns about their recurrence. School refusal and somatic complaints are symptoms commonly associated with several anxiety disorders (Albano et al., 2003).

It is important to note that anxiety is a normal emotional experience for all children and adolescents. Anxieties about specific events are considered normal and transient at each stage of development. During preschool years, children commonly experience anxieties about imaginary monsters and specific objects such as thunderstorms and bugs. School-age children often experience anxieties about physical health or being harmed (e.g., kidnapping). During the teenage years, adolescents typically report anxieties about social performances such as playing sports and giving presentations in front of the class. In general, most children experience normal levels of anxiety around specific events, which is considered developmentally appropriate. Normal levels of anxiety are usually described as mild to moderate, transient, and not interfering with daily functioning (Klein & Pine, 2002).

Because anxiety is a normal emotion in children, clinicians often struggle with distinguishing clinical levels that warrant an anxiety disorder diagnosis. Clinical anxiety differs from normal levels of anxiety on three dimensions: (1) intensity, (2) impairment, and (3) lack of flexibility (Klein & Pine, 2002). Intensity refers to whether a child's level of distress is disproportionate, given his or her developmental stage or the object or event. A good example of a clinical level of anxiety can be seen on the first day of kindergarten, which is typically a stressful event for most children entering school. A child who cries, complains of stomachaches, has a tantrum, and is inconsolable when parents leave is displaying greater intensity of anxiety as compared with a child who gets tearful when separating from parents but is able to calm him- herself in a short time period. The first child's reaction is disproportionate to other children's reactions, and that child is more likely to have an anxiety disorder.

The second dimension, impairment, refers to whether the child's level of distress interferes with his or her daily life. Examples include inability to make friends owing to social anxiety or receiving failing grades because of test anxiety. Both are suggestive of clinical levels of anxiety, inasmuch as the anxiety interferes with the child's social development. Finally, lack of flexibility refers to whether the child is unable to recover from his or her distress when the object or event is not present. Specifically, with clinical levels of anxiety, the child tends to be distressed about future occurrences of the event and to display the distress across multiple settings (e.g., home, school, camp). For example, a child with a clinical level of separation anxiety will be anxious about the next time his or her parent leaves and may have this difficulty when being left with a babysitter at home or when dropped off at school. Thus, as compared with normal levels of anxiety, clinical anxiety is more intense than experienced by other children of the same age, impairs the child's ability to achieve developmentally appropriate tasks, and prevents his or her ability to recover when the event or object is not present.

FEARS IN CHILDHOOD

Fears are a normal part of childhood. For most children, fears are mild, age-specific, and transient (King, Hamilton, & Ollendick, 1988). Most fears decrease with age and diminish without intervention. Some fears are considered developmentally appropriate. During the infant years, fears seem to be concrete and centered on the immediate environment, such as a fear of loud noises or a fear of strangers. Fears and scary dreams were found to be common among 4 to 6-year-olds, even more prominent in 7- to 9-year-olds, and to then decrease in frequency in 10- to 12-year-olds (Muris, Merckelbach, Gadet, & Moulaert, 2000). The frequency of certain fears changes across age groups, with fears of imaginary creatures decreasing with age (Muris et al., 2000). In general, even though there are common threads, each child's fears will be determined by his or her individual learning history. Children often learn to be fearful of objects or situations after experiencing unpleasant events associated with the stimuli. When the stimuli is presented later, fear may be evoked even without the unpleasant event.

Although mild, simple phobias are often transient fears that resolve over time (Silverman & Nelles, 1990), more complex fears are known as phobias and are often shortened by treatment (Agras, Chapin, & Oliveau, 1972; Hampe, Noble, Miller, & Barrett, 1973). Specific phobias are also included in the DSM-IV under "Anxiety Disorders." The core feature of such phobias is intense and persistent fear of specific objects/events. These fears are not developmentally appropriate and are irrational because no real danger exists. Phobias are evident in only a small sample of children, with prevalence estimates of only 3–8% of the population exhibiting excessive fears warranting clinical diagnosis (King et al., 1988; Silverman & Nelles, 1990). When phobic children are brought to treatment, it is usually because their fears are significantly interfering with everyday functioning or disruptive to the family. Examples include children who cannot separate from their parents, who are too fearful to ride elevators, or to attend school. Phobic children are often not brought for treatment at the onset of their fears. Strauss and Last (1993) found that children with simple phobias, on average, are brought to treatment approximately 3 years after the onset of their phobias. In addition, phobic children often have other presenting problems, with the fears being uncovered during a comprehensive evaluation.

ASSESSMENT OF FEAR AND ANXIETY IN CHILDREN

Assessment is a critical step to determining the developmental appropriateness of a child's anxiety and fears. Assessment of a child's fears and/or anxiety involves clinical interview with parents, behavioral rating scales, behavioral observation, parent monitoring forms, and play assessment with the child. Play interviews are used when necessary and can be helpful in understanding anxiety in preschool children. Based on a recent literature review, a multimethod assessment approach is recommended to obtain a comprehensive picture of symptoms across several contexts (for review, see Velting, Setzer, & Albano, 2004).

A developmental perspective is important to apply when assessing anxieties and fears in children. This is because most measures have been researched in specific age groups (Velting et al., 2004). In general, most assessment techniques have been validated for use with school-age populations. Therefore, clinical interview, behavioral observation, select behavioral rating scales, and parent monitoring forms are recommended for use with preschool and early school-age children.

Clinical Interview

Clinical interview is considered the most reliable assessment method for obtaining diagnostic accuracy with anxiety disorders. Clinical interviews may be either structured or semistructured. The most widely used instrument is the Anxiety Disorders Interview Schedule for DSM-IV: Child and Parent (ADIS-C and ADIS-P; Silverman & Albano, 1996a, 1996b). Both parent and child versions are used with children ages 7–17 years. The ADIS-P can be completed by parents of preschool-age children; however, there is currently no information on whether the reliability and validity are the same with this age group. The ADIS requires trained clinicians about 2–3 hours to administer. Therefore, it is more often used in research, rather than clinical settings, owing to the need for diagnostic clarity and greater flexibility with time.

With younger children and in clinical settings, semistructured interviews are recommended because of the age and time limitations of the structured interviews. Semistructured interviews allow clinicians to ask specific questions to obtain greater detail. These interviews should be conducted with parents. Several informative questions are suggested during the assessment to obtain details such as:

- How the child and family typically deal with the fearful object/event.
- How the anxiety and fear have interfered with the child's and family's life.
  - How does the fear impact the child's and family's day-to-day functioning?
  - Have family members changed their routines to accommodate the child's fears?

- Coping strategies (or lack thereof) for the child and family that have been developed (e.g., what efforts have the parents made to help the child, and how successful or unsuccessful have these been?).
- The extent and nature of the child's exposure to the feared stimuli, which are also important (e.g., a child who is afraid of roller coasters is not likely to need treatment, whereas a child who is afraid of elevators, and who lives in a high-rise apartment in a large city, will probably require some kind of intervention unless the fear is short-lived).

It is also important to assess and understand any changes in the family situation or environment that may have contributed to the child's fears. Lifestyle changes, such as a move to a new house, may prompt changes in the child's sense of safety or security and may thus contribute to changes in levels of fear. Traumatic events, such as divorce, abuse, or family illness/death must also be understood in terms of the impact they may have had on the child's fears.

Behavioral Observation

Behavioral observation is considered a useful assessment method in diagnosing young children. This assessment method is often supplemental to the clinical interview. Behavioral observation involves watching and recording the child's reactions to situations, for the purpose of understanding how the child's fear is connected to his or her environment. Clinicians take note of the child's body posture, facial expressions, and reactions to other people in various settings, such as in the clinic, home, and school.

Behavioral Rating Scales

The use of rating scales and self-reports is considered the most informative assessment method for understanding observable behaviors related to anxiety disorders. However, most of the commonly used measures are designed to assess anxiety symptoms in school-age children (Velting et al., 2004). These include the Multidimensional Anxiety Scale for Children (MASC; March, 1997). For assessment with young children, the Screen for Anxiety and Related Emotional Disorders—Parent Version (SCARED; Birmaher et al., 1997) is recommended. The recommendation is due to the strong empirical support of SCARED, which has been shown to be equally effective as the MASC in distinguishing clinical versus normal levels of anxiety.

Parent Monitoring Forms

Another supplemental assessment method is the use of parent monitoring forms, which are helpful for understanding anxieties and fears within a context.

With school-age children and adolescents, self-monitoring forms are used instead, on which children monitor and record their own behaviors. This is not possible for very young children; therefore, the forms are completed by parents, who are instructed to record anxiety-provoking situations, subsequent anxiety levels, cognitions, physical sensations, and behaviors. Parents are taught to use the "fear thermometer," on which 0 represents no fear and 10 represents extreme fear (originally introduced for use with adults by Walk, 1956). Such a task is not reliable, but helps the parents and the younger child quantify his or her fears in a concrete, understandable format. In addition, the parent monitoring forms are likely to provide valuable information on triggers and anxiety-related behaviors (Velting et al., 2004)

TREATMENT OF FEAR AND ANXIETY IN CHILDHOOD

Historically, even before short-term therapy was accepted, treatment for childhood fears and anxieties was typically described as brief (four to five sessions) (Ollendick, 1979). Early behavioral interventions included techniques of fear reduction, systematic desensitization, contingency management, modeling, and cognitive-behavioral techniques. Across orientations, most practitioners would agree that fearful/anxious children need to learn better coping skills to help them deal with the things that are worrying them. Recent literature supports cognitive-behavioral treatment as the most effective form of psychotherapy for anxiety disorders and phobias (Geddes, Reynolds, Streiner, & Szatmari, 1997; March & Wells, 2003; Ollendick & King, 1998). There is a large body of evidence to show that cognitive-behavioral approaches are effective in decreasing anxiety symptoms in children and adolescents. The reader is referred to several excellent, comprehensive reviews of the use of cognitive-behavioral therapy (CBT) for the treatment of anxiety disorders (Compton et al., 2004; Kazdin & Weisz, 1998; Ollendick & King, 1998; Turner & Heiser, 1999).

Cognitive-behavioral treatments that are considered to be effective forms of psychotherapy for anxiety disorders include five essential components (Albano & Kendall, 2002).

1. *Psychoeducation* refers to providing accurate information on anxiety, which is usually done by teaching children about the cognitive-behavioral model. The emphasis is on the child (a) learning the relationship between events, thoughts, feelings, and behaviors and (b) identifying his or her individual anxiety symptoms. This step is usually not done with preschool children and may be done with parents instead. The purpose is for the child to understand his or her diagnosis and how treatment will alleviate symptoms of fear and anxiety.

2. *Somatic management* primarily refers to relaxation training. Children

are taught techniques such as deep breathing and muscle relaxation for the purpose of reducing autonomic arousal and physiological responses associated with anxiety.

3. *Cognitive restructuring* is taught to identify, challenge, and change maladaptive thinking to positive, realistic thinking. Children are instructed on the techniques of "labeling thinking traps" (i.e., maladaptive thoughts) and "thought detective" (i.e., gathering the evidence). These techniques should be adapted to a child's developmental level. The purpose of these techniques is for children to develop skills in generating adaptive thinking for daily events.

4. *Exposure*, a critical component of cognitive-behavioral therapy, involves graduated, systematic, and controlled exposure to feared situations and stimuli. The technique usually occurs in two phases: (a) preparation (i.e., developing fear hierarchy and coping skills) and (b) active exposure (i.e., completing anxiety-producing tasks according to hierarchy). This component is particularly helpful with young children, for whom cognitive restructuring is not developmentally appropriate.

5. *Relapse prevention* is done with children of all ages to review and generalize therapeutic gains. They are taught to identify triggers and coping strategies and to review "lessons learned." Children are often asked to develop a plan to practice their anxiety management skills at home and at school.

One of the primary goals of CBT is to identify and modify maladaptive thoughts associated with the child's symptoms in order to develop more adaptive behavior (Bedrosian & Beck, 1980). Maladaptive thoughts are ideations that interfere with the individual's ability to cope with stressful experiences (Beck, 1976). With fears, maladaptive thoughts may include self-statements such as, "I am too fearful to do this" or "I cannot get over this fear."

A significant component of overcoming fear appears to be one's gaining control over a fear, especially through exposure. This may involve learning that one can deal with the feared stimuli, learning to manage feelings associated with the fear, and learning specific coping skills to deal with fear. Cognitive-behavioral interventions provide such learning opportunities, as well as the specific skills necessary to overcome fear. In play therapy, children may master a feared object by taking on the role of one who does not fear it. They may act in ways that suggest they are not afraid. By "pretending," and practicing, a child may overcome the feared stimuli.

Cognitive-Behavioral Play Therapy

Cognitive-behavioral play therapy (CBPT) is designed specifically for preschool and early elementary school-age children. It emphasizes the child's involvement in therapy by addressing issues of control, mastery, and responsibility for changing one's own behavior. CBPT is designed to be developmentally appropriate and to help the child become an active participant in change (Knell, 1993a, 1994, 1997, 1998, 1999). In addition to its use with children who have anxiety disorders and phobias (Knell, 1993a), CBPT has been used with children with a wide range of diagnoses, such as selective mutism (Knell, 1993a, 1993b) and encopresis (Knell & Moore, 1990; Knell, 1993a), as well as children who have experienced traumatic life events, such as divorce (Knell, 1993a) and sexual abuse (Knell & Ruma, 1996).

Setting/Materials

CBPT is usually conducted in a playroom with a wide array of play materials available. A typical play therapy room is well stocked with toys, art supplies, puppets, dolls, and other materials. The more directive and goal-oriented techniques of CBPT may require more materials to meet the needs of a child's specific problems. At times, the therapist may need to buy materials that meet the needs of a particular child. Sometimes it is not necessary to buy toys for specific situations because of the child's ability to be creative and flexible with existing toys. For example, a child fearful of sitting on the toilet may be able to play with a doll on a plastic bowl that resembles a toilet. However, the child may not be able to "pretend" in this way and may have an easier time using a specifically designed dolls' play toilet.

Although play therapy is usually conducted in a playroom, the fearful or anxious child may need to be treated *in vivo*. That is, the child may have to be seen in a setting that more closely resembles specific real-life situations. Thus, the child fearful of elevators may be seen in and around an elevator, the child who is school phobic may need to be treated at or around the school, and a child afraid of dogs may need to be seen in a setting where dogs are allowed. Children with social anxiety may have to be treated in group situations with other children; those with separation anxiety may be better treated in situations where they can separate from a parent gradually.

Treatment Stages

CBPT takes place as the child moves through several treatment stages, which have been described as the introductory/orientation, assessment, middle, and termination stages. After preparation for CBPT, the assessment begins. During the middle stage of CBPT, the therapist has developed a treatment plan, and the therapy is turning to focus on increasing the child's self-control, sense of accomplishment, and learning more adaptive responses to deal with specific situations. For fearful and anxious children, this will incorporate a wide array of cognitive and behavioral interventions specifically geared to helping the child with his or her specific concerns. Generalization and relapse prevention are incorporated into the middle stages of therapy, so that the child can learn to utilize new skills across a broad range of settings and begin to develop skills that will diminish the chance of setbacks after therapy is completed. During the termination phase, the child and family are prepared for the end of therapy (see Knell, 1999, for further description of these stages in CBPT).

Treatment Interventions

The main components of cognitive-behavioral interventions are incorporated into play therapy in various ways, with the primary concern being to present them to young children so that they are accessible and potentially useful.

A variety of treatment techniques are utilized in CBPT with fearful and anxious children. Given the limited cognitive abilities and anxieties of young children, play therapy offers fearful children an opportunity to express their feelings in a safe environment. Some of the most important interventions in cognitive-behavioral work with fearful children are behavioral interventions (e.g., systematic desensitization, contingency management, and modeling) and cognitive techniques. Some of the most common behavioral and cognitive interventions utilized in work with anxious and fearful children are described in the following paragraphs.

PSYCHOEDUCATION

Psychoeducation within a CBT model often teaches an individual about his or her disorder and about the CBT model. Some of the psychoeducation may be done with parents, rather than with the child. Another prominent aspect of CBPT is to teach skills or alternative behaviors. When the work is done with the child, modeling is often used. For example, the therapist may educate a puppet about the puppet's problems and how thinking affects feelings and behavior. The therapist may also teach skills or alternative behaviors. These can all be modeled for the child by the therapist in interaction with a puppet or another toy.

SOMATIC MANAGEMENT (OR RELAXATION)

Relaxation training can be part of CBPT by modeling a state of calm for the child. There are various ways in which this might be done, such as by teaching a puppet muscle relaxation or deep breathing and having the child observe. Books and tapes are often used with young children. An example is the book *Cool Cats, Calm Kids* (Williams, 1996), which models relaxation skills through the body posture and "self-statements" of cats. In addition, alternatives such as helping the child engage in relaxing activities and more calming play can be used in place of teaching specific relaxation skills.

COGNITIVE RESTRUCTURING

Cognitive restructuring techniques deal with teaching children skills to change their negative thinking to more positive, realistic thinking. The underlying theory for cognitive techniques is that anxiety is a result of maladaptive cognitions, or negative thinking about events in the environment. For example, before a birthday party a preschool child with maladaptive cognitions might think, "The kids won't like me" or "I'll be really bad at the party games," which leads to anxious feelings and behaviors (e.g., stomachaches, avoiding the party by hiding in the bathroom). Children can learn more adaptive thoughts, such as, "Birthday parties can be fun" or "No one will be good at *all* the party games." Thus, it is hypothesized that changes in thinking will produce changes in behavior. The therapist helps the child to identify, modify, and/or build cognitions. In addition to helping the child identify cognitive distortions and teaching the child to replace these maladaptive thoughts with more adaptive ones, the therapist also provides the child with an opportunity to test his or her new skills.

COGNITIVE CHANGE STRATEGIES AND COUNTERING IRRATIONAL BELIEFS

Once the child and therapist have identified maladaptive beliefs, the child can be taught to counter irrational or maladaptive beliefs through a number of different techniques. The cognitive change strategies used with adults usually involve a three-pronged approach: (1) look at the evidence, (2) explore the alternatives, and (3) examine the consequences. All three can be adapted for use with children. Beck, Rush, Shaw, and Emery (1979) developed the "What is the evidence?" technique. This technique helps fearful children identify their negative thoughts and develop more adaptive cognitions. In combination with this strategy, Beck et al. (1979) described the "What if?" technique. The therapist guides the child through a series of questions about the worst thing that could happen if the child's fears were to come true. Finally, teaching the child to examine alternatives (Beck et al., 1979), provides the child with alternative explanations and solutions.

These strategies are difficult to use with children because the hypothesis testing inherent in this approach is typically beyond the cognitive abilities of most children. Helping the child change cognitions will mean that the child will need assistance from an adult in generating alternative explanations, testing them, and changing beliefs (Emery, Bedrosian, & Garber, 1983). To challenge one's beliefs, it is usually necessary to distance oneself from the beliefs, a task that is beyond the grasp of most young children. In addition, the child needs an "accumulated history of events" to understand the ramifications of certain situations (Kendall, 1991). Children with limited life experiences, or those who have not formed beliefs about such experiences, often have not developed such an understanding. Despite these limitations in young children, Knell (1993a, 1993b, 1994, 1997, 1998, 1999) contends that cognitive change strategies can be adapted to the developmental levels of very young children. She argues that even preschoolers can benefit from cognitive interventions if they are presented in an age-appropriate way.

POSITIVE SELF-STATEMENTS

Individuals of all ages can be helped to develop adaptive coping self-statements. However, such positive self-statements must be adapted to the age of the child. Very young children can be taught clear, self-affirming statements that are linguistically and conceptually simple (e.g., "I am brave," "I can do this"). These statements contain an element of self-reward (e.g., "I am doing a good job"). Positive self-statements can be taught in therapy, but should be modeled by the therapist and parent alike. Turning praise into self-statements is not automatic, and the child must be helped to adapt positive, self-affirming comments. Children learn the positive value of what they do through specific labeling by significant adults, with positive feedback from those adults. Positive self-statements can teach coping strategies through active control ("I can walk past the dog whenever I feel like it"), reducing aversive feelings ("I will be able to go to school whenever I am ready"), reinforcing statements ("I am brave"), and reality testing ("There really are no monsters in our house") (Schroeder & Gordon, 1991).

In general, research suggests that cognitive interventions alone do not facilitate mastery over fear, although the combination of cognitive and behavioral interventions appear to help children cope with fearful situations and stimuli (Schroeder & Gordon, 1991). Therefore, CBPT treatment includes numerous behavioral interventions in addition to cognitive restructuring.

EXPOSURE

Exposure refers to the gradual and systematic confrontation of anxiety-provoking stimuli in real life so that habituation occurs (i.e, anxiety subsides or decreases owing to repeated exposure). Some researchers suggest that *in vivo* exposure is superior to imaginal exposure (Emmelkamp, 1982); others suggest that a blend of both imaginal and *in vivo* exposure should be used (James, 1985). When setting up *in vivo* exposure paradigms with a CBPT approach, it is important that the therapist has control over the feared stimulus (e.g., a cooperative dentist, an elevator that is not in a busy building and can be held at a floor for brief periods of time).

SYSTEMATIC DESENSITIZATION

Systematic desensitization is the process of reducing anxiety or fear by replacing a maladaptive response with an adaptive one (Wolpe, 1958, 1982). This is accomplished by breaking the association between a particular stimulus and the anxiety or fear response that it usually elicits. The stimulus is presented, but the anxiety is prevented from occurring. Systematic desensitization involves a person imagining a hierarchy of anxiety-provoking scenes in combination with these incompatible responses. Children over the age of 6 years can be taught modified relaxation techniques (e.g., Cautela & Groden, 1978), although some children may find other techniques more useful, such as calming play activities or visualization of calming scenes. Schroeder and Gordon (1991) even suggest the use of laughter, giving the example of a child imagining a feared monster dressed in red flannel underwear.

An example of systematic desensitization with a young child highlights the pairing of coping strategies with an anxiety-provoking situation. Liza was an 8-year-old girl who was fearful of small animals, including cats and dogs. She would panic if a dog came in view when she and her family walked on the sidewalk in their residential suburban neighborhood. In addition to screaming, she would often run to the other side of the street, or as far from the animal as possible. Her fears had interfered with her life in many ways. She avoided going to a friend's home to play if that friend had a pet. She avoided birthday parties and other social events if there might be an animal there. However, she was fine with pictures of animals, movies about animals, and any other representations of animals. In fact, she reported loving animals and even wishing that the family could have a cat or dog, if only she could get past her fear.

Liza was seen in play therapy, with a focus on developing a plan for dealing with her fears. Together with her parents and the therapist, a fear hierarchy was developed and a relaxation response, which included breathing and positive self-statements, was established. A list of self-statements was generated (e.g., "It's just my thought, it's not the nice dog"; "Just be brave and don't run away"; "I like animals"), mostly by Liza, but with the help of the therapist. Liza also made a list of comforting objects (e.g., a special necklace she had been given) that she could keep with her. A practice session included stuffed animals and pictures of animals, but this was easy for Liza as she experienced no fears with nonlive animals. In the first *in vivo* session, a calm, friendly small dog was introduced. The characteristics of the dog were important, as it was critical that the therapist have some control over the feared stimulus. If the dog had been loud, wild, or in any other way uncontrollable, Liza would have likely had a much more difficult time. During this session, Liza was reminded of her relaxation and self-statements, which she used throughout the session. She was able to approach the dog and eventually pet the dog, sitting on the ground next to the animal. She also practiced walking past the dog on the sidewalk (the dog was on a leash throughout the session, being walked by a graduate student therapist, while Liza's therapist stayed with her, coaching her through the techniques she had learned in the two previous in-office sessions). After this *in vivo* session, the family decided to try to help Liza without the therapist and later reported that she was approaching animals, petting them, and seemed to have gotten past her fears.

Exposure and systematic desensitization are powerful techniques with anxious and fearful children (Kendall et al., 2005). They are most useful when the child exhibits high levels of physiological reactivity (e.g., racing heart) and extreme avoidance (King et al., 1988). King and Ollendick (1997) report that there are numerous single-case studies, as well as several group studies, reporting that exposure and systematic desensitization are more effective than either no treatment or a waiting list control condition.

Other Behavioral Interventions in CBPT

CONTINGENCY MANAGEMENT

"Contingency management" is a general term that refers to techniques that modify a behavior by controlling its consequences. Positive reinforcement, shaping, stimulus fading, extinction, and differential reinforcement of other behavior (DRO) are all forms of contingency management. Management programs can be set up within the play therapy sessions or in the natural environment.

POSITIVE REINFORCEMENT

Positive reinforcement is an important component of almost every treatment for childhood fears. It is used with fears by specifying a target behavior, determining a reinforcer, and making the reinforcement contingent on the occurrence of the targeted behavior. It often involves social reinforcers (e.g., praise) or material reinforcers (e.g., stickers), and can be direct (e.g., praising a child with separation anxiety for venturing off to school without Mom) or more subtle (e.g., reinforcing independent play, which can ultimately lead to greater confidence in the ability to be away from a parent figure). Reinforcement can come from the therapist as well as the parents and significant others, who have been trained by the therapist to use appropriate reinforcement as the child conquers his or her fears.

For many children, chart systems that specify the desired behavior and reward can be extremely useful. Chart systems can help operationalize the desired behavior and ensure that the reinforcements are given in a systematic way. For example, a little girl fearful of sleeping in her own room can have a chart specifying that she will receive a sticker for going to bed within a certain time after being asked, will stay in her room without constantly complaining or leaving the room, and will stay in her bed all night. Such reinforcement also helps the child see that she can master the feared situation and provides the child fairly immediate feedback for her positive behaviors.

SHAPING

Shaping is a way of helping a child get progressively closer to a targeted goal. The child is given positive reinforcement for closer and closer approximations to the desired response. Eventually, the child reaches the desired behavior. One does not expect a fearful child to overcome his or her fears at once. Thus, a young boy who sleeps with his parents because he is fearful of sleeping in his own room could be shaped by providing reinforcement of his efforts in small steps (e.g., sleeping on the floor next to his parents' bed, sleeping on the floor in the hall toward his own room, sleeping on the floor in his room, sleeping in his own bed).

STIMULUS FADING

Stimulus fading is a technique designed to change behaviors by modifying their situational cues. A child may have some of the skills for a behavior, but may exhibit the behavior only in certain circumstances or with certain people (i.e., situational cues). In these situations, stimulus fading may be used. The therapist helps the child to use positive skills in one setting, and then helps the child transfer the skills to other settings. This is often seen when a child's responses may be different with each parent.

Stimulus fading was used with a 4½-year-old who was fearful of sleeping in her own room (see Case 1 later in this chapter for a more detailed description of the treatment in this case). At first the parents reported that she had not slept in her own bed since they moved into their new home 1½ years previously. In relating the history, the parents remembered that the child had stayed in her room approximately 1 year ago, when her father had been responsible for putting the child to bed. At that time, he had decided that "Mom was not allowed" around at bedtime (other than to say good night to the child), and the child had had no difficulty going to sleep under these circumstances. Unfortunately, she had gotten sick and regressed to her previous behavior. Treatment consisted, in part, of designating the father as the primary parent to get the child ready for bed. After a reasonable routine was established and the child was sleeping through the night in her room, the mother was gradually faded back into the bedtime routine.

EXTINCTION AND DIFFERENTIAL REINFORCEMENT OF OTHER BEHAVIOR

Some children exhibit fears because they have been (or are being) reinforced for performing them. In such cases, the reinforcing behaviors will have to be removed in order for the child to stop being fearful. A common reinforcing behavior is parental attention. After evaluation, it may become clear that the parent's attention is a causal factor or major contributor to the child's fear. Behaviors can be extinguished by withholding reinforcement. Extinction does not teach new behaviors, so it is frequently used in conjunction with a reinforcement program. A child can be reinforced for learning a new behavior at the same time that another behavior is being extinguished. This can be done through differential reinforcement of other behavior (DRO). Thus, behaviors that are different from or incompatible with the maladaptive behavior are reinforced.

MODELING

Modeling is well researched and used frequently with fearful and anxious children. Modeling allows the child to see nonfearful behavior in the anxiety-provoking situation and demonstrates for the child a more appropriate response for dealing with the feared stimuli. This approach provides the child with an opportunity to see a model learn new skills to deal with a feared stimulus, which may be particularly useful for a child who does not have the requisite skills to deal with his or her fears.

Modeling designed to enhance skills can involve either coping or mastery models. Coping models display less-than-ideal skills and then gradually become more proficient, whereas mastery models exhibit a "perfect" performance. Research has shown that the efficacy of modeling is improved by the use of coping models, which may be thought of as a way of shaping the model toward the desired goal (Bandura & Menlove, 1968; Meichenbaum, 1971). The child may observe the model in the model's efforts to learn more appropriate skills. It is felt that mastery models do not, in fact, model any skills for the child and are thus less likely to help the child acquire new behaviors. A systematic desensitization paradigm can be modeled for the child, for example, with the model gradually being exposed to a feared stimulus and learning to cope with it. Modeling can also take many forms, including symbolic modeling, whereby the models, often in stories, cope with feared stimuli, and participant modeling, in which the model and child directly interact, with the model guiding the child through steps to overcome fears.

Although studies show that modeling procedures have been used frequently and often successfully in treating fearful children, many of these studies have involved children with mild fears (King & Ollendick, 1997). Unfortunately, adequate studies of modeling with more intense fears and phobias have yet to be conducted.

SELF-CONTROL

Self-control is really not an intervention per se. Rather, it is a strategy geared toward teaching an individual to use new behaviors and ways of thinking that enhance the person's sense of control. Ollendick and Cerney (1981) outlined a number of reasons why teaching children to regulate their own behaviors has received increased interest. Evidence suggests that a child's controlling his or her own behavior may be more efficient (Lovitt & Curtiss, 1969) and more durable (Drabman, Spitalnik, & O'Leary, 1973) than programs initiated by significant others on behalf of the child.

Through cognitive self-control programs (e.g., Kendall et al., 1992), children are taught to monitor, evaluate, and reinforce themselves for using more adaptive coping skills. Silverman, 1989 (as cited in Eisen & Kearney, 1995) developed the STOP acronym to help children stop their anxiety (Scared, fearful Thoughts, Other thoughts [coping], Praise). Through self-control training and techniques such as utilization of the STOP acronym, fearful children can be taught to regulate their own behavior.

BIBLIOTHERAPY

Bibliotherapy is not technically a cognitive intervention, but is used increasingly as an adjunct to therapy. The focus of using self-help books with children is somewhat different than with adults. Most therapeutic books for children provide a story with a child (model) who copes with a situation similar to the one the child may be facing. Such stories may model a child's reaction to a particular situation, with the hope that the listener (or reader) will incorporate some of the ideas presented into his or her own approach to the problem. A separate reference section including appropriate published books for fearful children is included at the end of this chapter.

At times, published materials may not be available or appropriate, and in these cases it may be desirable to create books specifically for a particular child. A simple therapist-created book was used in the short-term intervention of a 2-year, 5-month-old child who was fearful of fires after experiencing several fires in abandoned homes in his neighborhood. He would become upset when he heard sirens or saw fire trucks. The therapist wrote a brief story about a child who experienced similar fires. The child in the story told his family about his fears, learned to talk about his feelings, and felt safe when he went to bed at night. Although the therapist wrote the book because of the age of the child in treatment, the child helped illustrate the book during treatment sessions, and it was read to him by the therapist over the course of several sessions and by his parents at home (Knell, 1993a).

With older preschool and school-age children, it can be helpful to create a book with the child during a treatment session. Often, the therapist may need to model much of the problem solving and creating of positive self-statements for and with the child. The advantages of working on the book together with the child are numerous. First and foremost, through such collaboration the child is a more active participant in change than if a previously published or therapist-written book is brought to the therapy session. As the child actively participates in the writing of the book, it is possible to incorporate spontaneous material brought to treatment by the child. Further, it is possible to involve the child in cognitive change strategies as the book is written. That is, if the child voices maladaptive thoughts, the child and therapist can collaboratively work on more adaptive, positive self-statements to include in the book.

A book written in therapy with a 7-year-old child who was experiencing depression and separation anxiety illustrates these points. The child was referred for treatment by her mother's therapist. The mother was being seen for depression and for her difficulty in parenting her two children. The child seemed to be mirroring her mother's sadness, fears, and need to be in constant contact with her child. In one session, the child expressed her concerns about being apart from her mother, but was also able to express things that helped her feel safe and comfortable when her mother was not near. Among the things that helped were hugging her dog and seeking comfort from her babysitter.

The therapist helped the child write a simple book entitled *Things to Do When I Miss Mom*. The child's own ideas were incorporated into the text, although new ideas and positive self-statements were added by the therapist. Each sentence was written on a separate page, which was illustrated by the child. Sample sentences included positive self-statements ("Say to myself, 'I miss Mom but she will be back soon,' 'Mom's OK, I'm OK, I will see Mom really soon'") and coping suggestions ("Look at a picture of Mom, look at this book") suggested by the therapist, as well as coping suggestions generated by the child ("I can give my babysitter a hug," "I can give my dog a hug").

PARENT INVOLVEMENT

Parents should be involved in both the assessment and intervention phase. Parents are always involved in the assessment phase of therapy, through clinical interview, behavioral rating scales, and/or behavioral observations at home. After the assessment is completed, it is often best to meet with the parents again to present the findings of the evaluation and agree on a treatment plan. The plan may involve individual play therapy with the child, work with the parents, or a combination of CBPT and parent work. Such decisions are based on the therapist's assessment of many factors, such as whether the parents will need help in modifying their interactions with the child and whether the child will need assistance in implementing a treatment plan outside therapy.

When the therapeutic work is primarily with the child, it is still important to meet with the parents on a regular basis. During these sessions, the therapist will gather new information about the child's progress, continue to monitor and intervene in relation to the parent's interaction with the child, and make suggestions on areas of concern.

A primary focus of parent work with fearful and anxious children involves helping parents to understand their role in their child's anxiety and to design an approach that will allow them to reinforce the child's ability to effectively manage his or her anxiety independently. The parents' behavior and responses to the child have served either to encourage, reinforce, and maintain or to exacerbate the child's symptoms. In the previous example of the almost 2½-year-old who was afraid of fire and fire-related objects and sounds (e.g., fire trucks, sirens), the therapist was able to observe the family interaction when a fire truck with siren blaring went by during a treatment session. In this unplanned but well-timed situation, the therapist observed the parents coddle the child the instant they heard the siren. In fact, the parents moved toward the child *before* it was clear that the child had even heard the siren. In this situation, it was helpful to instruct the parents not to assume that the child would react in a fearful way, and thus not to reinforce the response before it even occurred. Parents' behavior can serve to reinforce or encourage a child's fear.

Quite simply, a child who receives more attention for being fearful, than he or she receives for a more adaptive behavior, is likely to continue the fearful behavior because of the reinforcement received for the fearful response.

Parent involvement in intervention usually occurs in two phases: psychoeducation and skill building. During psychoeducation, clinicians help parents to understand their child's anxiety symptoms, by defining those symptoms. In addition, parents are asked to describe their responses to their child's anxiety and then identify the behaviors that are helpful and unhelpful.

The skill-building phase of parent involvement includes building parenting skills, with the goal of helping their child manage anxiety independently. Rapee, Spence, Cobham, and Wignell (2000) suggest that parents develop five strategies to accomplish this goal. First, parents are taught to communicate their empathy effectively. They are instructed to help their child feel listened to by labeling the emotion and validating his or her experience with statements such as, "Sounds like you are nervous about this visit" and "I can imagine that it is hard for you to face this fear." A second strategy is teaching parents to reward coping or "brave" behavior. After assisting parents in defining their child's brave behavior, the therapist instructs the parents to provide consistent and meaningful reinforcement, using verbal praise and stickers. In conjunction with the second strategy, the importance of decreasing attention for anxious behaviors (e.g., ignoring whining, tearfulness, tantrums) is explained to parents. In addition, parents are taught to prompt their child to use problem-solving skills. It is suggested that they use statements such as "What are some ways in which you can help yourself feel less nervous?" to coach their child to come up with their own solutions to problems. Finally, parents are encouraged to model brave, coping behavior for their children, as children tend to learn behaviors from adults.

In general, parents are consistently reminded that the goals of these strategies are (1) to help their child independently cope with his or her own anxiety and (2) to guide their child to use them as a support and not as a crutch. There is some research to suggest that cognitive-behavioral treatment is more effective when parent involvement is an additional component (Barrett, Dadds, & Rapee, 1996).

Relapse Prevention and Generalization

An important goal in the therapy of anxious and fearful children is for them to maintain adaptive behaviors after the treatment has ended, and to generalize these behaviors to the natural environment. Achievement of this goal means that if a child learns to overcome fears and anxieties during treatment, he or she will maintain this new ability after treatment ends, and that more adaptive behavior and thinking will be evident in all settings, not just the psychotherapy setting. Promoting and facilitating generalization should be part of the therapy;

it will not necessarily happen without such planning (Meichenbaum, 1977). Generalization can be dealt with through using real-life situations in modeling and role playing, teaching self-management skills, involving significant adults and caregivers in the treatment, and continuing with treatment past the initial acquisition of skills to ensure that adequate learning takes place.

In addition to generalization, therapy should be geared toward helping the child and family prevent relapse. High-risk situations should be identified, and the child and parents should be prepared for handing such potentially disruptive situations. In this way, the child is "inoculated" against failure (Meichenbaum, 1985; Marlatt & Gordon, 1985). High-risk situations may coincide with normal developmental tasks (e.g., starting a new school year) or with the child's life situation (e.g., coping with a divorce). In CBPT, the therapist may create play scenarios similar to those the child may face in the future, and include adaptive coping skills and positive behaviors as part of the play. An example of this approach occurred with a 4-year-old boy who was having difficulty in dealing with going back and forth between his newly divorced parents' homes. During the play, the child would have the child character swoop through the air between the homes in a frenzylike fashion. The therapist helped the child to "land" the male character at each home and deal more positively with each parent. This involved modeling both appropriate behavior (calm, not acting out) and positive self-statements ("I'm sad that they are divorced, but at least they aren't fighting anymore") about the divorce. In practicing anxiety management skills at each "home," the child was able to practice generalizing these skills to specific, real environments

CASE ILLUSTRATIONS

Case 1: Laura (Normal Developmental Fears, V Code)

The treatment of a 4½-year-old girl, fearful of sleeping in her own room, illustrates the use of the contingency management (positive reinforcement, shaping, stimulus fading, extinction, and DRO), bibliotherapy, modeling, and positive self-statements. Laura was brought to treatment by her parents, who reported that she had not slept in her own room since moving into their new home 1½ years ago. According to her parents, Laura would fall asleep in the family room and one of the parents would pick her up and put her in her bed. She would sleep for several hours, and then during the night she would get up and move to her parents' bed. If the parents insisted that she return to her own room, she would scream and cry. Laura reported being afraid of monsters in her room. The child had actually slept in her own room for a brief period of time approximately 1 year before the family sought treatment. According to her father, he had taken her to her room, told her that Mom was not allowed, read her a story, and put her to bed. She did extremely well with this until she became ill with the flu, and then the old pattern evolved again.

As part of the assessment, a Child Behavior Checklist (CBCL; Achenbach, 1991) was completed by each parent. The father's completed profile was non-clinical, with slight elevations (although still within normal limits) on the Anxious/Depressed and Social Problem scales. The CBCL completed by Laura's mother also provided a nonclinical profile, although with slight elevations (nonclinical) on the Social Problem and Thought Problem scales. The parental interview had taken place at the first appointment; at the second, Laura was seen. A Puppet Sentence Completion Task (Knell & Beck, 2000) was administered, and several of her responses suggested feelings/thoughts about her sleep difficulties. A few selections are listed here:

> I am afraid of *monsters.*
> The best secret is *that I sleep in my bed, that I should sleep in my bed.*
> I am happiest when *I wake up.*
> My biggest problem is *being afraid of the dark.*
> My room is *pretty.*

In discussion with Laura, she expressed her concern about monsters that are big and scary, with long teeth, who come out only at night, and only in her bedroom. She also spontaneously related that she was afraid of a poster in her room, didn't like her closet door open, and was able to sleep in her own room when she was 3 years old. She remembered that she felt good about being able to sleep there. Laura and the therapist made a list of everyone who would be happy if she slept in her own bed at night. The list consisted of her mom, dad, self, and family cat.

Recommendations were made to Laura and her parents at the end of the second appointment. The parents were given a list of suggestions, partly gleaned from Laura's own suggestions. They were instructed to keep her closet door closed and to remove the poster from her room that she had identified as frightening. Changing these small environmental stimuli gave Laura some control over how she wanted her room and potentially eliminated aspects of her room that she identified as frightening. The list of people who would be happy if she slept in her own room was to be taped next to her bed. This provided some immediate positive reinforcement, somewhat akin to the "friends who care list" developed by Azrin and Foxx (1974) to help children with toileting. Laura's parents were asked to buy a "special flashlight," one that she could keep next to her bed and could use herself whenever she became frightened. Finally, they were given a container of (imaginary) magic monster spray; Laura had "tried" this with the therapist and understood that when used, it could "magically keep the monsters away." Both the flashlight and the spray offered Laura some modicum of control over her environment and, potentially, her fears. At that point, it was decided that Laura's father would be the primary parent putting Laura to bed at night. This decision was based on the history that suggested that Laura's mother reinforced Laura's nighttime fears and had difficulty in insisting that Laura sleep in her own bed. (This stimulus-fading component of treatment is described in a previous section of this chapter). The parents were encouraged to continue with the program even if Laura had a difficult time the first few nights. The therapist explained to them that as the nighttime problem behavior gradually lessened, because it had been previously reinforced they could expect to see an increase in such behavior before it disappeared altogether (i.e., an increase in a previously reinforced behavior while it is being extinguished). Thus, the parents were told to expect that Laura might exhibit an increase in fear and/or crying when she was not receiving attention for not being in her bed (extinction). Laura and her parents left this session eager to try the new program.

The family was seen for the third session 1 week later. They reported that Laura cried for 2 hours the first night, and 1 hour the second night. By the third night of the program she fussed for only a few minutes, and by night 4 she slept in her own room without difficulty. At this session, Laura was given stickers for her positive accomplishments (reinforcement) and she and the therapist made a book (bibliotherapy) that consisted of simple positive self-statements on each page:

Laura's Book
One night, Laura slept in her own bed all night.
She used her flashlight.
She used her monster spray. Dad sprayed it all.
And she slept in her bed, ALL NIGHT.
YEAH.

They also made a special sign with stars on it to place on her wall. The sign said, "Good job Laura, for sleeping in your own bed" (positive reinforcement).

The family was seen for the fourth session 1 month later. At that time, Laura was sleeping in her own room, with either parent in charge of the bedtime routine. In individual play therapy with Laura, puppets were used to play out different bedtime scenarios. In response to a puppet who was fearful of the dark, Laura told him to "use his flashlight." Thus, she was able to "model" her own coping skills for the puppet. She also helped the therapist read the story they wrote at the last session, and drew pictures of herself in her own bed and her parents in their bed. These activities all served to reinforce her newly gained skills and thus provide a measure of relapse prevention for Laura.

Case 2: Cara (Separation Anxiety)

Cara was a 4-year, 9-month-old girl who was brought to treatment because of her difficulties in separating from her mother (a more detailed description of this case is provided in Knell, 1999). She would cry and sob for hours if left at preschool and would not separate from her mother at family gatherings and birthday parties. She had no specific traumatic experiences in early childhood, although she had certainly experienced much stress when away from her mother. This case is a classic example of Separation Anxiety disorder, but is presented here because of the efforts to deal with the child's fears associated with either the anticipation or actual event of separation from her mom.

Work with the mother included setting up a positive reinforcement chart on which Cara received a sticker for every day she was able to separate from her mom and play at school without crying. Her mother was encouraged to praise Cara's efforts (shaping) and ignore behaviors that interfered (extinction).

During play therapy, Cara was encouraged to express her feelings about separation through pictures, stories, and puppet play. In CBPT, the therapist introduced several puppets, including one who was afraid to go to school. Positive coping statements were modeled by the therapist for a bear puppet (e.g., "I can do this," " I will have a good time at school and not miss Mom too much"). Cara became interested in a puppet who seemed to "worry too much." Together with the therapist, she generated a list of things that would help the bear puppet entitled "Mr. Bear's List" (e.g., "Think of something happy," "Mom's coming back," "I think I can, I think I can," "Play with toys and have fun"). This list provided the bear with positive coping statements that he could use to alleviate his anxiety (modeling positive self-statements). Cara was guided through a series of discussions regarding a bear puppet's fears of being left at school. Through the "voice" of the puppet, the therapist modeled adaptive coping skills for the child. As therapy progressed, the child began to incorporate these skills into her stories and puppet play and, gradually, into her own coping behavior at school. The book *The Little Engine That Could* was used to model for Cara the idea that difficult things can be accomplished with lots of work and effort (bibliotherapy).

Cara and the therapist wrote and illustrated several books about her fears (bibliotherapy). For one book, she dictated a story of herself not crying at school and how proud she was ("Me not crying and I'm so proud of myself. One day I went to school, and I didn't even cry. At one point I started crying and then the teachers told me it's no problem to cry, and then I didn't not cry anymore [*sic*]. The end").

She also dictated a book about school titled, "Cara's Book about School." Pages in this book included statements such as "I think about the choo-choo train that could. . . . I picture things in my mind. . . . I think about coloring and that makes all the tears go away. . . . Sometimes I worry about if my Mom is OK. I remind myself, 'She's ok.'" During the course of treatment her mother expressed a new concern, that Cara was avoiding playing outside because of a fear of bugs. Cara and the therapist worked on a book about bugs:

One day, I looked at a bug and it scared me. Then it flew away, but it didn't bother me. The next day, I went outside. I walked past the bug. It saw me, but it flew by me, and didn't hurt me. It kept flying by me. One day, I went outside and I walked past a bug with a stinger. It watched me go by, and then it stinged me. It really hurt. Daddy took the stinger out. He carried me into the house, put a band-aid on, and fixed me up. Sometimes bugs can hurt, but it's OK, I don't need to be too afraid.

The treatment involved a total of nine sessions, which were typically spent partly with her mother, and then with Cara in CBPT. The sessions took place over the course of 6 months, with sessions purposely spaced out in order to accommodate changes in Cara's life (e.g., entering kindergarten). At termination, her mother reported that Cara was going outside and not showing any more fear of bugs. Peer interactions were increasing. Cara had begun kindergarten, was separating from Mom, and riding on the school bus without difficulty.

SUMMARY AND CONCLUSIONS

CBPT is designed specifically for preschool and early elementary school-age children. It emphasizes the child's involvement in therapy and addresses issues of control, mastery, and responsibility for changing one's own behavior. The child is helped to become an active participant in change (Knell, 1993a). By presenting developmentally appropriate interventions, the therapist helps the child benefit from therapy. A wide array of techniques and approaches can be incorporated into CBPT.

CBPT is solidly grounded in data-based psychological interventions, as delineated by the American Psychological Association's (APA) Task Force on the promotion and dissemination of psychological procedures (Chambless et al., 1996). CBT is well-established treatment for specific populations such as those with anxiety and depression; thus, the foundations of CBPT were developed by adapting empirically supported techniques for younger children in a play setting. Establishing the efficacy of CBPT is an important next step in the development of this therapy.

For CBPT to be effective, it should provide structured, goal-directed activities, at the same time allowing the child to bring spontaneous material to the session. The balance of spontaneously generated and more structured activities is a delicate one in CBPT. Unstructured, spontaneously generated information is critical to treatment, for without it the therapist would lose a rich source of clinical information. Yet when therapy is completely unstructured and nondirective, it is not possible to teach more adaptive behaviors, such as problem solving.

A significant component of overcoming fear and anxiety appears to be the child's gaining control and exposure to achieve mastery. Developing this sense of control may mean that the child learns to deal with the feared stimuli, to manage feelings associated with the fear, or to learn specific coping skills to deal with the fear. Similarly, specific anxieties (e.g., related to separation or social issues) may require developing a sense of control over the specific issues at hand. Cognitive-behavioral interventions provide such learning opportunities, as well as the specific skills necessary to overcome fears and anxieties. In play therapy, children may master feared objects by taking on the roles of those who do not fear these objects. They may act in ways that suggest they are not afraid. By "pretending," and practicing, a child may overcome the feared stimulus, and anxiety-provoking situations.

REFERENCES

Achenbach, T. M. (1991). *Manual for the Child Behavior Checklist 4–18 and 1991 Profile*. Burlington: University of Vermont, Department of Psychiatry.

Achenbach, T. M., Howell, C. T., McConaughy, S. H., & Stranger, C. (1995). Six-year predictors of problems in a national sample of children and youth: I. Cross-informant syndromes. *Journal of the American Academy of Child and Adolescent Psychiatry, 34*, 336–347.

Agras, W. S., Chapin, N. H., & Oliveau, D. C. (1972). The natural history of phobias: Course and prognosis. *Archives of General Psychiatry, 26*, 315–317.

Albano, A. M., Chorpita, B. F., & Barlow, D. H. (2003). In E. J. Mash & R. A. Barkley (Eds.), *Child psychopathology* (2nd ed., pp. 279–329). New York: Guilford Press.

Albano, A. M., & Kendall, P. C. (2002). Cognitive-behavioral therapy for children and adolescents with anxiety disorders: Clinical research advances. *International Review of Psychiatry, 14*, 129–134.

American Psychiatric Association. (1994). *Diagnostic and statistical manual of mental disorders* (4th ed.). Washington, DC Author.

Azrin, N. H., & Foxx, R. M. (1974). *Toilet training in less than a day*. New York: Simon & Schuster.

Bandura, A., & Menlove, F. L. (1968). Factors determining vicarious extinction of avoidance behavior through symbolic modeling. *Journal of Personality and Social Psychology, 8*, 99–108.

Barrett, P. M., Dadds, M. R., & Rapee, R. M. (1996). Family treatment of childhood anxiety: A controlled trial. *Journal of Consulting and Clinical Psychology, 64*, 333–342.

Barrios, B. A., & Hartmann, D. P. (1997). Fears and anxieties. In E. J. Mash & L. G. Terdal (Eds.), *Treatment of childhood disorders* (3rd ed, pp. 230–327), New York: Guilford Press.

Beck, A. T. (1967). *Depression: Clinical, experimental, and theoretical aspects*. NY: Harper and Row.

Beck, A. T. (1972). *Depression: Causes and treatment*. Philadelphia: University of Pennsylvania Press.

Beck, A. T. (1976). *Cognitive therapy and the emotional disorders.* New York: International Universities Press.

Beck, A. T., Rush, A. J., Shaw, B. F., & Emery, G. (1979). *Cognitive therapy of depression.* New York: Guilford Press.

Bedrosian, R., & Beck, A. T. (1980). Principles of cognitive therapy. In M. J. Mahoney (Ed.), *Psychotherapy process: Current issues and future directions* (pp. 127–152). New York: Plenum Press.

Birmaher, B., Khertarpal, S., Brent, D., Cully, M., Balach, L., Kaufman, J., et al. (1997). The Screen for Child Anxiety Related Emotional Disorder (SCARED): Scale construction and psychometric characteristics. *Journal of the American Academy of Child and Adolescent Psychiatry, 36,* 545–553.

Cautela, J. R., & Groden, J. (1978). *Relaxation. A comprehensive manual for adults, children, and children with special needs.* Champaign, IL: Research Press.

Chambless, D. L., Sanderson, W. C., Shoham, V., Johnson, S. B., Pope, K. S., Crits-Christoph, P., et al. (1996). An update on empirically validated therapies. *Clinical Psychologst, 49,* 5–18.

Compton, S. N., March, J. S., Brent, D., Albano, A. M., Weersing, V. R., & Curry, J. (2004). Cognitive-behavioral psychotherapy for anxiety and depressive disorders in children and adolescents: An evidence-based medicine review. *Journal of the American Academy of Child and Adolescent Psychiatry, 43,* 930–959.

Drabman, R., Spitalnik, R., & O'Leary, K. D. (1973). Teaching self-control to disruptive children. *Journal of Abnormal Psychology, 82,* 110–116.

Eisen, A. R., & Kearney, C. (1995). *Practitioners guide to treating fear and anxiety in children and adolescents.* Northvale, NJ: Aronson.

Emery, G., Bedrosian, R., & Garber, J. (1983). Cognitive therapy with depressed children and adolescents. In D. P. Cantwell & G. A. Carlson (Eds.), *Affective disorders in childhood and adolescence: An update* (pp. 445–471). New York: Spectrum.

Emmelkamp, P. M. G. (1982). Anxiety and fear. In A. S. Bellack, M. Herzen, & A. E. Kazdin (Eds.), *International handbook of behavior modification and therapy* (pp. 349–395). New York: Plenum Press.

Geddes, J., Reynolds, S., Streiner, D., & Szatmari, P. (1997). Evidence-based practice in mental health [Editorial]. *British Medical Journal, 315,* 1483–1484.

Gurley, D., Cohen, P., Pine, D. S., & Brook, J. (1996). Discriminating anxiety and depression in youth: A role for diagnostic criteria. *Journal of Affective Disorders, 39,* 191–200.

Hampe, E., Noble, H., Miller, L. C., & Barrett, C. L. (1973). Phobic children one and two years post treatment. *Journal of Abnormal Psychology, 82,* 446–453.

James, J. E. (1985). Desensitization treatment of agoraphobia. *British Journal of Clinical Psychology, 24,* 133–134.

Kazdin, A. E., & Weisz, J. R. (1998). Identifying and developing empirically supported child and adolescent treatments. *Journal of Consulting and Clinical Psychology, 66,* 19–36.

Kendall, P. C. (Ed.). (1991). *Child and adolescent therapy.* New York: Guilford Press.

Kendall, P. C., Chansky, T. E., Kane, M. T., Kim, R. S., Kortlander, E., et al. (1992). *Anxiety disorders in youth: Cognitive behavioral interventions.* Boston: Allyn and Bacon.

Kendall, P. C., Robin, J. A., Hedtke, K. A., Suveg, C., Flannery-Schroeder, E., & Gosch, E. (2005). Considering CBT with anxious youth? Think exposures. *Cognitive and Behavioral Practice, 12*, 136–150.

King, N. J., Hamilton, D. H., & Ollendick, T. H. (1988*). Children's phobias: A behavioral perspective.* New York: Wiley.

King, N. J., & Ollendick, T. H. (1997). Annotation: Treatment of childhood phobias. *Journal of Child Psychology and Psychiatry and Allied Disciplines, 38*, 389–400.

Klein, R. G., & Pine, D. S. (2002). Anxiety disorders. In M. Rutter & E. Taylor (Eds.), *Child and adolescent psychiatry* (4th ed., pp. 486–509). Oxford, UK: Blackwell.

Knell, S. M. (1993a). *Cognitive-behavioral play therapy.* Northvale, NJ: Aronson.

Knell, S. M. (1993b). To show and not tell: Cognitive-behavioral play therapy in the treatment of elective mutism. In T. Kottman & C. Schaefer (Eds.), *Play therapy in action: A casebook for practitioners* (pp. 169–208). Northvale, NJ: Aronson.

Knell, S. M. (1994). Cognitive-behavioral play therapy. In K. O'Connor & C. Schaefer (Eds.), *Handbook of play therapy: Vol. 2. Advances and innovations* (pp. 111–142). New York: Wiley.

Knell, S. M. (1997). Cognitive-behavioral play therapy. In K. O'Connor & L. Mages (Eds.), *Play therapy theory and practice: A comparative presentation* (pp. 79–99). New York: Wiley.

Knell, S. M. (1998). Cognitive-behavioral play therapy. *Journal of Clinical Child Psychology, 27*, 28–33.

Knell, S. M. (1999). Cognitive behavioral play therapy. In S. W. Russ & T. Ollendick (Eds.), *Handbook of psychotherapies with children and families* (pp. 385–404). New York: Plenum Press.

Knell, S. M. & Beck, K. W. (2000). Puppet sentence completion task. In C. E. Schaefer, K. Gitlin-Weiner, & A. Sandgrund (Eds.), *Play diagnosis and assessment* (Vol. 2, pp. 704–721). New York: Wiley.

Knell, S. M., & Moore, D. J. (1990). Cognitive-behavioral play therapy in the treatment of encopresis. *Journal of Clinical Child Psychology, 19*, 55–60.

Knell, S. M., & Ruma, C. D. (1996). Play therapy with a sexually abused child. In M. Reinecke, F. M. Dattilio, & A. Freeman (Eds.), *Casebook of cognitive-behavior therapy with children and adolescents* (pp. 367–393). New York: Guilford Press.

Lovitt, T. C., & Curtiss, K. A. (1969). Academic response rate as a function of teacher- and self-imposed contingencies. *Journal of Applied Behavior Analysis, 2*, 49–53.

March, J. S. (1997). *Multidimensional Anxiety Scale for Children.* Toronto: Mutli-Health Systems.

March, J., & Wells, K. (2003). Combining medication and psychotherapy. In A. Martin, L. Scahill, D. S. Charney, & J. F. Leckman (Eds.), *Pediatric pharmacology: Principles and practice* (pp. 426–446). London: Oxford University Press.

Marlatt, G. A., & Gordon, J. R. (1985). *Relapse prevention: Maintenance strategies in the treatment of addictive behaviors.* New York: Guilford Press.

Meichenbaum, D. (1971). Examination of model characteristics in reducing avoidance behavior. *Journal of Personality and Social Psychology, 17*, 298–307.

Meichenbaum, D. (1977). *Cognitive-behavior modification: An integrative approach.* New York: Plenum Press.

Meichenbaum, D. (1985). *Stress inoculation training.* New York: Pergamon Press.

Muris, P., Merckelbach, H., Gadet, B., & Moulaert, V. (2000). Fears, worries, and scary dreams in 4- to 12-year-old children: Their content, developmental pattern, and origins. *Journal of Clinical Child Psychology, 29,* 43–52.

Muris, P., Merckelbach, H., Mayer, B., & Prins, E. N. (2000). How serious are common childhood fears? *Behaviour Research and Therapy, 38,* 217–228.

Ollendick, T. H. (1979). Fear reduction techniques with children. In M. Hersen, R. M. Fisher, & P. M. Miller (Eds.), *Progress in behavior modification* (Vol. 8, pp. 127–168). New York: Academic Press.

Ollendick, T. H., & Cerney, J. A. (1981). *Clinical behavior therapy with children.* New York: Plenum Press.

Ollendick, T. H., & King, N. J. (1998). Empirically supported treatments for children with phobic and anxiety disorders. *Journal of Clinical Child Psychology, 27,* 156–167.

Rapee, R. M., Spence, S. H., Cobham, V., & Wignell, A. (2000). *Helping your anxious child: A step-by-step guide for parents.* Oakland, CA: New Harbinger.

Schroeder, C. S., & Gordon, B. N. (1991). *Assessment and treatment of childhood problems.* New York: Guilford Press.

Shaffer, D., Fisher, P., Dulcan, M., David, D., Piacentini, J., Schwab-Stone, M., et al. (1996). The NIMH Diagnostic Interview Schedule for Children, Version (DISC2.3): Description, acceptability, prevalence rates, and performance in the MECA study. *Journal of the American Academy of Child and Adolescent Psychiatry, 49,* 865–877.

Silverman, W. K., & Albano, A. M. (1996a). *The Anxiety Disorders Interview Schedule for DSM-IV: Child Interview Schedule.* San Antonio, TX: Psychological Corporation.

Silverman, W. K., & Albano, A. M. (1996b). *The Anxiety Disorders Interview Schedule for DSM-IV: Child Interview Schedule.* San Antonio, TX: Psychological Corporation.

Silverman, W. K., & Nelles, W. B. (1990). Simple phobia in childhood. In M. Hersen & C. Last (Eds.), *Handbook of child and adult psychopathology: A longitudinal perspective* (pp. 183–195). New York: Pergamon Press.

Strauss, C. C., & Last, C. G. (1993). Social and simple phobias in children. *Journal of Anxiety Disorders, 7,* 141–152.

Turner, S., & Heiser, N. (1999). Current status of psychological interventions for childhood anxiety disorders. In D. Beidel (Ed.), *Treating anxiety disorders in youth: Current problems and future solutions* (pp. 63–76). Washington, DC: Anxiety Disorders Association of America.

Velting, O. N., Setzer, N. J., & Albano, A. M. (2004). Update on and advances in assessment and cognitive-behavioral treatment of anxiety disorders in children and adolescents. *Professional Psychology: Research and Practice, 35,* 42–54.

Walk, R. D. (1956). Self-ratings of fear in a fear-invoking situation. *Journal of Abnormal and Social Psychology, 52,* 171–178.

Williams, M. L. (1996). *Cool cats, calm kids: Relaxation and stress management for young people.* San Luis Obispo, CA: Impact.

Wolpe, J. (1958). *Psychotherapy by reciprocal inhibition.* Stanford, CA: Stanford University Press.

Wolpe, J. (1982). *The practice of behavior therapy* (3rd ed). Oxford, UK: Pergamon Press.

Bibliotherapy–Books for Children

Dutro, J. (1991). *Night light: A story for children afraid of the dark.* New York: Magination Press.

Emberley, E. (1992). *Go away big green monster!* New York: Little, Brown.

Harrison, J. (1995). *Dear bear.* Lerner.

Lankton, S. R. (1988). *The blammo-surprise! book: A story to help children overcome fears.* New York: Magination Press.

Lobby, T. (1990). *Jessica and the wolf: A story for children who have bad dreams.* New York: Magination Press.

Marcus, I. W., & Marcus, P. (1990). *Scary night visitors.* New York: Magination Press.

Marcus, I. W., & Marcus, P. (1992). *Into the great forest: A story for children away from parents for the first time.* New York: Magination Press.

Penn, A. (1993). *The kissing hand.* Washington, DC: Child Welfare League of America.

Piper, W. (1950). *The little engine that could.* New York: Platt & Munk.

Weinstein-Stern, D. (1994). *Mira's month.* Highland Park, IL: BMT Newsletter.

Williams, M. L. (1996). *Cool cats, calm kids: Relaxation and stress management for young people.* San Luis Obispo, CA: Impact.

Bibliotherapy–Books for Parents

Chansky, T. E. (2001). *Freeing your child from obsessive compulsive disorder: A powerful, practical program for parents of children and adolescents.* New York, NY: Three River Press.

Manassis, K. (1996). *Keys to parenting your anxious child.* Hauppauge, NY: Barron's Educational Series.

Rapee, R. M., Spence, S. H., Cobham, V., & Wignell, A. (2000). *Helping your anxious child: A step-by-step guide for parents.* Oakland, CA: New Harbinger.

Websites for Parents

Anxiety Disorders Association of America (ADAA): www.adaa.org Nonprofit organization

Freedom from Fear: www.freedomfromfear.com National Nonprofit mental illness advocacy organization

CHAPTER 3

Short-Term Play Therapy for Children with Disruptive Behavior Disorders

SCOTT RIVIERE

In all of my years of working with children, the therapy of children with disruptive behavior disorders (DBDs) has always been a love of mine. I know many therapists who would rather refer a child with a DBD diagnosis than treat him or her. I believe this is because so many of the behavior interventions that are "supposed to work" seem ineffective with these children. In this chapter I hope to educate you on a *method* of working with children who have DBD diagnoses. Techniques will come and go, but having a solid method to operate from gives mental health professionals some parameters to design their own creative interventions to help such children. The method's primary function is to help parents, teachers, and mental health professionals get a glimpse of how these children see the world, as well as how their behavior affects others in their lives. I have found that this method can be applied to a variety of activities, games, and therapeutic interventions, as well as parenting skills. It can be equally effective in one session or over a period of time. I have discovered that most of the attention is given to the behavioral effects of a DBD diagnosis. So this chapter is also designed to assist mental health professionals in understanding the *emotional* effects of a DBD. By understanding the dynamics of how these children see their world, you will better be able to help them. The cornerstones of this method consist of three important concepts:

1. Buttons
2. Punishment/reward-based system
3. Self-confidence bucket

As you consider these concepts, it is important to remember that these children see the world very differently from most children. According to the DSM IV-TR (American Psychiatric Association, 2000) the disruptive behavior disorders can affect anywhere between 2 and 20% of school-age children. Although the techniques can be effective for all types of children, the concepts presented in this chapter are predominately for children with DBDs. The interventions discussed in the upcoming sections are most effective for children ages 5–12.

BUTTONS

The first concept to be considered is buttons (see Figure 3.1). Everybody has probably heard the phrase "Boy, that child really knows how to press my buttons." If you have children, you know full well that as early as age 2, they know how to press your buttons. So, as I talk about buttons, think a little about how humans react whenever their buttons are pressed.

The first thing most people do when their buttons are pressed is become defensive, and the first thing most of us do when we become defensive is begin to point the finger and blame somebody else. This is called *externalizing blame*, and children with DBDs are generally experts at it. A child may be asked, "Who left the toys on the floor?" with the child quickly responding, "Not me!" Maybe you ask your teenager, "Did you bring your permission slip home?" only to hear, "You were supposed to remind me!" So, what is the button for these children? For them, the button is a *fear* of incompetence or of not being "good." Thus, anything that points out that they are not good or that they are not "the

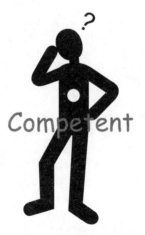

FIGURE 3.1. DBD button.

best" at something is going to press their buttons. For example, if they come in at second place in a game, for them that is just as bad as being in last place, because second indicates not being the best. Therefore, the first thing these children do is become defensive and blame somebody else: "Well, it's not my fault! Somebody tripped me up" or "So-and-so doesn't like me" or "They picked me last." Because the child does not take responsibility for his or her own behavior, the child feels there is nothing that has to change.

When a child makes a mistake, most parents want the child to accept responsibility for what he or she has done and to try to figure out how to do things differently so that he or she does not get in trouble again. So, as we work with these children in a helping environment, we design techniques and interventions to help them to avoid becoming defensive. If we can develop interventions that don't press the child's button, then the child will be better able to accept responsibility for his or her behavior and make the necessary changes. Therefore, by limiting the number of times we press the child's button, the child can spend more time learning about how to behave better.

Key Points 1

- Due to their fear of being incompetent, anything that points out children's mistakes is going to press their buttons.
- Pressing their buttons makes children defensive.
- When people are defensive, they blame others for their mistakes; because the child believes the misbehavior was not his or her fault, there is nothing for him or her to change.

PUNISHMENT/REWARD-BASED SYSTEM

The two main behavior modification theories can be categorized in either punishment-based systems or reward-based systems. How are most of us raised? What methods do we use in schools? What methods do we use in society? Think about what these two systems symbolize for a child. I use the chart shown in Figure 3.2 to help parents explore the expectations of each system and what the child "gets" from the adults.

In a punishment-based system, what do you think the expectation is— that the child will behave or that the child will not behave? In a punishment-based system, the expectation tends to be that the child will behave. The reason this is known to be true is that the only time the adult has to intervene is when the child misbehaves. So if I expect a child to pick up his or her shoes, if I expect a child to eat his or her dinner, or if I expect a child to follow what I say in class, the odds are that I am going to leave the child alone, because the child is doing what I expect him or her to do. The only reason I would need to intervene in a punishment-based system is if the child misbehaves. In other

Punishment-Based   Reward-Based

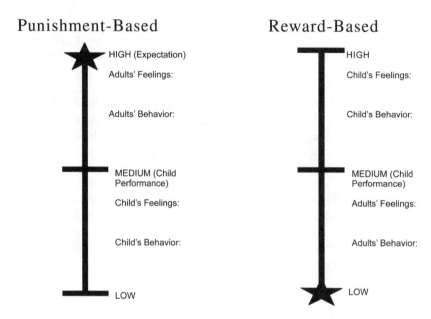

FIGURE 3.2. The punishment versus reward-based systems.

words, if a parent says, "Go pick up your toys" and the child picks up eight out of ten, in a punishment-based system the parent would say, "Why did you leave those two out?" Now assume in a punishment-based system that the expectation is that a child is going to do everything she is told to do that day. However, the child performs only half-way up to adult expectations. As an adult, how are you going to feel? Most parents say, "Well, I get frustrated, I get angry, and I start getting hopeless and more pessimistic about the future." If a parent is feeling that way, he or she is much more likely to be irritable with the child and point out more things that the child is doing wrong. Imagine implementing this approach for 1–2 years, with the child not living up to expectations and possibly misbehaving more. Most adults admit to beginning to feel incompetent in managing the child's behavior. Consider the same system from the child's point of view. If a child is fearful that she is not good, then what is her expectation of herself? High or low? If you said low, then ask yourself this question: what place do such children want to be in at the end of a game? Because of their insecurity about their performance, these children often need to win and expect themselves to be the best. Therefore, what we find is that children experience the same emotions as adults. Most children, believe it or not, want approval from the adults in their lives. So, if a child wants to impress parents or a teacher and is not able to, he or she is going to feel increasingly frustrated and angry. Even the child's own motivation to perform is going to drop. The child may begin to feel incompetent, which, as mentioned earlier, will continue to press his or her buttons.

To help you remember the needs of children with DBDs, I have developed what I call the "three-*A* model." More than anything else, these children seek *approval*. Approval helps to counterbalance a child's fear of incompetence. If the child cannot get approval, then he or she will work for *attention*. Attention is always negative. In other words: "If I can't show you I am good, I will show you I can be really bad." The final *A* is *alone*. Being ignored or left alone is very aversive for these children, because to them it confirms their inadequacies. Parents often report that when they ignore a child, the disruptive behavior escalates to a point where they can't ignore it and they have to intervene. Therefore, any system that is not designed to meet children's primary need for approval is not going to be effective.

Punishment-based systems are primarily designed to give the child adult attention—that is, the parent steps in when the child has not done what was expected. Because the child perceives that he or she cannot gain approval, the motivation to perform continues to drop and the behavior worsens. In contrast, a reward-based system is almost the exact opposite. In that system, the parent practically expects the child to misbehave the entire day. The parent wakes up in the morning thinking, "Little Johnny is going to be a nightmare. He is not going to get up when he is supposed to. He is going to fight me about getting out of bed. He is not going to eat breakfast. He is really not going to want to get dressed or brush his teeth and comb his hair. He is going to miss the bus, and I am going to have to take him. I am probably going to have three or four phone calls from the school, and when he gets home, it is going to be another fight to do his homework."

In a reward-based system, if the adult's expectations are quite low, and the child complies with some of the parents' requests (as on a punishment-based day) the parent, it is hoped, will have many positive things to point out to the child. Therefore, how is the parent going to feel? More optimistic, hopeful, empowered, and confident in his or her own ability as a parent? Because the parent feels that way, he or she is much more likely to be optimistic with the child, the parent's motivation to try harder increases, and he or she is going to be more diligent in finding the good things the child is doing. However, if I am a child in this system, imagine what it is like for me when I have my mom or my dad, or maybe even my teacher, pointing out all the great things I am doing. I am much more likely to want to perform for them, because I have found a way to receive my primary need for approval and show them that I am a good kid.

Key Points 2

- The first thing to remember about these children is that the button is that they are fearful that they are not good. Therefore, they want to be the "best" at what they do.

- Punishment-based systems point out what the child is not doing, thus, only giving them attention.
- Pointing out the child's mistakes makes the child defensive and causes him or her to blame others.
- Reward-based systems point out the good things the child is doing, thus giving the child approval.
- In reward-based systems, because the child is not defensive, he or she is more likely to see what he or she missed and want to correct it.

SELF-CONFIDENCE BUCKET

The final concept considered here is the child's self-confidence. Most children have a high degree of self-confidence. However, children with a DBD tend to be very insecure in their abilities. In order to visualize self-confidence, I use the image of a bucket (Figure 3.3). If you fill up the bucket of a typical child with praise, the child's confidence will rise and he or she will feel empowered. However, for a child with a DBD, the bucket is much different. This child's bucket is filled with holes. According to Hallowell and Ratey (1994) in their book *Driven to Distraction,* a primary symptom of adult attention-deficit-hyperactivity disorder (ADHD) is "a sense of underachievement regardless of how much one has actually accomplished." This symptom is very descriptive of the level of self-confidence of children with DBDs. Regardless of how well they perform, if they do not win, they do not feel successful. One way to deal

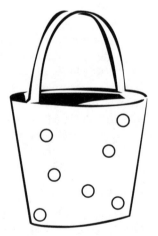

FIGURE 3.3. Self-confidence bucket.

with this "bucket full of holes" is to constantly praise the child. Therefore, if a parent gives the child a consistent stream of praise, the bucket will fill, but the minute the parent stops praising, what happens? The child's bucket empties and his or her confidence fades. Numerous parents have reported, "I just can't praise him enough! As long as I am praising him, staying on him, and telling him all the great things he is doing, he does fine, but, occasionally, I need a break." This approach is ineffective and often leads to parent burnout.

To better illustrate this point consider the analogy of two boys playing baseball: one child has DBD, and the other child is a typical laid-back, go-with-the-flow child. Both children go up to bat, and they both hit home runs. Both boys feel great. The next time they go to bat, the laid-back child strikes out, and although he may be disappointed, he still has confidence left over from the previous home run. However, if the child with a DBD strikes out, most parents indicate, the child breaks down emotionally and behaviorally, saying, "I hate this game," "I am never playing again," or "That was not a strike." Therefore, when designing an intervention, the primary goal is to show the child that he or she is successful. If the child feels competent, this will help to "plug up" those holes. When the child's self-confidence is higher, it should be apparent in the child's behavior. For example, when that child strikes out, he may still be upset but will not, it is hoped, have a melt-down. That child may even come in second place and not have a temper tantrum.

Key Points 3

- Children may or may not show that they feel insecure.
- The strong-willed or oppositional defiant child tends not to show that he or she feels insecure or incompetent on the inside.
- Occasionally, children with ADHD have their melt-downs and show their inadequacies.
- Generally, anxious/worry-type children frequently show that they feel insecure about their abilities.
- Because these traits are personality characteristics, for the most part these children will probably have them for the rest of their lives.

WORKING WITH PARENTS

When working with children with DBDs, it is very important not to neglect their parents. Most parents report that they bring many issues into the child's treatment. The child may be the identified patient, but the parents often struggle with parenting the child.

Kaduson (1996) identifies seven issues that parents bring to their children's treatment. It is important for parents to understand that it is common to struggle in parenting children with DBDs. To increase their awareness, parents can simply identify which of the following issues they may be bringing to their child's treatment.

Denial and Vain Hopes

The first thing parents tend to bring to their child's treatment is a combination of denial and vain hopes. Clinicians are familiar with the parent who says, "Oh, I was like that when I was a kid. He's just a little bit hyper. He is going to grow out of it." This can be an obstacle to treatment, just as much as the attitude of the parent who says, "All we have to do is this behavior plan, and he is going to be fine." Odds are that such parents are going to struggle with their children's behavior well into adulthood.

Guilt and Inadequacy

Because of their inability to help improve a child's behavior, parents often bring guilt and inadequacy to treatment. These are the parents who blame themselves for their children's behavior problems. They feel bad. They wish they had never had children. They do not know why God gave them a child, because they are just such incompetent parents. In time, these parents can become very permissive in their parenting, owing to their lack of self-confidence and self-defeating guilt.

Overinvolvement

Parents who are overinvolved in their child's life are easy to spot. These parents often blame others for the child's behavior and generally feel victimized. However, overinvolvement tends to have a good motive at its source. The parents' desire to shield the child from any kind of hurt tends to be the motive for overinvolvement. However, in shielding a child from hurt, what the parent is also shielding him or her from is the valuable learning of lessons they get when they experience hurt or painful feelings. This can also signal to the child that he or she cannot solve the problem on his or her own and needs outside help.

Fears and Worries

Fears and worries are often expressed by parents, which can also become an obstacle to progress. If parents have mapped out the next 10 or 15 years of their child's life, and it involves juvenile detention, failing, teenage pregnancy, or runaways, the parents may note such fears and worries to be discussed in their child's treatment.

Emotional Bankruptcy

Emotional bankruptcy is very common. Most parents report, when they come into treatment, that they are completely drained, they just do not have anything in them left to give to the child. This difficulty is similar to burnout, but is specific to the child and directly affects parenting.

Feeling Attacked and Not Understood

The next thing that parents tend to bring to treatment is a sense of being attacked and not understood by others, such as school personnel and in-laws. When a child is having a behavior problem, teachers may ask a parent, "Is there something going on at home?" and in-laws may be ready to step in: "You give him to me for one weekend, and I'll straighten him out." The reality is that most people do not understand how difficult it is to manage children with DBDs.

Anger and Resentment

Anger and resentment tend to result for most parents. They may be angry at God for giving them a child like this, angry at professionals for not being able to help, angry at teachers for not being able to teach their child, and generally angry at the child for being the way he or she is. These issues make it very difficult for a parent to find the motivation to enter treatment or to gain tools in parent training.

MAIN REASONS WHY CHILDREN MISBEHAVE

The next area covered in this chapter includes the main reasons why children misbehave. I give the chart shown in Figure 3.4 to parents and ask that they score the child "in general." It may also be helpful for both parents to score independently, as the child may behave differently with each parent.

Child Characteristics

When parents bring their child to treatment, I have found that they often ask, "Why does he (or she) act that way?" Kaduson (1996) offers several dynamics (as listed in Figure 3.4) for parents to evaluate in order to better understand what motivates children's behavior. I usually review each characteristic with the parent(s) and ask each one to evaluate every trait on a scale of 1–10, rating their child in general. This is very important, because these children can behave in a variety of different ways on different days.

Why Children Misbehave

1. Child characteristics

   a. Activity level   1 2 3 4 5 6 7 8 9 10

   b. Attention span   1 2 3 4 5 6 7 8 9 10

   c. Impulse control   1 2 3 4 5 6 7 8 9 10

   d. Emotionality   1 2 3 4 5 6 7 8 9 10

   e. Sociability   1 2 3 4 5 6 7 8 9 10

   f. Response to stimulation   1 2 3 4 5 6 7 8 9 10

   g. Habit regularity   1 2 3 4 5 6 7 8 9 10

   h. Physical characteristics

   i. Developmental abilities

2. Parental characteristics

3. Family stress

   a. Parents' emotional control   1 2 3 4 5 6 7 8 9 10

   b. Parental perceptions

   c. Direct effects on child

4. Learning history

FIGURE 3.4. The main reasons why children misbehave.

Activity Level

Activity level is the general level of physical energy or activity that the child demonstrates. Thus, a low number on this scale (1, 2, or 3) may indicate a child who is not active at all. This is a child whom you really have to get started because he or she does not have energy derived from the motivation to do things. A 9–10 on this scale may indicate a child who is incredibly active. From the moment of waking until the child goes to bed, he or she is always on the go.

Attention Span

Attention span reflects the child's ability to concentrate regardless of interest level. A low number on this scale suggests a child who is very easily distracted, even from things that he or she enjoys. A high number on this scale indicates a child who, regardless of what he or she is doing, even if it is something boring, can maintain concentration.

Impulse Control

Impulse control consists of the child's ability to manage and control his or her behavior. A high number on this scale indicates a child who thinks before he or she acts. This child learns quickly from consequences and typically does not need to be told more than once not to do something. A low number on this scale is typical of a child who tends not to learn from consequences and frequently does things without thinking about them (even when consequences have consistently been applied).

Emotionality

Emotionality basically reflects the child's ability to regulate and express emotions. A low number on this scale indicates a child who really does not show any emotions or does not express them. This is a child who is very flat in affect, and it is difficult to tell when the child is happy, sad, or mad. A high number on this scale indicates an unduly hypersensitive child, when he or she is angry, everybody knows it, and when the child is happy, everybody knows it as well.

Sociability

Sociability reflects how social the child is. Thus, a low number on this scale indicates a child who prefers to be by him- or herself, does not like being in groups, and tends not to feel comfortable when he or she is around people. The high end of this scale suggests a child who regards no one as a stranger, loves being in large crowds, and whose batteries are charged when he or she is around others.

Response to Stimulation

A low number on response to stimulation (1, 2, or 3) indicates a child whom you almost have to "crank start." This child does not get excited easily, even when for something he or she seems to enjoy; the child drags on and has to build up momentum. A high number on this scale suggests that all you have to do is say the word, and this child is ready to go.

Habit Regularity

Habit regularity reflects the child's need for a routine or schedule. A low number on this scale indicates a child who does not need a routine, does not need a ritual, is very flexible, and will go with the flow. A high number on this scale is typical of a child who needs ritual, who does not like it when things change, even something as simple as a departure from "We always have chicken nuggets every Monday." Even moving the furniture may upset this child.

Physical Characteristics

Physical characteristics include anything, whether it is an advance or a delay, that you would say distinguishes the child physically from other children. There may be nothing to score in this area, but it would include things like, "My child has a hearing aid" or "He's overweight for his age" or, perhaps, "She's taller (or shorter) than the majority of kids in her class."

Developmental Abilities

Developmental abilities include advances, as well as developmental delays, that make the child different from other children his or her age. Maybe the child is better coordinated or less coordinated. Maybe he or she is a better reader or a worse reader. This trait includes anything in the child's development that you would say separates this child from other children of the same age.

Parental Characteristics

The second section of the chart is Parental Characteristics. Reviewing parental characteristics allows parents to develop some insight into their parenting styles. I typically ask parents, "Take a few moments to write down words that you would say best describe your parenting style. Remember, do this for yourself and not for your spouse." It is usually a lot easier for a husband or wife to describe the other parent, but I want each of the parents to think about how he or she manages the children and what words would best describe his or her own style. Words that some parents have used include "permissive," "drill sergeant," "strict," "rigid," "absent parent," and "parenting out of guilt or fear."

Family Stress

Family stress, the third contributor to children's behavior, consists of three subcategories.

Parents' Emotional Control

A low number on this scale indicates parents who do not have much control over their emotions and may feel that their emotions are in control of them. So, if such a parent is angry, or is sad, or is happy, everybody knows it. Even when it is best to show a little restraint, these parents have a hard time. A high end number on this scale indicates parents who have almost too much control over their emotions. You never know how they feel because they tend to be so flat in their affect.

Parental Perceptions

The next item on the chart is the parents' true perceptions of the child. It is important that parents are given permission to put negative items in this section. Most parents report, "My child is a joy," "She is a blessing," or "I am so fortunate to have him." But it is also OK to admit that, at times, the child can be frustrating and annoying. Ask parents to take a few moments to write down their true perceptions of their child.

Direct Effects on Child

The last subcategory consists of things that have happened within the family that the parents think have had a direct effect on the child. These can be both positive and negative events. An example of a positive thing may be eating dinner as a family every night. An example of a negative event may be the separation of the child's parents or their divorce." Negative events can also include deaths in the family or frequent moves. The parents should include all the things that they would say have had a direct effect on the child.

Learning History

The final contributor to the child's behavior is learning history. This includes anything the child has learned within the home (such as on television), or outside the home, that the parent did not necessarily want him or her to learn. It can include things like the meaning of the "middle finger," mooning, and the curse words most children bring home from school. Obviously, parents are not going to be able to write down everything, because there are too many examples. Children have learned all kinds of things at home and in the larger world that we may or may not have wanted them to learn. So, in this section, parents are to write down a number of behaviors that they may or may not have wanted the child to learn.

Of the four items on the list, which two would parents say are the main reasons why children naturally misbehave? Most parents pick item 2, parental characteristics, and item 3, family stress. However, the main reasons why children *naturally* misbehave are item 1, the child's natural temperament, and item 4, the child's learning history. Most parents do not teach their children bad things, but a child's natural temperament can lend itself to behavioral problems. If the child ranks at 10 on activity level, that child is naturally going to misbehave because he or she is so active. If the child ranks very low on attention span, that child is naturally going to misbehave because he or she cannot concentrate. If the child ranks very low on impulse control, the child is naturally going to misbehave because he or she does not stop and think and tends not to learn from consequences. So the parent can breathe a sigh of relief learning that the predominant reason why the child misbehaves is usually a combination of the child's natural temperament in combination with his or her learning history.

Therefore, if 1 and 4 are the main contributors to why children misbehave, 2 and 3 must be the main contributors to why children can behave. This is really good news, because on this list, 2 and 3 are the only things we can truly change. A child's natural temperament is what God gave him or her, and parents are not allowed to lock their children in the basement and shield them from the effects of society. But a parent can change his or her parenting style, and a parent can change the family stress, which can have a powerful impact on modifying a child's behavior.

Now, if a parent rated a child at 10 or 1 on any of these scales, that child will probably never naturally be rated at the opposite number. Thus, a child who is naturally a 10 will probably never, barring some kind of brain injury, go to being a 1 or 2. However, parents can shape a child's behavior to the point at which they may rate the child as a 6 or a 7. Most parents say, "I can handle a 6. I just can't handle a 10." Or, "I can handle a 5. I just can't handle a 1."

GOALS OF TREATMENT

When designing a treatment program for a child with a DBD, the goals of treatment should be clear. Because such children have an inward sense of insecurity and incompetence, the first goal of any treatment plan should be to help the child succeed. Kaduson (1996) offers the following components to a successful treatment plan. After each component, I have included an intervention that the mental health professional can implement to greatly improve the effectiveness of treatment.

Have the Interventions Succeed

As you devise interventions, the primary goal is to make sure that those interventions are success-oriented. Fortunately, reward-based behavior modification systems meet this need.

Intervention: Reward-Based Play Therapy

The primary "reward" for children with DBDs is approval. Therefore, during their time together the therapist points out specific behaviors of the child that are acceptable. Pointing out specific behaviors, such as, "You hit the center of that target," versus indiscriminate praise like, "Great job," can be more beneficial for enhancing the child's self-concept. For young children, it can be helpful to provide a tangible reward throughout the session for good behavior; examples are small tokens, tickets, or stickers. The therapist gives these out frequently as a sign to the child that he or she was successful. I typically do not recommend allowing children to "turn in" their stickers or tickets for secondary rewards, but suggest allowing them to simply brag to parents or others about how many tickets they receive. You can also keep track of the number of stickers by placing them on a chart so that a child can see his or her improvement. I also recommend that parents be taught similar techniques to use at home so that the child can get their approval as well.

Build Self-Esteem

The second goal of a treatment program is to build the child's self-esteem. Some research indicates that as early as age 5, children with DBDs begin to realize that they are different from other children. So any treatment program needs to focus on the fact that these children need to have their self-esteem enhanced. The best way to do that is to point out the good things they do.

Intervention: Punch Cards

The use of punch cards can be an effective technique in a variety of settings. Both parents and teachers have reported that this simple intervention has proven effective with individuals and in group settings. The therapist simply draws graphics on 3 × 5 index cards and gives a card to the child. Graphics typically include smiley faces, stars, or circles. A punch card can have as many graphics on it as the therapist deems appropriate. Typically, each card includes at least 10 graphics Either in session or at home, the adult punches out one of the graphics for each good behavior. Once the child has received all of his or her punches, the child can hang up the card where people can see it. A tip that I learned early on is for the adult to obtain a specialty hole punch so that children are not able to punch out the graphics themselves with a standard hole punch. It is not uncommon for a child to loose a punch card. Simply give the child another one, but do not punch out the punches obtained previously. This holds the child accountable for losing the card and gives him or her an immediate opportunity to earn approval.

Teach On-Task Behavior

The next area to be addressed is teaching on-task behavior. Children with DBDs are notoriously off-track. Whether a task is something they enjoy or something they are somewhat bored with, they tend to be distracted very easily. Helping a child to build impulse control skills so that he or she can focus and concentrate is beneficial.

Intervention: Therapeutic Game Playing

Therapeutic game playing can be effective for a variety of treatment conditions. The first thing you need to decide is what skill to teach. For instance, suppose you want to teach a young boy on-task behavior. Then simply select a game that requires the child to have that particular skill in order to win. Next invite the child to play. Because children with DBDs are naturally competitive and enjoy winning, they often respond favorably. Prior to initiating this technique, prepare for the child to win, *but* keep the game competitive so that the child stays engaged. As the game begins, invite the child to go first in order to engage him in the intervention and lower his defenses. Observe the child's play and pay close attention to any incidents of being off-task. Once the child's turn is over, imitate the child's behavior that has caused him to lose a turn (or to be otherwise penalized) and simply announce the mistake out loud, using a casual tone—for example, "Oh man, I lost track of what I was doing," "I got too excited." Continue playing the game in this manner while imitating the child's off-task behavior, announcing the behavior out loud. However, also begin to demonstrate positive coping strategies and express these out loud as well—for example, saying to yourself, "OK, Scott, pay attention, pay attention." The primary thing you are looking for is the child's beginning to imitate your behavior. By using this technique, you are indirectly teaching the child the skill without having to point out his mistakes in the game. The reason this technique is very effective is that young children learn easily through observation and imitation. Remember to keep game competitive so that the child remains engaged. Examples of games that can be used are Concentration, card games, and board games involving taking turns.

Teach Self-Control

The fourth goal of a treatment program should be self-control. As discussed earlier, a child may be rated very low in the impulse control skill area. A treatment program can provide ways to help the child learn to stop and think and learn self-discipline.

Intervention: Therapeutic Game Playing

See description above. Examples of games to play are pick-up sticks, Jenga, and stacking cards.

Channel Aggression Appropriately

Another aim of a treatment program should be helping the child channel aggression appropriately. The reason that children with DBDs get very frustrated really makes sense. For instance, if all a little girl really wants to do is show Mom and Dad, and her teacher, that she is a good person, but she is in a punishment-based system that points out the things she does not do well, then in time that child is going to become aggressive because she is not able to reach her goal.

Intervention: "Shake 'Em Up"

The "shake 'em up" intervention is very helpful for children who externalize their anger and are generally aggressive. The supplies needed for this activity include an empty clear water bottle, children's paint, marbles, and superglue. Begin the activity by explaining to the child that anger is a normal emotion and that some children find that letting that anger out of their bodies helps them to feel better. Fill up the bottle three-quarters of the way with water, and then ask the child to pick a paint color that reminds her either of anger or of being relaxed. Once the child selects the color, allow her to pour a small amount of her color selection into the bottle. Next ask the child to pick between five and ten marbles, and encourage her to place the marbles into the bottle as well. After the paint and marbles are placed in the bottle, carefully put a small amount of superglue on the inside of the cap and tighten the cap onto the bottle; this helps to ensure that the contents stay in the bottle (and that parents stay happy). The game that can be played with this activity is called "shake 'em up." Set a timer for 1 minute, and challenge the child to shake the bottle as hard as she can until the buzzer goes off. Once the buzzer goes off, I find that the child is exhausted and smiling—all at the same time. This activity helps the child to externalize his or her anger in an appropriate manner, as well as metabolize the adrenaline produced when the child becomes angry. I have also found that the majority of school counselors are very receptive to keeping shake 'em up bottles in their offices for children to use when necessary.

Allow Expression of Anger through Play

The next thing a treatment program should do is help the child channel his or her anger. As discussed earlier, children with DBDs are always somewhat annoyed when they do not come in at first place. Unfortunately, that is not a reality for most children. There will be times when they lose or are not as successful as they want to be. Therefore, designing a program to help a child channel this anger can be beneficial, especially if it utilizes the child's natural language, which is play.

Intervention: Being the Boss

Suppose your client is a 5-year-old boy. In this intervention, inform the child that he is allowed to "be the boss" for the entire session. Use basic, nondirective play therapy skills such as tracking and attending, and encourage the child to express himself openly during this time. The only limits you set are that what is done cannot be dangerous or destructive. Define these words, but allow some latitude in your definition. Common experiences I have had during this "boss time" include being given time-outs, being fired, and playing the indentured servant. This intervention allows the child an opportunity to express his anger within predefined limits that help to ensure the safety of both parties. I frequently teach this intervention to parents and encourage them to give their child 5 minutes of boss time every other day. This helps the child to see that he does not have to fight his parents for "the power," because it will be given to him a few times a week. It also helps the child to work out his emotions toward a parent, *with* that parent.

Practice Patience

The next part of treatment is helping children to practice patience. Most of them are not very good at delaying gratification. They want what they want, when they want it, and what color they want it in. What I have tried to do is design a program that helps the children lean to delay gratification or to save up now for something better later on.

Intervention: Domino Stacking

I have always been fascinated by those contests that encourage an individual to stack a sequence of dominoes that will fall in a specific order once the first one is knocked down. This intervention not only helps a child to develop patience but also improves impulsivity the child's control. Suppose you are working with a 6-year-old girl. Divide a standard pack of dominos between the players (you and the little girl), and follow the rules of the game as outlined here: Each player is given 14 or more dominoes; the child is given the opportunity to go first and stack her dominoes on the table vertically. The therapist then has to place a domino either in front or behind the domino the child placed, making sure that it is close enough to make the other one fall. The child then places her dominoes either in front or behind one of the dominoes that are already in place. If at anytime during the game the dominoes fall, the game starts over. Once both players have stacked all their dominoes, the child is given the opportunity to knock down the first domino on either end. If all the dominoes do not fall, the game starts over. The purpose of this intervention is to help the child to develop the impulse control that is necessary to be successful, and to teach patience in a frustrating activity. You can model positive self-talk during the game, as well as offer frequent praise and encouragement.

Help Problem-Solve through Play

The final aim of any treatment program is to help children develop problem-solving skills. Children with DBDs are typically very creative problem solvers, but they are just not very functional. A story of one of children I have worked with in the past can help illustrate this point. This was a child whose parents had given him a key to let himself into the house when he got home every day after school. Within a year of doing this, the child had lost three or four keys because he had forgotten them or misplaced them. Of course, it was somebody else's fault. One day, the child got home and realized that he had once again lost the key. The last thing he wanted to do was to call his parents, because he knew he was going to hear a lecture about his having screwed up again. He remembered that his father had recently used a glass cutter to cut some glass, so he went into the garage and found his dad's tool chest. He took the glass cutter, went to his bedroom window, and cut out a little half-moon above the lock. He poked it through with his knuckle, turned the lock, and let himself into the house. He was so excited about what he had done that he could not wait for Mom and Dad to come home. He greeted them at the door with "I've got good news and bad news. The bad news is I've lost the key, but the good news is I've found a way to let myself in the house without having to call you." He excitedly took his mom and dad into his bedroom and showed them how he did it. Unfortunately, Mom and Dad thought it was not a great plan, because not only had he let himself into the house, but he had left the window open for other people to get in as well. This is an example of how children with DBDs are very creative problem solvers, but not very functional. Any treatment program should consist of helping them to develop problem-solving skills. A great opportunity for this is within their play.

Intervention: Ask the Expert

I have found that most people are effective at solving other people's problems but often get stuck when they are in similar situations. In the "ask the expert" activity, a young boy, for example, is given an opportunity to explore his current dilemma from "the expert" perspective. To setup this activity, write the child's problem on an index card and place it in the center of the room. Then help the child to figure out his current perspective on the problem and write that on the card—for example, "I don't know what to do." Then place that card on the floor a few feet away from the problem card. Direct the child to either stand or sit behind his current perspective card and help the child to explore his thoughts, feelings, and options. Once the child has explored this perspective, invite the child to explore his problem from another perspective. Then write "The Expert" on a card and place that card a few feet away from the center card, but on the other side of the room. Direct the child to stand or sit behind the expert card. The therapist may provide costumes or props to help the child to dress or act the part so that he can fully embrace this perspective. Then encourage the child to explore his thoughts, feelings, and options from this perspective. Next, write on a card all of the options the child expresses, helping him to brainstorm as much as possible. Once the child has identified several options, ask him to select the one or two options he is willing to implement. After the child has selected his choice(s), explore ways to build in accountability for completion—for example, e-mailing the therapist when completed, behavior charting, or leaving a voice mail.

SUMMARY

Although dealing with children who have DBDs can be challenging, using the method described here can bring about a positive change in a child's life. In a perfect world the therapist would also train the child's parents and teacher in this method, so that all of the adults are on the same page. Techniques will have to be modified for each setting, and I encourage you to develop your own interventions that focus on acknowledging the child's successes. However, if you are unable to engage parents and/or teachers in this method, do not get discouraged. Even one person in the child's life who gives him or her a place where he or she is acknowledged and accepted can have a profound impact on that child's future. I hope that this information has given you insight into how children with DBDs see the world. In applying this method, I hope you find the success and fulfillment you are looking for in your work with children.

REFERENCES

American Psychiatric Association. (2000). *Diagnostic and statistical manual of mental disorders* (4th ed., text rev.). Washington, DC: Author.

Hallowell, E. M., & Ratey, J. (1994). *Driven to distraction.* New York: Pantheon Books.

Kaduson, H. (1996). *Play therapy for children with ADHD.* Workshop presented in New Orleans, LA.

CHAPTER 4

Short-Term Play Therapy
for Children with Mood Disorders

ERIK NEWMAN

Mood disorders are believed to affect up to one-third of the general population during the course of their lives. Despite this high prevalence, there is controversy over the diagnosis of such disorders in children. There is a growing
collection of literature on the treatment of depression in children and adults,
but a body of literature on bipolar disorder is just beginning to emerge. The
text revision of the fourth edition of the *Diagnostic and Statistical Manual,
Fourth Edition* (DSM-IV-TR; American Psychiatric Association, 2000) does not
classify mood disorders under "Disorders Usually First Diagnosed in Infancy,
Childhood, or Adolescence." However, the diagnosis of depression in children
has become more commonly accepted in recent years, and the DSM-IV-TR
does indicate that depression can occur at any age.

Much more controversy surrounds the diagnosis of bipolar disorder in
children (Biederman et al., 2000). Research in this area began to emerge in the
1980s and 1990s, but most of the literature that exists today was published since
the year 2000. Although clinicians are regularly reporting cases of children who
appear to display manic episodes, many researchers argue that mania cannot be
diagnosed in children, and therefore a diagnosis of bipolar disorder cannot be
made. Several reasons are cited throughout the literature as to why bipolar disorder is so difficult to diagnose in children. The first reason is comorbidity with
externalizing disorders such as attention-deficit/hyperactivity disorder (ADHD),
oppositional defiant disorder (ODD), and conduct disorder (CD) (Wozniak,
2005). Second, these manic states described in children have no clear onset or
offset points (Findling et al., 2001; Kowatch et al., 2005). Third, one cardinal
symptom of a manic episode in adults is an elevated mood characterized by

euphoria. Children are much more likely to display (or at least report) irritability than euphoria (Findling et al., 2001; Geller, Zimerman, & Williams, 2000). Finally, DSM-IV-TR requires that the full criteria for depression, mania, or hypomania be met for a period of 2 weeks, 1 week, and 4 days, respectively, for a diagnosis to be made. The manic and depressive symptoms that occur in these children often occur simultaneously, as in a mixed state, or they cycle several times within a day. This type of cycling is known as ultradian cycling (Geller et al., 1998b). All of these points are revisited later in this chapter.

For the reasons cited here, it is still unclear whether the children currently being classified as bipolar are indeed bipolar. That is, it is not known whether this cluster of symptoms translates into bipolar disorder as it is seen in adults. What is clear is that there is an increasing number of children being diagnosed with this disorder, and very little is known about effective psychotherapeutic interventions for them. For this reason, most of this chapter focuses on what is known about the assessment and treatment of these children, and treatment of depression is integrated when appropriate. The term "pediatric bipolar disorder" (PBPD) is used to describe these symptoms, and a play therapy treatment program is laid out to meet these children at their developmental level in a fun and nonthreatening environment.

Before considering the characteristics of PBPD in detail, it is first necessary to understand the criteria and associated behavior patterns for both depressive and manic episodes.

CHARACTERISTICS OF DEPRESSION

Depression is believed to occur in 2–8% of children and adolescents (Garrison et al., 1997; Kessler & Walters, 1998). Although depression may not appear as serious as many of the externalizing disorders, it can be very debilitating. In the most severe cases, it can even result in suicide if not treated (Brent, Baugher, Bridges, Chen, & Chiappetta, 1999).

In order for an individual to be verified as having a depressive episode, the DSM-IV-TR requires that he or she display at least five of nine criteria: depressed mood, diminished interest in previously pleasurable activities, significant change in weight or appetite, insomnia or hypersomnia, psychomotor agitation or retardation, fatigue, feelings of worthlessness or guilt, diminished ability to concentrate, and recurrent thoughts of death. At least one of the symptoms experienced must be either depressed mood or diminished interest, and the symptoms must represent a change from previous functioning (American Psychiatric Association, 2000).

Despite the recent acceptance of the notion of childhood depression, it is difficult to diagnose (Kerns & Lieberman, 1993). Because of developmental factors, children may display depression differently than adults (Dulcan &

Popper, 1991). Young children often lack the necessary communication skills to let others know how they feel. DSM-IV-TR allows for depressed mood and diminished interest to be assessed not only by self-report, but also by observation. DSM-IV-TR also notes that depressed mood in children can manifest as irritability. Still, it is not always easy to tell when a child is depressed just by looking at him or her. Irritability combined with psychomotor agitation, lack of sleep, and feelings of worthlessness often result in frustration that can lead to behavioral problems. These behavior problems have the potential to "mask" an underlying depression when they become the most salient features (Briesmeister, 1997). Another developmental consideration noted by DSM-IV-TR has to do with changes in weight. In adults, a 5% change in either direction meets this criterion as long as it is not due to dieting. In children it is also necessary to consider failure to gain weight as expected.

Depression is often associated with a lack of social skills (Segrin, 2000). As noted earlier, depressed children may exhibit poor communication skills. These deficits are manifested by an inability to make conversation, eye contact, and appropriate gestures and facial expressions. In addition, they tend to lack skills associated with assertion (Segrin, 2000).

Suicide is a serious risk associated with depressed children. Although many children harbor thoughts of death in general, some depressed children have suicidal ideations and even a plan to carry out such an idea. Any assessment should address this possibility so that a child can be hospitalized if necessary.

CHARACTERISTICS OF MANIA

As previously noted, the idea that children can have a manic episode is relatively new to modern psychology. According to DSM-IV-TR, a manic episode is "a distinct period of abnormally and persistently elevated, expansive, or irritable mood, lasting at least 1 week (or any duration if hospitalization is necessary)." For such a diagnosis, the episode should consist of at least three of seven criteria, or four if the mood is only irritable. The seven criteria listed are grandiosity, decreased need for sleep, pressured speech, flight of ideas or racing thoughts, distractibility, increase in goal-oriented activity or psychomotor agitation, and constant involvement in pleasurable activities that could result in harmful consequences. If these criteria are met for a period of at least 4 days, but less than a week, the episode is referred to as hypomania. For hypomania, these symptoms should mark a significant change from normal functioning, be observable by others, and not be so severe that they cause marked impairment in functioning or require hospitalization (American Psychiatric Association, 2000).

As noted earlier, the symptom profile for a manic episode in a child often differs from that in an adult. In adults, the elated mood experienced is often described as euphoric. This is not necessarily the case with children. Children often display intense irritability instead (Findling et al., 2001; Geller et al., 2000; Wozniak, 2005). In addition, many of the criteria for a manic episode overlap with those for ADHD (Papolos & Papolos, 1999). Indeed, many children who are later determined to have a manic episode are first diagnosed with ADHD. Symptoms such as irritability, pressured speech, distractibility, and increased energy are evident in both disorders (Wozniak, 2005). For this reason, emphasis is often put on the other symptoms of mania as the "cardinal symptoms" for a diagnosis of a manic episode. These symptoms include elated mood, grandiosity, and decreased need for sleep (Geller et al., 2003). It is important to note that decreased need for sleep means that the child can sleep 4 or 5 hours per night and be completely energized the following day. A child who is tired the following day should not be considered for this criterion.

The last criterion listed for a manic episode is excessive involvement in pleasurable or risky activities. In adults, this often takes the form of spending sprees, gambling, or sexual indiscretions. A common display of this type of behavior in children is hypersexuality (Kowatch et al., 2005); this is also a possible indicator of sexual abuse. However, the sexual behavior displayed by a manic child is often erotic, seductive, and pleasure seeking. Hypersexuality resulting from sexual abuse often takes a compulsive form (Kowatch et al., 2005). Other types of risky behaviors in which manic children tend to engage include daredevil acts and uninhibitedly seeking out the company of strangers (Geller et al., 2003).

PEDIATRIC BIPOLAR DISORDER

Because of the controversy over what, if anything, constitutes PBPD, determining its prevalence rate is difficult. However, researchers have found that the heritability for bipolar disorder is extremely high. In 1921, Emil Kraeplin (1921) noted that approximately 80% of offspring he observed with bipolar disorder had a family history of mood disorders. A meta-analysis of offspring studies concluded that children with bipolar parents are more than two and a half times more likely to have a disorder in comparison with the control subjects, and approximately four times more likely to have an affective disorder (Lapalme, Hodgins, & LaRoche, 1997). Twin studies indicate that the concordance rate for bipolar disorder ranges from 50 to 67% in monozygotic twins, and from 17 to 24% in dizygotic twins (Badner, 2003). Furthermore, DSM-IV-TR states that 10–15% of adolescents diagnosed with major depressive disorder go on to develop bipolar disorder (American Psychiatric Association, 2000). In light of the strong heritability of this disorder, this statistic makes one wonder if earlier detection is possible with more developmentally sensitive assessment tools.

In the current classification system, bipolar disorders are broken down into bipolar I, bipolar II, and bipolar disorder not otherwise specified (BPD-NOS). A diagnosis of bipolar I disorder requires the presence of at least one manic episode. It can also include the presence of one or more depressive episodes or mixed episodes. A diagnosis of bipolar II disorder requires the presence of at least one depressive episode combined with at least one hypomanic episode. BPD-NOS is reserved for disorders with bipolar features that do not meet full criteria for the other types.

As noted earlier, PBPD is a controversial diagnosis. In addition to the similarities between mania and ADHD, there are other problems in the identification of bipolar disorder in children. In adults, manic and depressive episodes usually occur at separate and distinct times and are separated by a period of euthymia, or good mood. Indeed, the definition of a manic episode begins with the phrase "a distinct period" (American Psychiatric Association, 2000). Rapid cycling is generally defined as having four episodes within the period of 1 year. Children cycle multiple times in a day. Because of this ultradian cycling, there is not always a clear distinction between episodes. Many children exhibit mixed episodes, which is characterized by symptoms of both depression and mania occurring simultaneously (Findling et al., 2001; Geller et al., 2000). It is less common to find a child who meets the full criteria for either a depressive episode or a manic episode for the full duration indicated in DSM-IV-TR. The only acceptable diagnosis for these children in the current classification system is BPD-NOS. For this reason, many researchers and clinicians have argued for a revamping of the classification system to include a diagnosis of PBPD (Biederman et al., 2000; Findling et al., 2001).

In addition to the symptoms discussed here, a few other characteristics are common in children with PBPD. Many of these children also have learning disabilities. Cognitive deficits in verbal learning and recall are common (Cavanagh, Van Beck, Muir, & Blackwood, 2002; Fleck et al., 2003; McClure et al., 2005). Such children often begin to brainstorm ideas while following a specific train of thought, but within a very short period of time, they will have forgotten the original topic. Poor judgment has frequently been observed, as evidenced by many of their risky and inappropriate behaviors (Geller et al., 2003). Executive functioning is greatly compromised (Shear, DelBello, Rosenberg, & Strakowski, 2002). Many lack the skills to plan their actions or anticipate the consequences of those actions. Shifting attention is also a common problem (Dickstein et al., 2004). Although these children may be fine as long as they are concentrating on a task, they may be unable to efficiently shift their attention when they are asked to focus on a new task. Finally, PBPD is commonly associated with anxiety disorders, including panic disorder (Chen & Dilsaver, 1995; Simon et al., 2003), as well as night terrors (Papolos & Papolos, 1999).

With all the cognitive, emotional, and behavioral problems exhibited in children with PBPD, one might expect that a number of neurological differences can be found. Although the exact cause of the disorder is unknown, subtle abnormalities in the structural, functional, and neurochemical systems of patients with bipolar disorder have in fact been reported. It is believed that parts of the limbic system and prefrontal cortex are associated with this disorder (Blumberg et al., 2003; DelBello, Zimmerman, Mills, Getz, & Strakowski, 2004). Limbic structures such as the thalamus and the amygdala are responsible for interpreting sensory stimuli and assigning emotional meaning to them. The prefrontal cortex is thought to be responsible for executive functions such as planning behavior. A number of different neurotransmitters are also thought to be important in this disorder. Norepinephrine and serotonin are believed to be associated with arousal, alertness, attention, and sleep–wake cycles. Dopamine is likely associated directly or indirectly with reward-related behavior, mood, speech, and motor activity. These neurotransmitters also likely interact with second messenger systems that amplify their signals (Papolos & Papolos, 1999). One theory about how mood-stabilizing medications work is that they block second messenger systems, thereby dampening these signals (Papolos & Papolos, 1999).

FAMILY ISSUES IN PBPD

PBPD is clearly a difficult disorder for a child to live with. However, it is easy to overlook the possible effects of this disorder on parents and siblings of the affected child. PBPD can potentially destroy an entire family if its members are not properly educated.

Most parents know how difficult a job they have, regardless of how well their child behaves. However, parenting a child with PBPD presents a whole new list of problems that can make life seemingly unbearable. Effective parenting of such children requires a great deal of time, money, and effort. Treatment, which is discussed in detail later in this chapter, requires a multimodal approach, and parents are likely to have to bring their child to several appointments a week, not to mention the school meetings to discuss the child's behavior and individualized education plan (IEP). Each mode of treatment is costly. All this effort and financial strain can result in the sheer exhaustion of the parents (Fristad & Goldberg-Arnold, 2003).

Parents may also experience high levels of anxiety, fear, and uncertainty about their child's future. Despite their best efforts to improve their situation, they are still living with a terrible disorder. If the situation does not improve significantly, they may feel like failures as parents. Feelings of powerlessness are common. Even more harmful are the feelings of guilt and/or blame that parents may harbor for passing on the genes for this disorder. Many parents, out of frustration, begin to blame each other for the disorder, which takes a serious toll on the relationship (Fristad & Goldberg-Arnold, 2003).

One of the most straining issues that threatens the family structure is lack of equality and consistency of parenting roles. When the majority of the parenting responsibilities are accepted by one parent while the other works outside the home, exhaustion is the common result for the parent who remains at home. Resentment of the parent who is "slacking" often follows. In addition, parents often argue over the best way to discipline their children. Although positive parenting strategies are optimal, consistency is absolutely essential. Research has shown that when parents are not "on the same page" with their parenting styles, their child's behavioral problems get worse (Jouriles et al., 1991) and the quality of their marriage decreases, along with their general effectiveness as disciplinarians (Deal, Halverson, & Wampler, 1989; Lamb, Hwang, & Broberg, 1989).

The parents of a child with PBPD do not have an easy task ahead of them. However, the family picture becomes even more complicated when the afflicted child has siblings. The child with PBPD often consumes all the parents' attention. Siblings are left to vie for attention from parents who can't find enough time in the day to effectively manage the child with bipolar disorder. These siblings often perceive their parents as displaying favoritism toward the afflicted child. This commonly results in behavioral problems, because these children have learned that the way to get attention from Mom and Dad is to act out like their brother or sister. If they continue to feel neglected, they often look for their emotional needs to be met elsewhere, which can potentially lead to negative outcomes such as gang involvement and drug use (Fristad & Goldberg-Arnold, 2003). Asessing these problems and addressing them in therapy are critical components of effective treatment for PBPD.

ASSESSMENT OF PBPD

A thorough assessment is absolutely critical to the effective treatment of children with PBPD. As previously mentioned, the cognitive and social deficits suffered by such a child may be many, and early detection and attention to these deficits is crucial in order to optimize the child's functioning. In fact, one theory of mood disorders posits that these deficits are not only due to current symptoms of the disorder, but also due to a disruption in the developmental process that prevents the child from acquiring the necessary skills (Goldberg-Arnold & Fristad, 2003).

A second reason for the importance of a thorough assessment is its implication for pharmacological treatment. PBPD is a disorder in which an accurate diagnosis is absolutely critical. In the absence of a manic episode, PBPD can look like depression. With the display of mania, children with PBPD can look very similar to those with ADHD and ODD and are sometimes treated with stimulant medications. These stimulants can have severe adverse effects on a child with PBPD. This subject is revisited in greater detail in the section on treatment in this chapter. It has even been questioned whether part of the reason clinicians are seeing an increase in the number of children with PBPD is that children who display symptoms of these other disorders are being treated with stimulant medications, which are, in turn, precipitating an earlier onset of the disorder.

Assessment of PBPD should begin with a detailed family history. A genogram that spans at least three generations is advisable so that the clinician can have a graphic representation of the family unit. Once all family members are mapped out with their names and ages, the clinician can begin to get a sense of the kind of support structure the child has, as well as target areas in which problems can potentially arise, such as the parent and sibling issues discussed earlier. It is important to find out if any of the family members listed have a history of mental disorders, diagnosed or otherwise. This information is important, because the heritability of these disorders is high and parents often neglect to mention chronic problems with anxiety or depression just because they have never been diagnosed or treated for them. Finally, questions about substance abuse and physical or sexual abuse are necessary. Substance abuse has long been associated with mood disorders. Although physical or sexual abuse can have an impact on anxious, aggressive, or hypersexual behavior, and is detrimental to a child's wellbeing, such abuse should be viewed as a separate issue.

A detailed medical history is also essential to a comprehensive evaluation. This should include chronic conditions, past medical procedures, and methods and medications used in the treatment of these conditions. Many medical conditions can result in behavioral patterns that mimic bipolar disorder. Head trauma, hyperthyroidism, and multiple sclerosis are just a few of these disorders. In addition, many of the medications used to treat other medical problems can have an effect on behavior (Kowatch et al., 2005).

The next step in the assessment process should be a series of parent and child interviews to determine the child's past and present levels of functioning. These interviews should minimally address academic functioning, home and family functioning, and peer functioning. This will help determine the child's developmental progress, as well as the social and coping skills that he or she lacks. Several standardized semistructured interviews have been developed by researchers to aid in this process. The most commonly used of these are the Schedule of Affective Disorders and Schizophrenia for Children (K-SADS) (Kaufman, Birmaher, Brent, & Rao, 1997) and the Washington University in St. Louis Kiddie Schedule of Affective Disorders and Schizophrenia (WASH-U-KSADS) (Geller, Warner, Williams, & Zimerman, 1998a).

Once an assessment of functioning has been completed, the clinician can focus on symptom presentation. Assessment of symptoms can be based on self-reports, parent and teacher reports, and observations made directly by the clinician. Youngstrom et al. (2004) examined the diagnostic accuracy of several rating scales as compared to that of the K-SADS. For children and adolescents between the ages of 11 and 17, they found the most powerful test to be a parent rating scale called the Parent General Behavior Inventory (P-GBI) (Youngstrom, Findling, Danielson, & Calabrese, 2001). For 5- to 10-year-olds, the most powerful predictor of PBPD was a parent report called the Parent Young Mania Rating Scale (P-YMRS) (Gracious, Youngstrom, Findling, & Calabrese, 2002). Also effective was the externalizing scale on Achenbach's (1991) Child Behavior Checklist (CBCL). However, the CBCL was much more effective in ruling out a diagnosis of PBPD than ruling it in (Youngstrom et al., 2004). That is, if a child rates low on that scale, the likelihood of such a diagnosis is small. However, a high rating on that scale is not as powerful a predictor as the P-YMRS.

In assessing bipolar symptoms, it is important to consider the severity as well as the presence of symptoms, especially in light of the developmental process. Kowatch et al. (2005) suggest the application of what they call the FIND method. FIND is an acronym for frequency, intensity, number, and duration. *Frequency* pertains to how many days in a week a symptom is present. These authors suggest that it should occur most days in a week before it is considered to meet the criteria for a diagnosis. *Intensity* refers to the qualitative severity of the symptom. It should cause impairment or disturbance in at least two areas of functioning. *Number* refers to the number of times in a day the symptom is present. Three to four times a day is considered adequate to meet the criteria. *Duration* refers to the number of hours in a day that the symptom is present in total. Four or more hours is suggested as the cutoff point. Consideration of developmental and environmental factors is also crucial when assessing the severity of symptoms. For example, a certain level of irritability may be considered normal in a young child. The same applies for grandiosity. When lost in fantasy play, a child is more likely than an adult to make claims of a grandiose nature. Moreover, pressured speech, racing thoughts, and distractibility may all be normal to a certain extent in a young child who is introduced to novel stimuli (Kowatch et al., 2005).

After the severity of the symptoms involved in PBPD is assessed, a neuropsychological assessment should be conducted. This should begin with tests of intelligence and academic achievement. It should also include tests of language, executive, and motor functioning. As noted earlier, learning disabilities are very common in children with PBPD. A determination of cognitive strengths and weaknesses can guide the clinician toward an appropriate intervention program (Papolos & Papolos, 1999).

Continual input from the child's school is an important component in the assessment of a child with PBPD. Although teacher reports do not necessarily add to the strength of a PBPD diagnosis (Youngstrom et al., 2004), communication with teachers and counselors can be a large part of ongoing assessment. Their input can help identify a functional baseline from which progress can be assessed. An IEP can then be developed and modified according to the child's progress.

Finally, a number of play therapy techniques can be used in the assessment of children. Puppet interviews are popular assessment tools. An example is the Berkeley Puppet Interview (Ablow & Measelle, 1993). Using this technique, the therapist has two puppets that make a series of statements, and the child has a puppet that answers. In this way, children are able to communicate their views of themselves and the world through their puppets' responses to the therapist's statements. Having children create sandtrays using miniatures provides another way for them to communicate their perceived places in the world. Finally, various artistic techniques can be used to elicit valuable information about the emotions a child is experiencing. Kevin O'Connor's (1983) Color-Your-Life technique is an example of this type of assessment tool. Using this technique, the therapist gives the child a box of crayons and a sheet of paper with a large circle on it. The child is instructed to identify different emotions and to give each emotion a color. He or she is then asked to color in the circle using different amounts of each color to represent the different amounts of each emotion he or she is experiencing.

TREATMENT

Despite the difficulties involved in diagnosing and treating depression in children, psychotherapy is generally considered the first-line treatment for this disorder. Cognitive-behavioral therapy has proven very effective, and pharmacological treatment, although common, should be administered in conjunction with psychotherapy (Birmaher, Brent, & Benson, 1998). However, this is not the case with PBPD. The symptom profile and unpredictability of PBPD make it so impairing that little, if any, therapeutic benefit results from psychotherapeutic interventions if the child is not in a state of euthymia. For this reason, medication is considered the first-line treatment for children with PBPD (Kowatch et al., 2005; Pavuluri et al., 2004). Indeed, for a long period of time, pharmacological treatment was considered the only appropriate treatment for bipolar disorder because of its strong biological base (Craighead & Miklowitz, 2000). Many clinicians and parents hate to see children treated with medication unless it is absolutely necessary, but in this case it is almost always necessary in order to make gains in other areas.

The treatment of PBPD requires a multimodal approach. Because pharmacology is the cornerstone of this treatment, this section begins with a review of the different types of medication used in the treatment of depression and PBPD, as well as their side effects and adverse effects. Following this review, the therapeutic process is discussed, along with a template for a short-term play therapy program. Psychoeducation and basic parenting strategies are incorporated along the way. More comprehensive forms of these types of strategies may be more beneficial, but the basic approaches are presented here in conjunction with individual play therapy due to the time limitations of the 12-session intervention described later in this chapter. Finally, this section closes with a few words on group therapy for PBPD.

Medication

The most popular antidepressant medications include tricyclic antidepressants (TCAs) and selective serotonin reuptake inhibitors (SSRIs). The former are the older antidepressant medications and include drugs such as amitriptyline and imiprimine. The mechanisms of action of these drugs are not fully understood. They appear to have a significant antidepressant effect, but they also have potentially serious side effects, including cardiovascular problems (Bezchlibnyk-Butler & Jeffries, 2004). More commonly used now are the SSRIs, which, as the name suggests, selectively inhibit the reuptake of serotonin. This results in downregulation of receptors and higher levels of serotonin available in the synapses for communication with adjacent neurons, effectively increasing transmission (Bezchlibnyk-Butler & Jeffries, 2004). SSRIs include such popular drugs as Prozac, Paxil, and Zoloft. They are about as effective as the TCAs, but are generally considered to be safer. One of the most important reasons for a comprehensive assessment and accurate diagnosis of PBPD is the implication of this diagnosis for pharmacological treatment. Antidepressant medications, especially the SSRIs, are considered relatively safe and are sometimes used to augment treatment of acute phases of depression in patients with bipolar disorder. However, they can still have adverse effects when taken by a child with PBPD. It is believed that these medications enhance the activity of neurons that are already prone to firing erratically, and can therefore induce a manic episode. Papolos and Papolos (1999) reported that when children with PBPD were given SSRIs, more than 90% of them switched into a manic episode. This also holds true for those with a diagnosis of ADHD. The first-line pharmacological treatment for children with ADHD is stimulant medication. Such medications are sometimes used in conjunction with mood stabilizers for children who have comorbid PBPD and ADHD, but these stimulants also have potential to bring on a manic episode. One study reported that 65% of children with PBPD who were originally diagnosed with ADHD and given stimulant medications subsequently switched into a manic phase (Papolos & Papolos, 1999).

Pharmacological treatment for PBPD usually involves mood stabilizers, neuroleptics, or a combination of both (Kowatch et al., 2005; Wozniak, 2005). Mood stabilizers include lithium and anticonvulsant medications such as Depakote and Tegretol. Lithium has long been considered the standard by which to compare other drugs. It is used in higher doses for the treatment of acute manic phases, as well as in lower doses for maintenance phases of bipolar disorder. It is thought to exert its effect by blocking second messenger systems, thereby reducing neurons' responsiveness to neurotransmitters (Bezchlibnyk-Butler & Jeffries, 2004). Although lithium has long been recognized as having a mood-stabilizing effect, recent research has shown that it is only minimally effective in many children (Kowatch et al., 2000). Furthermore, lithium toxicity is of concern. Because the doctors prescribing these medications are not those who are seeing the children on a weekly basis, the therapist should be aware of the signs of potential toxicity. These may include fatigue, slurred speech, tremors in the hand or jaw, muscle twitches, stomach problems, and tinnitus (Papolos & Papolos, 1999).

Although lithium tends to be effective in adults, anticonvulsants may be better for children. They are indicated for rapid cycling more than lithium (Papolos & Papolos, 1999). They are believed to exert their effects through the body's primary inhibitory neurotransmitter, GABA. These medications are often used in combination with each other, or with lithium, to optimize treatment effects (Kowatch et al., 2005).

Even these anticonvulsants, as effective as they are, do not demonstrate the effect size that many would hope for (Kowatch et al., 2000; Wagner et al., 2002). Recent research has shown that another effective pharmacological treatment may be the use of the atypical antipsychotic medications, or neuroleptics, such as Risperdal and Zyprexa (Wozniak, 2005). The primary site of action of these drugs is thought to be at dopamine receptors in the limbic region and the prefrontal cortex. These drugs produce a calming or tranquilizing effect. They are especially effective in the treatment of acute mania and may be combined with other medications during maintenance and depressive phases (Papolos & Papolos, 1999). The most common side effect of these drugs is weight gain, especially with Risperdal. Cardiovascular problems and tardive dyskinesia are also of concern, but the risk for these serious side effects is significantly lower in atypical antipsychotics than in their predecessors, the conventional antipsychotic medications (Bezchlibnyk-Butler & Jeffries, 2004).

Although nobody likes the idea of medicating children, the presence of PBPD is one instance in which it is absolutely necessary. Without it, such children cycle so fast that they cannot function appropriately in most domains. Once a child is stabilized with medication, he or she will be much more receptive to psychotherapeutic interventions.

Psychotherapy

Goals of Therapy

Because of the debilitating nature of PBPD, the goals of therapy are many. Depending on a child's individual strengths and weaknesses, some or all of the goals discussed in the following paragraphs may apply. In addition, some, but not all, of these goals apply to depression. It is important to note that not all of these goals will be fully met through individual psychotherapy alone. Some will be met through the combined efforts of the child and the parents, whereas others will be met primarily through group therapy.

The first goal of therapy for children with PBPD is *psychoeducation*. There are many psychological disorders for which the prevailing thought is that the child does not need to be aware of his or her own illness, because this is irrelevant to treatment. However, children with PBPD are likely very much aware that something is wrong with them. In addition, they are often led to believe that they are to blame for their symptoms. It is very important that the child and the parents become aware of the symptoms of this disorder. They should be presented with the notion that the symptoms are not the child's fault, but that the child does have the challenge of managing those symptoms (Goldberg-Arnold & Fristad, 2003). The family should be educated about the possible symptoms of the disorder and the importance of compliance with medication in the management of these symptoms. In addition, the child must learn to separate the symptoms from the self (Goldberg-Arnold & Fristad, 2003). That is, the child should learn that the negative thoughts and feelings the child has about him- or herself should be redirected at the symptoms and the disorder.

The second goal of therapy with these children is *affect regulation* (Pavuluri et al., 2004). This begins with regularly monitoring moods. Such monitoring should be done by both children and parents and should focus on what moods the child experiences at different parts of the day, how long those moods last, and what triggers them. Once awareness of these factors grows, the child can begin to learn how to anticipate mood changes before they occur and make use of appropriate coping skills to regulate them. Monitoring of mood changes is an important part of ongoing assessment in both children with depression and those with PBPD.

The third goal in treating PBPD is *emotional regulation*. This refers to the more general level of emotions experienced by the child. Many children with PBPD have extremely high levels of anxiety, frustration, and anger (Greene & Ablon, 2004). They spend so much energy throughout the day trying to control these emotional states that by the time they get home, they explode all over their parents and siblings. Part of this difficulty will, it is hoped, be alleviated as coping skills increase. However, it is important to provide these children with an opportunity for cathartic release—an outlet for their built-up emotions. Several techniques that are discussed later allow the child to pair this outlet with an identified trigger in order to further associate the way he or she feels with the things that make him or her feel that way. This can be a powerful tool in treating children with depression as well as those with PBPD.

Coping skills have been mentioned twice in this section in association with other therapeutic goals. The fourth goal of therapy is to strengthen these skills. The cathartic release mentioned earlier can be extremely effective in a therapy setting, but children with PBPD need to have a repertoire of their own for dealing with environmental stressors. Therapy should aim to help these children develop methods of coping that span several types of activity, such as through physical outlets, creative outlets, social outlets, and ways to isolate themselves in order to "cool down" (Goldberg-Arnold & Fristad, 2003). A specific coping skill that will probably have to be developed in children with PBPD is how to deal appropriately with a shifting mental set. These children have a sufficiently difficult time following instructions because of problems with executive functioning, such as planning and sequencing. When they are finally engaged in an appropriate task and are doing exactly what they are supposed to do, someone eventually asks them to turn their attention to another task. This often results in a "meltdown," due to a lack of coping skills. Strengthening their coping skills is also important for children with depression, because it focuses attention on more productive acts in which they can take pride.

Improving *problem-solving* skills is the fifth goal of therapy for these children. Once a child has an awareness of his or her problems and the skills to deal with them, the child can learn how to evaluate alternative solutions based on risks and benefits, choose the best solution, and implement it (Goldberg-Arnold & Fristad, 2003; Pavuluri et al., 2004). The child can then learn to evaluate the success of his or her solution and determine whether that is a solution to be used again in the future. Children with bipolar disorder often have problems anticipating the consequences of their actions. Practicing this process can teach that skill. In addition, both children with PBPD and those with depression tend to lack a sense of mastery and control. Teaching them how to solve problems effectively is a great way to address this issue.

A sixth goal of therapy, and one that certainly applies to children with depression as well as children with PBPD, is to improve *social skills*. A great many skills are included under this umbrella. Starting or joining a conversation is a skill that many of these children lack. Such children, and those with PBPD in particular, often do not have the skills necessary to recognize social cues in themselves or in others. A child may make a gesture that others find offensive, but have no idea he is doing it. Alternatively, another child may make a kind gesture toward him, and he may ignore it, not because he was not paying attention, but because he did not recognize the cue. Reciprocity is another skill often lacking in these children. Concepts such as sharing, gratitude, and support need to be explored, and the accompanying skills practiced (Goldberg-Arnold & Fristad, 2003). Finally, a depressed child in particular may have difficulty with assertion skills and allow others to walk all over her (Segrin, 2000). These skills can be taught and practiced in individual therapy, but are much more effective when practiced in a group.

All the goals discussed thus far can be addressed in multiple formats, including play therapy. However, play therapy's most fundamental power is utilized in the seventh goal—*increasing positive experiences and thoughts*. Both children with depression and those with PBPD have a need for more positive experiences in their lives. These can take the form of success, praise, or just sheer fun. The therapist is benefiting the child if he or she is providing these qualities during the course of a session (although this should usually occur within the context of striving to meet other goals).

The final goal of therapy, but certainly not the least important, is to establish a consistent *routine* with the child and family (Pavuluri et al., 2004). Children with PBPD have a difficult time dealing with change. They can be gradually desensitized to change in therapy, but they should not be expected to function at home or at school with unnecessary changes. The establishment of a routine should involve the parents and the school as well as the child. This should start with consistent times to go to bed and wake up. It should also include specific times for homework and meals. The purpose of the routine is to avoid as many unnecessary and unpredictable environmental stressors as possible, and the focus should be on sticking to this routine regardless of anything that may get in the way.

The Therapeutic Process

Cognitive-behavioral therapy (CBT) is a well-established and empirically validated treatment for depression (Curry, 2001). However, much less is known about the treatment of bipolar disorder. As noted earlier, it was only recently that researchers pointed to any need for psychosocial interventions for bipolar disorder. Preliminary research supports the use of interpersonal, family-focused, and cognitive-behavioral interventions for this disorder (Miklowitz, George, Richards, Simoneau, & Suddath, 2003; Swartz & Frank, 2001). Pavuluri et al. (2004) outlined a child- and family-focused cognitive-behavioral treatment plan for PBPD using a program they termed the RAINBOW program. The name is an acronym for the active ingredients they point to in their program, which include many of the goals discussed earlier. Goldberg-Arnold and Fristad (2003) also proposed a group therapy program with many important goals in mind. Some of their strategies are incorporated into the program outlined in the following discussion.

Play therapy presents an ideal format through which the treatment goals discussed earlier can be accomplished. Children with PBPDs are identified as having problems in executive function and verbal communication. Children with no developmental or learning problems do not always have the verbal capacity of adults to express ideas through words. Children with PBPDs have it even worse. Play therapy attempts to teach them the skills they need through a "language" in which they are fluent. The play therapy setting is also nonthreatening and, above all else, fun.

The therapeutic process detailed in the next section is an application of the play therapy template to the cognitive-behavioral strategies that researchers have found important in the treatment of PBPD. It is a 12-session program. The goals discussed earlier do not necessarily apply to every child with PBPD. Individual differences in strengths and weaknesses determine which goals should be the primary focus for each child.

Therapy begins with a parent intake in the first session and a child intake in the second session. The third session is an educational session for both parent and child. Beginning in the fourth session, the parent is seen alone for the first 10–15 minutes, and the rest of each session is spent with the child only. The only exceptions to this pattern are the ninth session, which is a parent-only session, and the twelfth session, which is the termination session. The parent joins in for the last part of that session. A number of techniques are presented to meet new goals as therapy progresses. These techniques are chosen because of their specific therapeutic powers, but any techniques with similar powers may be substituted. The clinician is encouraged to adapt this program in any way that makes it more suitable to the therapist or the patient. Instituting a reward system in which the child earns tokens upon completion of each technique may increase incentive. The child can then trade the tokens for a prize at the end of the last session.

Play Therapy

SESSION 1: THE PARENT INTAKE

In session 1, the therapist spends the entire time with the parents for the initial assessment described earlier. The clinician should gather all relevant information, including a detailed family history, medical history, developmental information, and social and academic functioning. Information about the child's favorite toys and games is also useful for breaking the ice in the child intake. In addition, the parents should be given rating scales to fill out, such as the P-GBI, the P-YMRS, or the CBCL. These forms should be completed and returned by the second session.

SESSION 2: THE CHILD INTAKE

In session 2, the entire time is spent with the child. In order to complete the assessment process, the therapist may decide to interview the child or have him or her complete a rating scale. If this is the case, the therapist brings the child into the playroom and says something like, "I can't wait to show you this cool toy I got, but before we get to the fun stuff, I just want to get a few boring things out of the way quickly." After the "boring" part of the assessment is out of the way, the therapist can then decide whether to use play assessment tools to get more information from the child. This can involve a puppet interview such as the Berkeley Puppet Interview (Ablow & Measelle, 1993) or the Puppet Sentence-Completion Test (Knell, 1993). In addition, the therapist might have the child complete a sandtray or a Color-Your-Life drawing. Alternatively, the therapist may choose to break the ice with specific toys and games that the parent indicated as favorites of the child, or may spend the rest of this session in a child-centered format in which the child is safe to explore as he or she sees fit, in which case the therapist might just reflect. Before the child leaves the office, the therapist should be sure to get any rating scales from the parents that have not yet been returned.

SESSION 3: PSYCHOEDUCATION

Session 3 involves the child and parents together. The purpose of this time is to discuss problems and symptoms they are experiencing or are likely to experience, the goals of therapy, the limitations of therapy and of the client, and the expectations of everyone involved.

The first piece of information that must be conveyed here is that the symptoms the child is experiencing are separate from the child. That is, the family must learn to externalize blame by separating symptoms and behaviors from personality. It is not the child who is bad, it is these terrible symptoms. This can be stressed through a technique that Goldberg-Arnold and Fristad (2003) call "Naming the Enemy." This technique involves drawing a chart with two columns. The first column is labeled "Things I Like about Me" and the second column is labeled "My Symptoms." Before each symptom is listed in the second column, the child generates positive self-thoughts. The line separating the two columns separates "good self" from "bad symptoms." This allows a discussion to take place about various symptoms of bipolar disorder. It also gives the therapist an opportunity to educate the family on any common symptoms they have not already listed.

Once the symptoms are listed and separated from the child, the therapist asks the family, "Who is to blame for these symptoms?" After a short discussion, the therapist should make it clear that nobody is to blame. Instead, the disorder is to blame. Next, the therapist asks, "Who is responsible for managing these symptoms?" The child may feel pressured to answer that he or she is responsible. The therapist should then respond by saying, "Yes, that's true, but who else is responsible?" This discussion should eventually lead to the conclusion that everyone in the room, including the therapist, is responsible, but that because the disorder takes its greatest toll on the child, a goal of therapy will be to help the child learn to take more responsibility for symptom management (Goldberg-Arnold & Fristad, 2003).

The session then progresses with a discussion about how difficult it is to manage these symptoms when new and unpredictable situations arise. This leads to a conversation about the importance of establishing a routine. Any routine established should be followed as strictly as possible in the home so the child learns exactly what to expect at different times. This routine should include specific times for taking medication each day. In addition, the parents should be encouraged to bring as many people on board with this plan as possible. This means that the parents should be in contact with teachers and counselors at the child's school about the best ways to make the school day more predictable.

This session ends with a discussion of the goals of therapy. The therapist should begin by saying, "There are several goals of this program, and for the most part, we're going to address them one at a time. However, there is one goal that we want to accomplish in every session. Can you guess what that is?" The therapist should give the family a chance to respond, and then say with enthusiasm, "No matter what else we do in the playroom, the one thing we're going to do every day is have fun, because I don't want to be bored any more than you do!" A brief discussion of the goals of affect regulation, emotional regulation, coping skills, and problem-solving skills should ensue. A quick introduction to affect regulation should be given, with an example of a monitoring technique such as the Color-Your-Life technique described earlier. The therapist should discuss with the parents the importance of constant self-monitoring, and the child should be given an assignment: complete this technique a few times each day as practice, and label each drawing with the time of day (morning, noon, or night). The therapist can provide several copies of a template to make this assignment easier for the child. Parents should also be given a more adult-friendly template for monitoring the symptoms they observe at specific times of the day.

SESSION 4: AFFECT REGULATION AND EMOTIONAL REGULATION

Time Spent with the Parents. Session 4 should include a brief discussion of the homework assignment. How difficult was it to get the child to do this? What patterns arose? The therapist should begin to address the establishment of a routine with the parents. If the parents are stuck, the therapist should offer suggestions, beginning with times for going to bed, waking up, eating meals, taking medication, and doing homework. The parents should be introduced to the concept of emotional regulation with a description of how the child spends so much effort throughout the day trying to control emotional outbursts that the child often explodes once he or she gets home. They should be encouraged to keep a journal such as the Good Behavior Book (Kaduson, 1997), in which they keep track of all the times they notice the child doing what he or she is supposed to do and following the routine. This allows them an opportunity to realize that the child often acts appropriately, as well as to praise the child when this occurs so that these behaviors are positively reinforced. The therapist should also warn the parents that although positive reinforcement is essential, they should be aware of the pitfalls of assuming that the child is always capable of doing what is asked of him or her. Often parents believe that the child can do what is asked but just does not want to. They need to be reminded that their child may or may not be capable, and that the reason they are with the therapist is to work on the necessary skills.

Time Spent with the Child. The therapist should begin this session by praising the child for doing the homework. The rest of the session focuses on various techniques the child can use to monitor his or her feelings. The use of simple monitoring techniques, like Color-Your-Life, will begin every session with the child from this point forward. Monitoring is reinforced with several techniques that serve the same basic purpose. Another technique that is useful in this regard is the RAINBOW technique laid out by Pavuluri et al. (2004). In this technique, the child is given (or can draw) a picture of a rainbow with parts that range from ultraviolet to infrared and everything in between. The various colors are associated with different levels of moods. For example, blue is sad, ultraviolet is very depressed, red is irritable, infrared is explosive, and the colors in the middle represent happiness, or a euthymic state. These are just examples of the many different monitoring techniques available to the therapist.

The child should then be reminded that he or she is not to blame for the symptoms, but rather has the challenge of managing them, and the first step in doing that is to identify what triggers those symptoms. One way of doing that is to use the Anger Wall technique (Sribney, 2003). The therapist draws a wall with three different levels, each level representing a degree of anger, such as "frustrated," "mad," and "steaming." The child then writes several things that make him or her angry (triggers) on individual cards or sticky notes and decides which anger category to place them in.

The session then progresses toward an introduction to emotional regulation. The child is offered a cathartic release for his or her anger and frustration, while pairing that release with various triggers so that the child "releases" that anger from inside him- or herself. This was done by the therapist of a young boy by using a plastic gun that shot foam darts. The therapist drew a target on a white board and told the child to shoot the darts as he yelled out something he hated or something that made him mad. Silly String guns can also be used for a longer release. Another variation of this technique that has great sensory appeal is the Angry Kleenex Game (Filley, 2003), in which the therapist has the child draw what makes him or her mad on a large sheet of paper and attaches it to the wall. The therapist then gives the child wads of tissue or toilet paper and a small bucket of water. The child is instructed to get the tissue wet, squeeze it out just a little, and throw it as hard as possible at the drawing. The child gets to feel the release and watch the wet tissue splat all over the drawing. An activity of this type should be chosen to use for a short period of time in order to illustrate to the child that there are certain ways to let out that intense emotion (and the implication may be that the child does not have to take it out on his or her parents).

Because this type of activity can often make children with PBPD excitable, this session should close with at least 5 minutes of calm and nonthreatening play. This play does not have to be therapeutic. It is only meant to calm the child before leaving the playroom.

SESSIONS 5, 6, AND 7: COPING SKILLS

Time Spent with the Parents. In the fifth session, parents are introduced to the idea of coping skills. The therapist should discuss the different types of coping skills and ways in which they are tools for regulating emotion and solving problems. Goldberg-Arnold and Fristad (2003) suggest using a drawing of a toolbox for the child, with different compartments for four different types of coping skills (physical, social, creative, and relaxation-type skills). The parents should be familiarized with this technique so that it can be used in homework assignments for sessions 5, 6, and 7. To elaborate on this model even further, the therapist might have the parents get a toy toolbox for the child that he or she can bring to each session. The homework assignment should consist of adding one of each type of "tool" to the box before the next session.

The time spent with the parents in session 6 should build on the discussion in session 5. The therapist should review the homework and focus on the fact that the child is adding tools to his or her toolbox. The parents should be told that, in the meantime, they should focus on ways to strengthen the family and avoid common problems. They should be urged to take care of themselves, because an unhappy or unhealthy parent does not benefit the child. If the child has siblings, a discussion should ensue about ways to maximize their happiness and minimize their behavior problems. The therapist should suggest that each parent spend regular one-on-one time with each sibling. If the situation with the child's siblings is already a problem, the therapist may suggest that the parents seek filial therapy to learn how to effectively use the skills involved in nondirective interventions.

Session 7 with the parents should begin with a review of what has been addressed thus far. At this point, the focus turns to problem solving. Parents should be introduced to parenting strategies such as those outlined by Ross W. Greene and J. Stuart Ablon (2004) in their video *Parenting the Explosive Child.* Most of the discussion in the next few sections of this chapter focuses on the rationale for, and the implementation of, these types of techniques. This session introduces the approach by identifying the three ways in which problem solving can take place within the parent–child relationship. A problem can be solved the parents' way (imposing adult will), the child's way (parents drop expectations of the child), or collaboratively. Most parents either know what they want done and are not willing to listen to input from the child, or conversely, they are so frustrated that they drop all expectations. According to

Greene and Ablon (2004), if parents learn to work in a truly collaborative fashion with their child, they are able to reduce meltdowns, achieve stability, pursue their own expectations of the child, and teach the child effective ways to solve problems.

Time Spent with the Child. Each of these sessions (5, 6, and 7) should begin with a simple self-monitoring technique like those described earlier.

Session 5 should then move to another cathartic activity like those described previously to reinforce that concept of emotional regulation. The child should be introduced to the idea of coping skills and the toolbox described earlier. The therapist should remind the child of all the triggers that were put up the Anger Wall, explain how the cathartic activities were ways of dealing with those feelings, and note that there are many other ways as well. The therapist can begin the toolbox by putting the activities in the "physical" compartment. The child should then be asked to think of more problems that make him or her angry, which the child can work on in subsequent sessions. A great technique for this is the Garbage Bag Technique (Kaduson, 2001c). The therapist begins by describing what garbage is and identifying the negative feelings within the child as the child's "garbage." The child then decorates his or her own brown paper bag and writes down problems on note cards to be placed in the bag. The therapist does the same, and in subsequent sessions they work on identifying and choosing ways to solve each problem. This technique is often time-consuming, so in session 5 it may consist only of decorating the bag. The child can then be told that before they jump to solving these problems, child and therapist are going to work on identifying different options for dealing with them (coping skills).

The remaining time of these three sessions is spent using multiple techniques that demonstrate coping skills, except the end of session 7, which focuses on an introduction to problem solving by revisiting the Garbage Bag. An effective technique for generating coping skills is Relaxation Training: Bubble Breaths (Cabe, 2001). Using this technique, the therapist shows the child how taking deep, slow breaths through a wand results in blowing one big bubble, whereas blowing hard and fast results in lots of little bubbles. The therapist then challenges the child to see who can make a bigger bubble. The therapist should be sure to fix the game so the child wins. This not only demonstrates relaxation skills like deep breathing, but it makes the child feel good about him- or herself for winning.

Another effective technique is Balloons of Anger (Horn, 1997), in which the therapist demonstrates the benefit of letting out anger slowly through various physical and social outlets. The therapist has the child blow up a balloon and tie it off (the therapist can tie it off if the child is unable). The air inside this balloon represents the child's anger that has no place to go. The balloon must be stomped on and broken for the air to come out (an explosion). The child blows up a second balloon, but does not tie this one off. Instead, this balloon is held closed, and as the therapist describes different outlets such as talking to someone, going to karate class, and singing a song about it, the child lets the air out little by little. In this way, the air can come out without an explosion. Another balloon technique developed by Kaduson (2001a), called Balloon People, involves dressing up balloons with cutout accessories and having a balloon fight with them. This is helpful in illustrating the use of humor to deal with problems.

A number of artistic techniques can be used to allow the child to "blow off steam" in a creative outlet. An interesting technique is one called Tune It In, Tune It Out (Linden, 2003). Using this technique, the therapist describes how radio stations work and notes that if you tune the radio in clearly to one station, you hear one song or message, and if you tune it to a different station, you hear a different message. The child then creates two different radio stations with different formats and commercial messages by drawing two radio towers on opposite sides of a piece of paper and a dial in the middle that can be tuned to either side. These messages can be in the form of negative thoughts and positive thoughts. The child is then able to tune out the negative messages and tune in the positive ones. In addition, signal boosters can be added to the stations that the child would prefer to hear, and "ask the expert" role plays can be broadcast on these stations.

As each session progresses, the child should be adding more "tools" to his toolbox through homework assignments and ideas that come up in therapy. As previously mentioned, session 7 ends with a revisiting of the Garbage Bag for an introduction to problem solving.

SESSION 8: PROBLEM SOLVING

Time Spent with the Parents. Session 8 should consist primarily of reviewing the parent–child problem-solving methods discussed earlier and how they are most effectively used. The parents are told that although the collaborative method is generally the best method, there are times when they can use the other methods. For instance, when there is a safety issue that requires immediate attention, the parents' way can be used, but a collaborative discussion should then take place about how best to avoid that situation in the future. Similarly, it is not always bad for parents to lower their expectations of the child. It can become very difficult to work on many problems at once. Sometimes, if a problem is not very high on the list of priorities and there are too many other problems to deal with, expectations can be dropped temporarily. Should the parent decide to revisit that problem later, a collaborative effort should be used (Greene & Ablon, 2004).

The parents should then be told what sort of problem-solving activities the child will be doing in that session, and they should be given an assignment that requires the child (with the parents' help if needed) to use the problem-solving strategy learned during the session to solve a problem before the next week's session. This strategy is outlined in the description of the following technique.

Time Spent with the Child. Session 8 begins with a self-monitoring technique and a review of the toolbox. Problem solving is then addressed, using the problems from the Garbage Bag. Problems can be added to the Garbage Bag as needed. The technique to be used in this session is called Problem-Solving Play Therapy (Swearer, 2003). This is a simple technique that makes use of puppets or dolls to act out the process of solving a problem. The therapist writes the acronym POWER for the child, explaining that the acronym stands for the five things that should be addressed in problem solving: the *problem,* the *options, which* option is best, *execute* the option, and *rate* the option on how well it worked. The puppets present the problem and decide to use their POWER to solve it, and the process is acted out. The child is instructed to use the five items as questions to solve a problem as a homework assignment.

SESSION 9: PARENTS ONLY

Session 9 provides the therapist and the parents with an opportunity to discuss progress, express concerns, and make suggestions for modification of the last few sessions if needed. The remainder of this session focuses on the skills the parents need to develop in order to make the parent–child problem-solving process effective. Parents are reminded that because of the child's lack of executive functioning skills, they will likely have to act as the child's "surrogate frontal lobe" and aid in the planning of ideas and anticipation of consequences.

The three main skills needed by parents, as laid out by Greene and Ablon (2004), are empathy, defining the problem, and inviting the child to join in the process. Empathy keeps the child calm because the parents are first addressing his or her concerns. Children often feel that their concerns are dismissed by their parents. The problem is defined when the parents present their concerns. The parents tell how the child wants to solve the problem and how they want to solve the problem, and then ask, "What are some ways we can work this out together?" The solution should be satisfactory to all parties involved. This process should be used to address a problem when it comes up, but should also be used proactively when the child is calm to address how they will solve that problem again when it comes up in the future. The first solution the family comes to is often not the optimal solution. The same process should be used to reevaluate the situation (Greene & Ablon, 2004).

SESSIONS 10 AND 11: PROBLEM SOLVING, CONTINUED

Time Spent with the Parents. Sessions 10 and 11 should be used primarily to practice the skills learned in session 9. In addition, homework assignments should be explained, based on the techniques described in the following section.

Time Spent with the Child. Sessions 10 and 11 begin with self-monitoring techniques and then continue to address problem solving. The therapist should review the Problem-Solving Play Therapy technique used in session 8. Three other techniques are described here that can be used throughout the course of these sessions to enhance problem solving.

Kaduson's (2001b) Broadcast News technique is one in which the therapist plays the role of a news anchor and the child plays an expert being interviewed for a specific type of problem. The therapist also pretends to be various callers asking the expert for advice. The therapist, through the roles of the anchor and the callers, can help with appropriate questions and suggestions when needed, but the child ultimately determines the solution. This is also a wonderful tool because, in giving the callers advice, the child is solving someone else's problem instead of his or her own, which is always easier.

The next two problem-solving techniques were developed by Judith Bertoia (2003a, 2003b). The first technique is called Hand-ling the Decision-Making Process (Bertoia, 2003a). In this technique, the child traces a hand on a piece of paper and writes the problem in the middle of the hand. He or she then writes an option for solving the problem on each of the five fingers. Outside each finger, the child writes the pros and cons of each option. The child is empowered with the responsibility of choosing an option, and then the child and therapist role-play the execution and evaluate the outcome. Bertoia's (2003b) second technique is called The Storyboard. This involves creating a series of television or comic book frames that represent the problem broken down into small chunks. This is similar to the "divide and conquer" strategy in which a problem is broken into smaller parts because it seems overwhelming in its whole form.

At the end of each of these sessions, the child is asked to use the corresponding technique to solve a problem at home. The child is also told at the end of the tenth session that there are only two remaining sessions. At the end of the eleventh session, the therapist reminds the child that the next session will be their last time together.

SESSION 12: TERMINATION

Session 12 begins by giving the parents a chance to express any final concerns. After these are addressed, the parents are given rating scales to complete. The therapist tells them that he or she will now go in with the child, but that they will be invited into the room toward the end of the session. In the meantime, the parents are to complete the forms. These forms should be the same as those administered prior to treatment so that a comparison and an evaluation of treatment can be made.

The therapist reminds the child that this is their last session together, and begins with a self-monitoring technique. Next, the therapist introduces the concept of the Support Tree (Goldberg-Arnold & Fristad, 2003). This is a technique that involves drawing a tree on a large piece of paper or a white board. Each large branch on the tree is to represent an area to which the child can turn for support if he or she needs it. Each smaller branch should correspond to a specific person. The purpose of this exercise is to show children that even though they are ready to take more responsibility for managing their symptoms, they are not on their own.

The parents are then invited into the room. The therapist goes over the Support Tree with them and to see if they have anything to add. Next, the therapist reviews with the family everything that has been accomplished in therapy. Finally, if a reward system has been used, the child should be given an opportunity to trade in tokens or points for a prize.

Group Therapy

The one goal not directly addressed in the individual play therapy program outlined here is social skills training. This goal is much more efficiently accomplished in a group therapy setting. In addition, many of the other goals that were addressed previously can be addressed as well, or better, in group therapy. The main drawbacks to group therapy are the lack of personal attention and the inability to tailor a session to the needs of one child. However, one of the main benefits of a group setting is that the children can see that other children have similar problems, and they have support from each other in addressing these problems. In addition, each child will undoubtedly have a different set of strengths and can model these strengths for other group members. For a detailed outline of a group therapy format for children with PBPD, see Goldberg-Arnold and Fristad (2003).

CONCLUSION

Despite the high prevalence of mood disorders in the general population, the idea that bipolar disorder can afflict young children is very controversial. Bipolar disorder is not as common as depression, but it is a much more debilitating condition. Whether due to increasing incidence or better recognition, more people are being diagnosed with bipolar disorder now than ever before. A great number of children are being diagnosed as such because of their mixed episodes of depression and mania along with their ultradian cycling between states. Whether this truly represents a pediatric form of bipolar disorder is unknown. However, these children are in desperate need of effective treatment.

Diagnosis of PBPD is difficult owing to a number of issues. The states described here do not represent the classic presentation of depressive and manic episodes. They do not last for the duration specified by the DSM-IV-TR. In addition, the comorbidity rates with ADHD and ODD are extremely high. A thorough assessment is needed before a diagnosis can be made and strengths and weaknesses can be identified. Once these steps are taken, a treatment plan can be developed.

PBPD is a relatively new topic, and most of the research available in this area focuses on assessment and pharmacological treatment. Very little is available on empirically validated psychosocial interventions. The program outlined in this chapter attempts to apply the therapeutic change mechanisms in play to the needs of children with PBPD, based on what is available in the literature. Much more research is needed in this area so these children can get the most effective treatment possible, as early as possible.

REFERENCES

Ablow, J. C., & Measelle, J. R. (1993). *Berkeley Puppet Interview: Administration and Scoring System Manuals.* Berkeley: University of California.

Achenbach, T. M. (1991). *Manual for the Child Behavior Checklist/4–18 and 1991 Profile.* Burlington: University of Vermont.

American Psychiatric Association. (2000). *Diagnostic and statistical manual of mental disorders* (4th ed., text rev.). Washington, DC: Author.

Badner, J. A. (2003). The genetics of bipolar disorder. In B. Geller & M. P. DelBello (Eds.), *Bipolar disorder in childhood and early adolescence* (pp. 247–254). New York: Guilford Press.

Bertoia, J. D. (2003a). Problem-solving techniques: Hand-ling the decision-making process. In H. G. Kaduson & C. E. Schaefer (Eds.), *101 favorite play therapy techniques* (Vol. III, pp. 14–18). Northvale, NJ: Aronson.

Bertoia, J. D. (2003b). Problem-solving techniques: The storyboard. In H. G. Kaduson & C. E. Schaefer (Eds.), *101 favorite play therapy techniques* (Vol. III, pp. 19–25). Northvale, NJ: Aronson.

Bezchlibnyk-Butler, K. Z., & Jeffries, J. J. (Eds.). (2004). *Clinical handbook of psychotropic drugs* (14th rev. ed.). Cambridge, MA: Hogrefe & Huber.

Biederman, J., Mick, E., Faraone, S. V., Spencer, T., Wilens, T. E., & Wozniak, J. (2000). Pediatric mania: A developmental subtype of bipolar disorder? *Biological Psychiatry, 48,* 458–456.

Birmaher, B., Brent, D., & Benson, R. S. (1998). Summary of the practice parameters for the assessment and treatment of children and adolescents with depressive disorders. *Journal of the American Academy of Child and Adolescent Psychiatry, 37,* 1234–1238.

Blumberg, H. P., Kaufman, J., Martin, A., Whiteman, R., Zhang, J. H., Gore, J. C., et al. (2003). Amygdala and hippocampal volumes in adolescents and adults with bipolar disorder. *Archives of General Psychiatry, 60,* 1201–1208.

Brent, D. A., Baugher, M., Bridges, J., Chen, T., & Chiappetta, L. (1999). Age- and sex-related risk factors for adolescent suicide. *Journal of the American Academy of Child and Adolescent Psychiatry, 38,* 1497–1505.

Briesmeister, J. M. (1997). Play therapy with depressed children. In H. G. Kaduson, D. Cangelosi, & C. Schaefer (Eds.), *The playing cure* (pp. 3–28). Northvale, NJ: Aronson.

Cabe, N. (2001). Relaxation training: Bubble breaths. In H. G. Kaduson & C. E. Schaefer (Eds.), *101 more favorite play therapy techniques* (pp. 346–349). Northvale, NJ: Aronson.

Cavanagh, J., Van Beck, M., Muir, W., & Blackwood, D. (2002). Case-control study of neurocognitive function in euthymic patients with bipolar disorder: An association with mania. *British Journal of Psychiatry, 180,* 320–326.

Chen, Y.-W., & Dilsaver, S. C. (1995). Comorbidity of panic disorder in bipolar illness: Evidence from the Epidemiologic Catchment Area Survey. *American Journal of Psychiatry, 152,* 280–282.

Craighead, W. E., & Miklowitz, D. J. (2000). Psychosocial interventions for bipolar disorder. *Journal of Clinical Psychiatry, 61*(Suppl. 13), 58–64.

Curry, J. F. (2001). Specific psychotherapies for childhood and adolescent depression. *Biological Psychiatry, 49,* 1091–1100.

Deal, J. E., Halverson, C. F., & Wampler, K. S. (1989). Parental agreement on child-rearing orientations: Relations to parental, marital, family and child characteristics. *Child Development, 60,* 1025–1034.

DelBello, M. P., Zimmerman, M. E., Mills, N. P., Getz, G. E., & Strakowski, S. M. (2004). Magnetic resonance imaging analysis of amygdala and other subcortical brain regions in adolescents with bipolar disorder. *Bipolar Disorders, 6,* 43–52.

Dickstein, D. P., Treland, J. E., Snow, J., McClure, E. B., Mehta, M. S., Towbin, K. E., et al. (2004). Neuropsychological performance in pediatric bipolar disorder. *Biological Psychiatry, 55,* 32–39.

Dulcan, M. K., & Popper, C. W. (1991). *Concise guide to child and adolescent psychiatry.* Washington, DC: American Psychiatric Press.

Filley, D. K. (2003). Angry Kleenex game. In H. G. Kaduson & C. E. Schaefer (Eds.), *101 favorite play therapy techniques* (Vol. III, pp. 336–338). Northvale, NJ: Aronson.

Findling, R. L., Gracious, B. L., McNamara, N. K., Youngstrom, E. A., Demeter, C. A., Branicky, L. A., et al. (2001). Rapid, continuous cycling and psychiatric comorbidity in pediatric bipolar I disorder. *Bipolar Disorders, 3,* 202–210.

Fleck, D. E., Shear, P. K., Zimmerman, M. E., Getz, G. E., Corey, K. B., Jak, A., et al.(2003). Verbal memory in mania: Effects of clinical state and task requirements. *Bipolar Disorders, 5,* 375–380.

Fristad, M. A., & Goldberg-Arnold, J. S. (2003). Family interventions for early-onset bipolar disorder. In B. Geller & M. P. DelBello (Eds.), *Bipolar disorder in childhood and early adolescence* (pp. 295–313). New York: Guilford Press.

Garrison, C. Z., Waller, J. L., Cuffee, S. P., McKeown, R. E., Addy, C. L., & Jackson, K. L. (1997). Incidence of major depressive disorder and dysthymia in young adolescents. *Journal of the American Academy of Child and Adolescent Psychiatry, 36,* 458–465.

Geller, B., Craney, J. L., Bolhofner, K., DelBello, M. P., Axelson, D., Luby, J., et al. (2003). Phenomenology and longitudinal course of children with a prepubertal and early adolescent bipolar disorder phenotype. In B. Geller & M. P. DelBello (Eds.), *Bipolar disorder in childhood and early adolescence* (pp. 25–50). New York: Guilford Press.

Geller, B., Warner, K., Williams, M., & Zimerman, B. (1998a). Prepubertal and young adolescent bipolarity versus ADHD: Assessment and validity using the WASH-U-KSADS, CBCL, and TRF. *Journal of Affective Disorders, 51*, 93–100.

Geller, B., Williams, M., Zimerman, B., Frazier, J., Beringer, L., & Warner K. (1998b). Prepubertal and early adolescent bipolarity differentiate from ADHD by manic symptoms, grandiose delusions, ultra-rapid or ultradian cycling. *Journal of Affective Disorders, 51*, 81–91.

Geller, B., Zimerman, B., & Williams, M. (2000). Diagnostic characteristics of 93 cases of a prepubertal and early adolescent bipolar disorder phenotype by gender, puberty and comorbid attention deficit hyperactivity disorder. *Journal of Child and Adolescent Psychopharmacology, 10*, 157–164.

Goldberg-Arnold, J. S., & Fristad, M. A. (2003). Psychotherapy for children with bipolar disorder. In B. Geller & M. P. DelBello (Eds.), *Bipolar disorder in childhood and early adolescence* (pp. 272–294). New York: Guilford Press.

Gracious, B. L., Youngstrom, E. A., Findling, R. L., & Calabrese, J. R. (2002). Discriminative validity of a parent version of the Young Mania Rating Scale. *Journal of the American Academy of Child and Adolescent Psychiatry, 41*, 1350–1359.

Greene, R. W., & Ablon, J. S. (2004). *Parenting the explosive child: The collaborative problem solving approach*. Newton Corner, MA: Center for Collaborative Problem Solving.

Horn, T. (1997). Balloons of Anger. In H. G. Kaduson & C. E. Schaefer (Eds.), *101 favorite play therapy techniques* (pp. 250–253). Northvale, NJ: Aronson.

Jouriles, E. N., Murphy, C. M., Farris, A., Smith, D. A., Richters, J. E., & Waters, E. (1991). Marital adjustment, parental disagreements about child rearing, and behavior problems in boys: Increasing the specificity of the marital assessment. *Child Development, 62*, 1424–1433.

Kaduson, H. G. (1997). Play therapy for children with attention-deficit hyperactivity disorder. In H. G. Kaduson, D. Cangelosi, & C. Schaefer (Eds.), *The playing cure* (pp. 197–227). Northvale, NJ: Aronson.

Kaduson, H. G. (2001a). Balloon people. In H. G. Kaduson & C. E. Schaefer (Eds.), *101 more favorite play therapy techniques* (pp. 231–235). Northvale, NJ: Aronson.

Kaduson, H. G. (2001b). Broadcast news. In H. G. Kaduson & C. E. Schaefer (Eds.), *101 more favorite play therapy techniques* (pp. 397–400). Northvale, NJ: Aronson.

Kaduson, H. G. (2001c). Garbage bag technique. In H. G. Kaduson & C. E. Schaefer (Eds.), *101 more favorite play therapy techniques* (pp. 3–7). Northvale, NJ: Aronson.

Kaufman, J., Birmaher, B., Brent, D., & Rao, U. (1997). Schedule for Affective Disorders and Schizophrenia for School-Age Children—Present and Lifetime Version (K-SADS-PL): Initial reliability and validity data. *Journal of the American Academy of Child and Adolescent Psychiatry, 36*, 980–988.

Kerns, L. L., & Lieberman, A. B., (1993). *Helping your depressed child: A reassuring guide to the causes and treatments of childhood and adolescent depression*. Rocklin, CA: Prima.

Kessler, R. C., & Walters, E. E. (1998). Epidemiology of DSM-III-R major depression and minor depression among adolescents and young adults in the National Comorbidity Survey. *Depression and Anxiety, 7*, 3–14.

Knell, S. M. (1993). *Cognitive-behavioral play therapy.* Northvale, NJ: Aronson.

Kowatch, R. A., Fristad, M., Birmaher, B., Wagner, K. D., Findling, R. L., & Hellander, M. (2005). Treatment guidelines for children and adolescents with bipolar disorder. *Journal of the American Academy of Child and Adolescent Psychiatry, 44,* 213–235.

Kowatch, R. A., Suppes, T., Carmody, T. J., Bucci, J. P., Hume, J. H., Kromelis, M., et al. (2000). Effect size of lithium, divalproex sodium, and carbamazepine in children and adolescents with bipolar disorder. *Journal of the American Academy of Child and Adolescent Psychiatry, 39,* 713–720.

Kraeplin, E. (1921). *Manic-depressive insanity and paranoia.* Edinburgh, UK: Livingstone.

Lamb, M. E., Hwang, C. P., & Broberg, A. (1989). Associations between parental agreement regarding child-rearing and the characteristics of families and children in Sweden. *International Journal of Behavioral Development, 12,* 115–129.

Lapalme, M., Hodgins, S., & LaRoche, C. (1997). Children of parents with bipolar disorder: A metaanalysis of risk for mental disorders. *Canadian Journal of Psychiatry, 42,* 623–631.

Linden, C. (2003). Tune it in, tune it out. In H. G. Kaduson & C. E. Schaefer (Eds.), *101 favorite play therapy techniques* (Vol. III, pp. 102–105). Northvale, NJ: Aronson.

McClure, E. B., Treland, J. E., Snow, J., Dickstein, D. P., Towbin, K. E., Charney, D. S., et al. (2005). Memory and learning in pediatric bipolar disorder. *Journal of the American Academy of Child and Adolescent Psychiatry, 44,* 461–469.

Miklowitz, D., George, E., Richards, J., Simoneau, T., & Suddath, R. (2003). A randomized study of family-focused psychoeducation and pharmacotherapy in the outpatient management of bipolar disorder. *Archives of General Psychiatry, 60,* 904–912.

O'Connor, K. J. (1983). The Color-Your-Life technique. In C. E. Schaefer & K. J. O'Connor (Eds.), *Hanbook of play therapy* (pp. 251–258). New York: Wiley.

Papolos, D. F., & Papolos, J. D. (1999). *The bipolar child: The definitive and reassuring guide to one of childhood's most misunderstood disorders.* New York: Broadway Books.

Pavuluri, M. N., Graczyk, P. A., Henry, D. B., Carbray, J. A., Heidenreich, J., & Miklowitz, D. J. (2004). Child- and family-focused cognitive-behavioral therapy for pediatric bipolar disorder: Development and preliminary results. *Journal of the American Academy of Child and Adolescent Psychiatry, 43,* 528–537.

Segrin, C. (2000). Social skills deficits associated with depression. *Clinical Psychology Review, 20,* 379–403.

Shear, P. K., DelBello, M. P., Rosenberg, H. L., & Strakowski, S. M. (2002). Parental reports of executive dysfunction in adolescents with bipolar disorder. *Child Neuropsychology, 8,* 285–295.

Simon, N. M., Smoller, J. W., Fava, M., Sachs, G., Rachette, S. R., Perlis, R., et al. (2003). Comparing anxiety disorders and anxiety-related traits in bipolar and unipolar depression. *Journal of Psychiatric Research, 37,* 187–192.

Sribney, K. M. (2003). Anger wall. In H. G. Kaduson & C. E. Schaefer (Eds.), *101 favorite play therapy techniques* (Vol. III, pp. 118–121). Northvale, NJ: Aronson.

Swartz, H. A., & Frank, E. (2001). Psychotherapy for bipolar depression: A phase-specific treatment strategy? *Bipolar Disorders, 3,* 11–22.

Swearer, S. M. (2003). Problem-solving play therapy. In H. G. Kaduson & C. E. Schaefer (Eds.), *101 favorite play therapy techniques* (Vol. III, pp. 171–174). Northvale, NJ: Aronson.

Wagner, K. D., Weller, E. B., Carlson, G. A., Sachs, G., Biederman, J., Frazier, J. A., et al. (2002). An open-label trial of divalproex in children and adolescents with bipolar disorder. *Journal of the American Academy of Child and Adolescent Psychiatry, 41,* 1224–1230.

Wozniak, J. (2005). Recognizing and managing bipolar disorder in children. *Journal of Clinical Psychiatry, 66*(Suppl. 1), 18–23.

Youngstrom, E. A., Findling, R. L., Calabrese, J. R., Gracious, B. L., Demeter, C., Bedoya, D. D., et al. (2004). Comparing the diagnostic accuracy of six potential screening instruments for bipolar disorder in youths aged 5 to 17 years. *Journal of the American Academy of Child and Adolescent Psychiatry, 43,* 847–858.

Youngstrom, E. A., Findling, R. L., Danielson, C. K., & Calabrese, J. R. (2001). Discriminative validity of parent report of hypomanic and depressive symptoms on the General Behavior Inventory. *Psychological Assessment, 13,* 267–276.

CHAPTER 5

Short-Term Play Therapy for Children with Attention-Deficit/ Hyperactivity Disorder

HEIDI GERARD KADUSON

Attention-deficit/hyperactivity disorder (ADHD) is a chronic condition and the most commonly diagnosed behavioral disorder among children and adolescents (Wender, 1987; Barkley, 1990). In the past decade alone, there has been a tremendous upsurge of scientific and public interest in ADHD. This interest is reflected not only in the number of scientific articles, but also in the explosion of books and articles for parents and teachers. Although great strides have been made in the understanding and management of this disorder, there is still much more to be learned. Numerous types of therapies have attempted to manage this condition with limited success. Play therapy has been a successful technique because it involves the child in the process while it teaches the him or her life management techniques.

Childhood cognitive and behavioral problems categorized as disorders of attention, impulsiveness and hyperactivity, present a challenge for the play therapist. The cluster of problems includes inattention, excessive stimulation, hyperactivity, impulsiveness, irritability, and inability to delay gratification. These conditions are diagnostically referred to as ADHD (American Psychiatric Assocaition, 1994), one of the most complex disorders of childhood. These problems affect children's interaction within their own environment and result in an inability to meet situational demands in an age-appropriate manner (Routh, 1978). Children with ADHD typically experience behavior difficulties at home, in school, and within their community. Peer interaction, academic achievement, and overall adjustment are affected. Children with ADHD are frequently enigmatic to their parents and teachers. Their sporadic, unpredictable behavior creates addition stress, leading to the erroneous belief that these are problems of motivation and desire rather then physically driven disabilities. Although we know that all children, from time to time, are inattentive, impulsive, and too active, for children with ADHD these behaviors are the rule—not the exception.

ADHD symptoms typically cause significant pervasive impairment to a child's daily environmental interaction. Although this condition begins at birth, prognosis at an early age is impossible. The familial, social, and academic demands placed on children are determined primarily by the adults in their lives (Goldstein & Goldstein, 1990). Whereas adults can minimize the negative impact of these problems on their lives, children cannot do so. They feel different and do not understand the reason. ADHD appears to significantly impact a child's emerging personality and cognitive skills. These skill deficits result in negative feedback in various areas of their environment. For example, a child may feel that he or she never does anything right, senses the family's displeasure with negatively exhibited behavior, and experiences a lot of negative interactions with others while feeling helpless to remedy the situation. Skill deficits result in years of suffering negative feedback and lack of positive reinforcement, as well as an inability to meet the reasonable demands of family, friends, and teachers. These behaviors can cause a child to have real problems at home, at school, and with friends. As a result, many children with ADHD feel anxious, unsure of themselves, and depressed. These are not symptoms of ADHD, but they come from having these problems over and over again in school, in social situations, and at home. As a result, the child is affected for life. Play therapists must be concerned with both the core symptoms of this disorder and the significant secondary impact they have on the child and associated family members.

ADHD confronts many practitioners, including physicians, psychologists, educators, social workers, speech pathologists, and play therapists. For years each discipline worked in isolation, developing its own set of definitions and ideas for assessment and intervention. The short-term approach introduced in this chapter is a combination of various clinically tested, state-of-the-art techniques with multimodal approaches to give the child with ADHD the most effective treatment possible.

This multimodal approach requires the education of parents regarding ADHD facts and prognoses whenever possible, training of parents on a weekly basis, medication referrals when necessary, classroom intervention, social skills training, and individual play therapy. Such an approach helps the child and the family to take ownership of the disorder and develop coping skills. This chapter focuses on the parent training and individual play therapy that can be accomplished in a short-term format. Classroom intervention and social skills training are separate parts of the total program and are not covered in this chapter.

In this short-term approach, the parents of the child become cotherapists, capable of continuing treatment when the short-term intervention is completed. For a variety of reasons, it is not always possible for parents to act in such a role. To get the best results, parent, teacher, and child interventions should be carried out at the same time (American Academy of Pediatrics, 2001). It is imperative to educate parents about the significance of their participation. When a child is referred, the therapist is frequently confronted with complex problems, further complicated by a variety of social and nonsocial problems. Having the parents as cotherapists helps the child continue to get the necessary understanding and assistance so that he or she can flourish in whatever environmental situation occurs.

PARENTAL ISSUES

It is extremely important to realize that parents of children with ADHD are dealing with several issues at the same time. First, they have to mourn the loss of the "normal" child. This is a process that requires support and guidance. Although the child's physical appearance may be normal, a good deal of the child's behavior is not. Children experiencing paralysis require a wheelchair for mobility and are not expected to walk. Children with ADHD have a behavior disorder—a conceptual "wheelchair" is mandatory for the brain to function in a normal fashion. Therefore, one cannot expect the child to behave.

Therapists may encounter a variety of issues when dealing with parents. These include denial and false hopes. The parents must recognize that ADHD is not a temporary problem and that the child will not outgrow it. They must be trained to effectively improve their child's behavior (Hartman, Stage, & Webster-Stratton, 2003). This process is quite possible. Therapists should advise the parents to maintain a realistic attitude and stay open-minded to additional approaches. Difficulties prevail with a child who has ADHD, but there are numerous coping techniques. Parents need to be open to all possible strategies to treat ADHD (medication, child and associated family therapy, and communication with school personnel). Parents must learn all they can about ADHD in order to teach other family members the necessary coping skills. In addition, therapists should teach the parents about child development norms in order for them to adjust their expectations of the child with ADHD. Although many studies have shown that children with ADHD have age-appropriate cognitive skills, their social and emotional maturity is about one-third their chronological age (Barkley & Murphy, 1998; Barkley, 2000; Wodrich, 2000; Mrug, Hoza, & Gerdes, 2001).

Parents of children with ADHD should understand that feelings of guilt and inadequacy are natural. They must accept negative and ambivalent feelings and gain a better perspective of the child by avoiding perfection as a goal.

The child must be educated to accept this perspective as well. Working to accept mistakes and exercising the courage to be imperfect can assist parents to function effectively with the daily problems that can occur. Therapists must also try to help the parents realize and appreciate small gains and improvements in the child's behavior in order to develop a stronger parent–child relationship. Reminding parents to compare their child with him- or herself at different stages, rather than with the "norm," will help everyone in the family feel more positive. Unconditional love of the child should be displayed at all times, not just as a reward for positive behavior. Parents should learn to create situations for positive interaction with the child. These productive steps should incorporate positive feedback for the parents, resulting in a stronger sense of confidence and self-worth. Parents of children with ADHD tend to be excessively critical of themselves as people. The therapist should continue to stress for parents the importance of self-appreciation as a person and not just as a parent.

Another prevalent issue with the current population of parents is their tendency toward overinvolvement. Many children, including those with ADHD, love to help out at home when they are toddlers. At this time in their lives, however, parents may be worried about what the child might do when using paper towels, folding the laundry, or whatever task the child is interested in. Therefore, the child is encouraged to do something else. As children grow to elementary school age, the parents may begin to expect them to complete chores just as typical children do. For elementary school age children, however, there is now much less interest in doing chores. So, when the child neglects to follow through with chores, and so on, the parents tend to do the chores themselves and the child never learns how to do the skills needed. Instead, they should back off somewhat and enjoy sharing in the child's life experience. Allowing the child the freedom to accomplish something on his or own produces a sense of competency that cannot otherwise be taught. Once the child assumes responsibly and experiences his or her own life, the parents should express faith in the child's ability to handle difficult situations. If problems occur, parents can *assist* the child in generating solutions to these difficulties, rather then solving them for the child. It is beneficial for the child to deal with the natural consequences of his or her behavior to a certain degree. Displaying sympathy for the child causes the child to experience negative feelings about his or her own situation. Parents must strive to overcome feelings of pity for their child. It is vital for them not to dramatize the situation but to organize events with the proper perspective in order to help the child to handle difficult situations more effectively.

The therapist must remember that parents of children with ADHD have many fears and worries. Some will ask for a guarantee that they are not raising a juvenile delinquent. Although no guarantees can be made, the therapist can teach the parents to distinguish between concern (a warm expression of interest in potentially dangerous or stressful situations) and worry (a weak, nonproductive state of anxiety about a person's ability to contend with difficulties). Concern may be helpful; worry is not. Guide parents to analyze a problematic situation to determine the best course of action. One of the most difficult parts of parenting a child with ADHD is the parents' need to control what happens. If the family has had a negative experience, they are trying their best to avoid its ever happening again. Past experiences cannot be changed, so parents should concentrate on the future. There are so many wonderful ways to encourage parents to remove their fear and worry, and instead focus on the pride and joy of having a child with such creativity, energy, and charm.

Parents of children with ADHD often experience ridicule and criticism from people with no understanding of the condition. Therapists can help parents to realize that there may be some credibility in the advice they receive from others. They should anticipate such advice and consider it harmless. Usually they have heard these opinions before and, although it may not be constructive, it is well intended. They may misinterpret the advice as criticism. It is very difficult for parents of typical children to understand how the world of a family of a child with ADHD functions. Thus, the therapist must help parents to let go of the embarrassment they may feel when others are observing them. Guide parents to sift through the words of advice to discover substance. This process can alleviate resentment and defensiveness. Advise parents to accept suggestions based on empathy and insight, and ignore all others.

Parents often come to your office full of anger and resentment. They had never expected to give birth to or adopt a child with ADHD. They can spend a lifetime questioning why this happened, but there will be no answer. Help parents to avoid anger displacement toward others, especially the child with ADHD. No one can force anyone else to feel angry. People *choose* to feel and express anger. When parents acknowledge this fact, the power to control and channel their anger is possible. It is also important for parents to realize that anger is a secondary reaction to other primary emotions, such as stress, disappointment, frustration, anguish, and sadness. It is more productive to decrease the effects of the primary emotion rather than the anger. When embarrassment is transformed into anger because of a misbehaving child, parents should not attempt to control their child. In addition, they must not fault themselves for the child's negative behavior. It is not a reflection of the parents' personal worth or value as parents. "I" statements can help parents to locate the source of their anger. In many instances, the anger is self-directed for what they consider to be ineffective and impulsive behavior. Have them explore and discuss their frustration. Educate them to differentiate between their relationship with the child and their reaction to the child's experiences, and to provide unconditional support.

Children with ADHD have so many difficulties with people who do not understand the biological basis for ADHD. It has, however, been found that even with children who have conduct problems, early intervention through parent training and teacher training can produce more positive outcomes (Webster-Stratton, Reid, & Hammond, 2004).

Parents must be prepared to accept the toll that years of living with ADHD will have on their child as an adult. The prognosis appears to be better if (1) the parents use effective parenting skills, (2) the child gets along with other children, and (3) the child succeeds in school.

PREDICTORS OF ADULT OUTCOME

There are a number of general variables that predict adult outcome for children with ADHD. These predictors are generally independent of specific types of childhood problems.

Socioeconomic Status

The higher the parents' socioeconomic status (SES), the better a child's chances. Parents of higher SES are more likely to be aware of behavior problems, more likely to receive pre- and postnatal care, and more likely to be able to afford professional help, as well as able to introduce their child to many activities, hoping to find the child's passion.

Intelligence

Higher intelligence levels can help children with ADHD to compensate for their distractibility and lack of self-control. However, the gifted ADHD child seems to live with the burden of feeling that he or she should know something more but cannot retrieve, visualize, or define it. In general, anyone with higher intelligence makes a better adjustment to adult life.

Aggressiveness

Often, the controlling attitude of a child with ADHD moderates as the years pass. However, aggression is closely related to parenting style and SES (Conners & Wells, 1986). One of the best single predictors of antisocial behavior and poorly adjusted emotional status in adolescence is a history of aggressive behavior in younger childhood (Loney, 1980). This is a very stable characteristic, and once established, it is very difficult to extinguish. Research has focused on this problem for years, and it is possible to do preventive interventions for aggressive elementary school children (August, Realmuto, Hektner, & Bloomquist, 2001).

Activity Level

Certain studies have suggested that there is an inverse relationship between the degree of hyperactive behavior in elementary school and academic achievement in high school. The more hyperactive the elementary school child, the more likely high school achievement will be negatively affected (Loney, Kramer, & Milich, 1981). Channeling the hyperactivity seems to help in the prognosis for the success of a child with ADHD. However, because nonhyperactive children with ADHD are easier to control, these children may slip through the cracks of the educational system. Therefore, they are not likely to be seen at an earlier age, and therefore no preventive measures can be taken.

Social Skills

Milich and Landau (1981) have reported that the best single predictor of adequate emotional adjustment in adulthood is the ability to develop and maintain positive social contacts and friendships during childhood. Although many children with ADHD have social problems, children who have a history of positive social interaction frequently adapt better to their attention deficit disability and to daily frustrations in the home and at school. Early intervention in this part of a child's life has shown some promising results, allowing for the education and training of children with social skills deficits (Webster-Stratton, Reid, & Hammond, 2001; Blachman & Hinshaw, 2002; Houk, King, Tomlinson, Vrabel, & Wecks, 2002).

Delay of Gratification

It is suggested that children who are more competent at delaying rewards tend to develop into adolescents who perform more effectively on intelligence tests, resist potentially problematic temptations more successfully, demonstrate more appropriate social skills, and have higher achievement desires (Mischel, Shoda, & Rodriguez, 1989). Certainly the ability to delay gratification can be taught, but it is not intrinsic in many children with ADHD.

Family Mental Health

In many of the families of children with ADHD, one of the parents exhibits the same syndrome. Families with multiple generations of people with ADHD tend to be difficult to treat in therapy. Although such parents certainly want their child to change his or her behavior, their follow-through is weak. Sometimes they lack the skills, persistence, and ability to stick with therapy and a treatment program. A history of psychiatric problems in a family increases the likelihood that the child with ADHD will grow up and be presented with a similar or related set of problems (Weiss & Hechtman, 1986). When such a possibility is evident, therapists can assist and work with the parents by problem solving with them so that they can make the change in parenting more conducive to success by individualizing the treatment.

Acquainting parents with these predictors can assist them in a motivational way. It is rare for a child not to exhibit some of these variables that predict a positive outcome in adulthood.

SHORT-TERM PLAY THERAPY APPROACH

The basic assumption of a short-term play therapy program is that children with ADHD need intensive treatment in order to learn skills to manage their world better and enhance relationships with others. In today's managed health care environment, it is important to find ways to help the child with ADHD within a short-term format. This multimodal approach includes the combined use of play therapy and participation by school personnel and parents to create a more well-rounded treatment protocol. Empirical research has found that children who participate in a multidisciplinary intervention program demonstrate better adjustment than children receiving no intervention or a single intervention (Satterfield, Satterfield, & Cantwell, 1981).

The following 10-week program presents the treatment protocol, with many updated techniques to use for success. This protocol includes meeting with the parents separately for 15 minutes, and then meeting with the child separately in the playroom for 35 minutes, or the rest of the 50-minute session. The procedure is very direct and teaches both parent and child improved ways of handling ADHD.

Treatment focuses on the primary components of ADHD; namely, attention (short attention span, approximately one-third of agemates; Barkley, 1990), hyperactivity (restlessness, fidgeting, difficulty in staying seated, etc.), and impulsiveness (acting before thinking, poor planning ability, low frustration tolerance, etc.). Treatment goals focus on building the child's self-confidence in specific areas of deficiency, increasing the child's ability to stay focused on tasks, encouraging the child to demonstrate self-control, and teaching the child to consider consequences before acting.

Session 1: Intake

Probably one of the most important aspects of treatment is the process of the intake session. The therapist should make sure that a complete family developmental history is taken. Figure 5.1 is a genogram that is used at the time of intake. Including the names and ages of everyone is important as well. In a classic interview, one would ask the names and ages of the child's siblings,

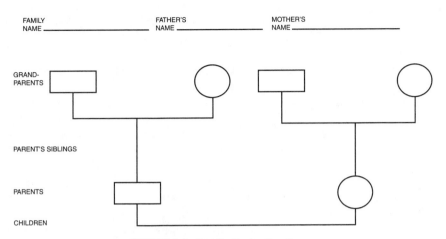

FIGURE 5.1. Family Evaluation Form.

parents, grandparents, aunts, uncles, and cousins. In addition, the parents' educational achievements and professions (outside the home) are documented, as well as how each parent was disciplined (especially important to know, inasmuch as when parents are overwhelmed or at the "end of their rope," they are more likely to use their automatic style—the one with which they were reared). Once the information is obtained, the following questions are asked of maternal and paternal relatives:

- Has there been any drug abuse?
- Has there been any physical or sexual abuse?
- Has anyone had emotional disorders—diagnosed or otherwise?
- Has anyone had a chronic physical illness?
- Has anyone had any learning problems or attention-deficit disorders?

In most cases, one or more of those questions will be answered in the affirmative. In the case of an adopted child, there may not be any biological history available. The therapist should seek this information anyway, because it gives insight into the parent's upbringing, any learning disabilities, and their importance in the treatment protocol.

Discipline is an important part of parenting, and the therapist needs to explore (nonjudgmentally) disciplinary techniques in the home. Time-out, spankings, yelling, and the like, tend not to work with children who have ADHD because of their impulsivity. Generally, when punishment is used, it is effective because the child can learn to think of the punishment he or she has just received for doing the behavior, and therefore will not do it again. Impulsivity is doing something "without thinking," and so the punishment is not remembered at all the next time the behavior is done. Once disciplinary techniques are established, the therapist should determine from the parents whether these methods are successful.

The therapist must obtain specific information about the child:

- *School, teacher, grade, academic problems.* Determine learning problems (mathematics, reading), homework issues, etc.
- *Biological habits.* Establish whether there is a sleep disorder (trouble falling asleep, staying asleep, nightmares, etc.), eating pattern problem (finicky eater, overeater, etc.) unusual toileting pattern (late toilet training, bed wetting, primary or secondary enuresis, encopresis, etc.), or self-care issue (dressing self, brushing teeth, etc.).
- *Sensory issues.* Asking parents about sensory issues may easily be done by just checking to see if their child is bothered by (1) certain textures of food,(2) bright lights, (3) loud sounds, (4) types of clothing, or (5) light touch.
- *Social problems.* Determine problems in relationships in the child's environment (inability to make or maintain friendships, controll play, etc.).
- *Gross motor abilities.* Gather insights into the child's physical abilities (sports oriented, fear of sports or organized sports, problems with riding a bike, etc.).
- *Fine motor abilities.* Gather insights into child's finer physical skills (trouble with drawing and/or writing, pencil grasp, etc.).

After this information has been retrieved, the therapist conducts a play history with the parents. Figure 5.2 is a Play History Questionnaire that includes some of the questions the therapist might ask to determine the child's response in the playroom and in other parts of the treatment protocol.

The parents are then given the following rating scales to provide baseline data on the child.

Conners' Parent Rating Scale

Conners' Parent Rating Scale (CPRS-R), developed by C. Keith Conners (1989) and revised in 1998 (Conners, Sitarenios, Parker, & Epstein, 1998), is the most widely used rating scale of parental opinion concerning ADHD (Barkley, 1995, 1998). It lists items that rate the child, using descriptors such as excitability, impulsiveness, excessive crying, anxiety, oppositional, restlessness, inability to complete tasks, and so forth. The scale is simple for parents to complete. The items are rated on a 4-point scale (Not at all = 0; Just a little = 1; Pretty much = 2; and Very much = 3). The long form is used so that parents will have more

1. What are the child's favorite playthings?
2. How long does the child play with one toy?
3. Is your child responsible for keeping his or her toys in order?
4. Does the child play with a toy or take it apart?
5. Does your child collect anything?
6. Does your child have a favorite game?
7. How does your child play the game—can he or she finish the game; can he or she lose?
8. If your child is given a choice, what would he or she choose to do?
9. How much time does your child watch TV?
10. What is your child's favorite program?
11. Does your child play video games? How much time does he or she spend doing it?
12. Does your child like to draw or color?
13. Does your child join in with others when at a playground?
14. Would your child prefer to play alone or with others?
15. What sports, if any, does your child enjoy?

FIGURE 5.2. Play History Questionnaire.

items to consider. The therapist should require that each parent fill the form out separately so that there is a more complete perception of what the parents feel is most difficult.

Achenbach Child Behavior Checklist

The Achenbach Child Behavior Checklist (CBCL) was created by Thomas M. Achenbach (1978) and revised in 1982. Although this is a more lengthy scale (113 items), it helps with differential diagnoses because it asks questions regarding internalizing (depressed, anxious) and externalizing (hyperactive, aggressive) behaviors. Parents rate their child's behavior on a 3-point scale (0 = Not true; 1 = Somewhat or sometimes true; 2 = Very true, or often true). This checklist is also given to each of the parents, and they are asked to complete the form separately (comparing their notes afterward if necessary).

Behavior Rating Inventory of Executive Function

The Behavior Rating Inventory of Executive Function (BRIEF; Gioia, Isquith, Guy, & Kenworthy, 2000) is filled out by both parents individually so that they can assess the behaviors they notice with specific regard to the executive function deficiency of children with ADHD. The executive function is what controls inhibition, shifting ability, organizing and planning, and self-monitoring.

Barkley Home Situations Questionnaire

The Barkley Home Situations Questionnaire was developed by Russell Barkley (1987) as a means of assessing the impact of a child's attention deficit and related deficits on home and community-based situations. This also gives the therapist qualitative data, as opposed to quantitative data, to use in assessment of the child.

Child and Family Interview Questionnaire

Figure 5.3 is the Child and Family Interview Questionnaire that is given to parents to take home to complete. It gives a more detailed accounting of the child's developmental history and family problems. It reduces the time needed to obtain this information by the therapist during the intake, and allows the parents time to analyze occurrences within the family that are the result of the child's participation.

Session 2: Child Intake

In the second session, the child is seen alone. The therapist greets the child in the waiting room and invites him or her to play in the playroom. The child most likely will enter the playroom without hesitation. If the child is cautious, the parent can walk him or her to the door, where the therapist engages the child in conversation about the toys, and the parent departs.

The first part of the session is conducted with the child drawing a person. If this child is a young boy who has fine motor problems and cannot draw, the therapist takes out a set of shoe boxes, each filled with a different part of the body (usually collected from magazines) and faces showing various feelings. One box contains faces and hair of different colors, one has body types, and one box has clothing cutouts. The child then selects the pictures to put together as his "drawing." While the child draws or puts together his drawing, the therapist can praise the work or ask questions about the picture ("How old is this person?", "What is this person doing?", "Does this person go to school or work?", "What does this person like to do best?", or "What does this person like to do least?", etc.). Because the first drawing of a person is usually a representaton of the child himself, the therapist can gather information without directly asking the child.

After the "person" drawing exercise, the therapist asks the child to draw a house and a tree. The therapist can make a judgment on whether the child

Date:_____

Child Name:_____   Date of birth:_____

Present address:_____

_____

Home phone:_____   Bus. phone:_____

Race:_____   Religion:_____

Sex: M   F   Birthplace:_____

Annual income:_____

No. of persons dependent on this income:_____

School attending:_____Grade:_____

Name of adult(s) completing this form_____

Relationship to child:_____

Who referred you? _____ Address: _____

How long has the child had the problem that help is being asked for? _____

_____

What is the main problem for which you are seeking help? _____

_____

_____

Why did you seek help at this time?_____

_____

_____

Has the child been seen previously for psychological or psychiatric consultation?

Yes _____ No _____

If yes: Name of professional:_____

          Dates of service:_____

          Place of service:_____

          For what purpose:_____

Is the child adopted: Yes _____ No _____ Date:_____

Is the child a twin?   Yes _____ No _____ Identical_____

Was the child ever placed away from family, or has the child ever boarded or lived away from family?   Yes_____ No_____

If yes, with whom?_____Dates:_____

Has the child ever had difficulty or contact with police?   Yes_____ No_____

If yes, describe circumstances:_____

_____

_____

continued

FIGURE 5.3. Child/Family Questionnaire. © Heidi Gerard Kaduson, PhD.

List all those living in child's home.

Name   Relationship   Date of Birth   Occupation

_____

_____

_____

_____

List other persons closely involved with the child but not living in the home (e.g., older brothers, and sisters, grandparents, sitter, teacher, religious leader, etc.)

Name   Place of residence

_____

_____

_____

If the child is not currently living with both natural parents

      Is either natural parent deceased?_____

      If so, when?_____

      Were natural parents married?_____

Explain briefly any special living circumstances (foster care, custody arrangements, visiting rights, etc.).

_____

_____

_____

Who financially supports the child?_____

How long has child resided at present address?_____

With whom does the child share a bedroom, if anyone?_____

How would you describe the child as a person?_____

_____

_____

_____

Has your child had problems in school? Describe briefly:_____

_____

_____

_____

Has your child repeated any grade?_____

Briefly discuss progress and behavior in school._____

_____

_____

Does your child have many friends?_____

FIGURE 5.3. *continued*

Does your child have difficulty making or keeping friends?_____

Difficulty with brothers and/or sisters?_____

Family concerns: (X if appropriate)

Marital difficulties _____	Death in family _____
Aging grandparents _____	Drug addiction _____
Alcoholism _____	Financial problem _____
Serious illness _____	Single parent _____
Birth of new child _____	Job loss _____

Other: Please specify:_____

Describe briefly any special interests, hobbies, and recreational activities in which family members participate.

Child   Mother   Father

_____

_____

_____

_____

_____

FIGURE 5.3. *continued*

can do this, but even with fine motor difficulties, it can be usually be done. According to Lord (1985), the following questions can be asked at this time:

1. What's the one special thing about this house?
2. What's the worst thing about this house?
3. What kind of tree is this?
4. What's the one thing you would change about this house?
5. Is there a scary place in this house?

The next drawing (or pasting of pictures) is of the entire family. Ask the child the following questions about the drawing or montage of a family (Lord, 1985):

1. What is each family member's name?
2. What is this family doing?
3. What is the one best thing about this family?
4. What is the one bad thing about this family?
5. Does this family have any secrets?
6. What kinds of things do the members of this family do together?
7. Who is the favorite person in this family?
8. How does everyone get along?

It is important to keep all questions in the third person so that they can be less threatening to the child. If there is no answer to a question, the therapist should just move on to the next.

Following the drawings, a Puppet Sentence Completion Test (Knell, 1993) is given. Many children with ADHD find this to be fun and participate willingly. The therapist allows the child to choose a puppet. Then the therapist chooses two puppets; one for each hand. Puppet A and Puppet B are on the therapist's hands, and Puppet C is on the child's hand. Puppet A states its name, Puppet B states its name, and then the child is prompted to have Puppet C to give its name. After these introductions, several nonthreatening stems are presented. When the child understands the task, more stems are presented to access the child's thinking on various issues ("I am saddest when . . . ," "I am happiest when . . . ," etc.). The stems can be modified to fit each child's issues, based on the initial input from the parents ("I get yelled at when . . . ," "I need more self-control when . . . ").

The next portion of the session is structured with several games to check the child's ego stability, concentration, self-control, and auditory processing. Guess Who? (by Milton Bradley) is a very useful tool in assessing the child's ability. Many children with ADHD respond impulsively to board games and will not wait for the answer to a question before proceeding. The therapist can intervene and assist the child when that occurs. However, during the assessment process, it is better to allow the child to continue playing without intervening. This game has, in addition, been useful as a "red flag" to signal auditory processing difficulties. If the child cannot follow the questions and answers of the game, the therapist can see what difficulties seem to be presented (e.g., child didn't hear the question, child responded opposite to what the answer was, etc.).

The second game which can be used to assess self-control, is Rebound (by Mattel). This game is simply played, with instructions given before the play begins. Then the child goes first, and the therapist can determine whether the child has any self-control ability and/or awareness (the child moves the marker too fast at first, but then controls the second move, or the child is too cautious to move the piece at all, etc.). Trouble (by Milton Bradley) or Sorry! (by Hasbro) can also be used to measure the child's response in taking turns, winning, and losing. Once again the therapist does not intervene during the intake session. The gathering of information will help formulate the treatment plan.

It is important to observe the child at play to analyze his or her style of interactions with play materials. During this last unstructured playtime, the therapist notes the child's approach and attitude toward the toys, any response latency, frequent changes, creativity, aggressive style, or inability to play without structure. It is important to determine if the age level of playing is appropriate for the diagnostic criteria, inasmuch as children with ADHD tend to play at a more immature level than their peers. The therapist should determine if there are any repetitious themes in the play, and whether the child has trouble initiating or finalizing play.

Session 3: Meeting with the Parents

When meeting with the parents, several important factors must be noted. The therapist must keep parents focused on the parent training only in order to learn the skills necessary to manage their child. Parents may insist that the therapist recommend another type of punishment for their child, because previous methods have been unsuccessful. The therapist should emphasize that parents know best which punishments can work. A positive parenting program is recommended, because it focuses on positive reinforcement that encourages better behavior and stronger relationships. It takes time to develop, but it has promising results.

The therapist should teach the parents the four reasons children misbehave (Barkley, 1990). The therapist gives the parents a characteristic sheet (Figure 5.4), which requires the mother and father to respond to the following topics about their child and themselves:

- Activity level
- Attention span
- Stimulation response
- Impulsiveness
- Sociability
- Habit consistency
- Physical characteristics
- Developmental abilities

Although parents cannot change the "wiring" of the child (Reason 1), the "wiring" of themselves (Reason 2), or family stressors (Reason 3), there is an ability to change the learning history that the child and parent have developed (Reason 4). These behavior patterns have developed over time and can be changed by focusing on the positive.

It is also helpful if the therapist changes the subject a bit in order to offer the parents a more realistic view of parenting a child with ADHD. This is done by drawing a vertical line down a piece of paper for each parent, one side indicating the characteristics the parent found to be attractive in his or her boss at the best job he or she ever had, and the other column indicating the characteristics of the boss in the worst job he or she ever had. By visually presenting this comparison on a piece of paper, it allows the parents to see whom they wanted to do more for, wanted to please, or whom they wanted to do nothing for. When all is listed, the therapist defines ADHD and specifically notes that it is a behavior disorder. Therefore, good behavior is hard to do. The therapist

Child	Mother	Father
Activity level	Activity level	Activity level
Attention span	Attention span	Attention span
Impulse control	Impulse control	Impulse control
Emotionality	Emotionality	Emotionality
Sociability	Sociability	Sociability
Response to stimulation	Response to stimulation	Response to stimulation
Habit regularity	Habit regularity	Habit regularity
Physical characteristics	Physical characteristics	Physical characteristics
Developmental abilities	Developmental abilities	Developmental abilities

FIGURE 5.4. Parent–child fit. © 2005 Heidi Gerard Kaduson, PhD.

next asks, "Which type of parent are you (pointing to the two columns)?" This is just a moment for awareness, not to be discussed or answered aloud.

The "Good Behavior Book" is then presented (Kaduson, 2000). This is a stenographer's pad in which the parents record all of their child's good behavior during the day. All good behavior is defined as behavior that is not "bad." The therapist illustrates a sample page and tells the parents to say aloud and write the behaviors, such as "got up, dressed, put on underwear, put on shirt, put on shorts, put on socks, put on shoes, went to bathroom, combed hair," etc. Each positive behavior is communicated and listed on a separate line so that by the end of the day, a full page of good behaviors has been recorded. Each entry should be only two to four words. The parent recording this information should share it with the significant other in the child's life either after school or at dinnertime. "You won't believe the day Joey had today! He got up. He got undressed!" Whenever possible, the child should overhear the parents praising his or her positive behavior, which will reinforce its importance. More sharing and positive reinforcement occurs at bedtime when the parent reads the book again, outlining the positive behaviors of the day. The parents know the child is hooked when he or she makes a statement such as, "I picked up my clothes—did you write that in the book?"

Session 3: Meeting with the Child

In the playroom, the therapist can have the child play the Feeling Word Game (Kaduson, 1993a). The therapist needs four pieces of 8½" × 11" blank paper—

torn in half to create eight pieces, a marker, and a bag of bingo chips. Then the child is asked, "What feelings does a [age of child]-year-old have?" Each feeling is written on a piece of paper and placed in front of the child. A feeling word poster should be placed on the wall so that the child can refer to it. Children often resist contributing specific words. In order for the therapist to model this technique, basic feeling words such as "happy," "sad," "mad," and "scared" must be introduced. If the child does not produce these, the therapist asks, "Do you think that child would be happy?" This allows the word to be written on one of the papers for the game.

Once all of the feelings are listed, the therapist tells a personal, nonthreatening story that includes several of the feelings listed by the child. After telling the story, the therapist discloses that the bag of Bingo chips is a bag of feelings, and puts down a number of chips, representing the feelings the therapist has about the story just told. The number of chips indicates the intensity of the feeling. For example:

> "I went to the mall to get my favorite toy. I got the toy and then came outside, and my car was missing. I might feel happy because I got the toy I wanted. But I might also feel scared because my car was missing, and mad because someone might have taken it. I could have different feelings all at the same time, and different amounts of those feelings [represented by the number of Bingo chips put down]. Now let me tell you a story, and you put your feelings down."

The therapist then tells a nonthreatening story that includes both negative and positive feelings, represented by the child's list of feeling words. After the child lays down the Bingo chips, the therapist explores the associated feelings.

The last part of this process requires the child to tell a story while the therapist associates feelings with Bingo chips. This telling technique is a valuable therapy tool. The technique can be repeated several times to encourage verbal expression of the child's unconscious mind.

The second technique to use is self-control training. This is done with the use of the game Rebound (which is also used in the intake), but now, while the child plays the game initially, the therapist just sits by and lets the child practice. While the child practices, the therapist encourages the child with positive or corrective statements about self-control. If the child moves the marker too fast, the therapist says, "Wow, you're going to need more self-control on that one," and when that trait is exhibited, the therapist follows with, "Now, look at all that self-control you have!" In this way, the game becomes the mechanism to allow the child to understand what self-control is and what it feels like. This game is played every week to increase the child's monitoring of self-control.

The next process introduces the Beat the Clock game (Kaduson, 1993b). In this game, the child is taught to focus on a project without interruption, thus increasing the child's attention span. The therapist gives the child 10 poker chips, a paper to color, and the following instructions:

"We are going to play the Beat the Clock game. I am giving you 10 poker chips. You must keep your eyes on your work for 2 minutes [or whatever is the baseline attention span of the child], without looking up and without paying attention to anything else. If you do that, you will earn an additional 10 chips. If you look up, however, I will have to take a chip away. After we have done this 3 times, and you have accumulated 25 chips" [allowing for five mistakes], you can pick a prize from the treasure box [simple, inexpensive toys from a dollar store or warehouse sale]."

The child must be successful in all the techniques and interventions performed in the play session. The timing of the Beat the Clock game is done with a wristwatch, so if the child is having significant difficultly, the therapist can shorten the time and begin again. After successful completion, the child can choose from the treasure box immediately.

The last part of the session is a strategic board game. Suggestions for this section include Trouble (by Milton Bradley), Sorry! (by Hasbro), Connect Four (by Hasbro), or checkers. They are all commercially available. During these games, the therapist plays along with the child, but also speaks all of his or her thoughts about what move he or she is taking and why. Illustrating how the therapist uses strategies will be less threatening to the child than correction or instruction during the child's turn. This allows the child to observe the therapist problem solving, taking turns, decision making, and using strategies to win. Once the child is willing, the therapist helps him or her to make appropriate strategic moves and to learn the "stop and think" method.

Session 4: Meeting with the Parents

In session 4, the Good Behavior Book is reviewed and inappropriate entries in the book are corrected. For instance, negative statements like "He didn't hit his sister" are replaced by "Kind to his sister." Because the book is read to the child, only positive statements are helpful. The next portion of parent training involves a nondirect, client-centered approach to playtime. Although it is certainly not as extensive as "filial therapy" (Van Fleet, 2005), this training teaches parents to play with their child without giving directions, making demands, or initiating commands. The therapist can demonstrate this technique to the parents by allowing the parents to play on the floor while the therapist models the tracking of play skills. This is a difficult task, and the parents should know this so that their expectations are not unrealistic. It is helpful if they spend 10 minutes a day doing this special play. The only question parents should ask is, "What do you want to play?" The parents can guide the child to figurines, dolls, blocks, drawings, and so on. This will promote creative play by the child so that the parent can follow the play by what he or she sees.

During this session, parents are also formally taught the Beat the Clock Game so that they can start playing it at home for short periods of time.

Session 4: Meeting with the Child

The therapist reads the Good Behavior Book to the child, with heavy emphasis on how terrific the behavior has been. The child is asked whether it is hard to display good behavior all the time. Whatever response is given, the therapist guides the child into another Feeling Word Game, with different stories based on the initial intake and information provided by parents via subsequent telephone calls.

The next technique introduced to the child is the "Garbage Bag technique" (Kaduson, 2000). The child and the therapist each have a brown paper bag (used for sandwiches) and begin drawing whatever they want on the outside. While drawing, the therapist describes how garbage is collected in the house, the smell and look of the garbage, and the dirt all over the garbage—hooking the child on the subject. The therapist then states:

> "What if there wasn't any garbage collection, and the garbage had to stay in the house? It would probably gather into huge piles. These piles would be so heavy that they could not be moved, and finally all the garbage would have no place to go, so it would have to be carried around on people's backs from our house to our friend's house, from home to school, and so on. If we never disposed of the garbage, we would always have to worry about where to store it."

This metaphor is then compared to the type of garbage that we as people carry around.

> "Garbage for us is all that yucky stuff that we think about all the time, that bothers us when we try to go to sleep, that interferes with our thinking pleasant, happy thoughts. So let's get some of that garbage out of ourselves and stick it in the garbage bag."

The child is then given six slips of paper to jot down personal "garbage"—one item per piece of paper. The therapist writes six items as well, and each person places the papers into his or her own garbage bag and closes it. The garbage bags remain with the therapist for each subsequent meeting.

The Beat the Clock game is played again, increasing the time slowly by 1 minute a week until the child reaches 5 minutes without looking up. The child is given the instructions and rules again prior to the start of the game. Three trials are played again. The child is told that this game will also be played at home.

The end of the session is centered on playing Rebound, to again focus on self-control. The competitive nature of a child with ADHD is used in teaching the child self-control capabilities in order to win the game. Moving the game pieces quickly will result in a loss, but demonstrating self-control will result in a win. The therapist must play this game well enough to be able to win or lose at will. The object is to keep the game relatively even until the last move.

Session 5: Parents and Commands

In session 5, a review of the special playtime between parents and child is conducted to determine if any problems occurred. The therapist then helps the parents to understand the needs of the child, and offers positive interaction scenarios as examples. After review, the parents are taught how to give effective commands. Many parents of children with ADHD have been "asking" the child to do chores rather then directly commanding. When parents ask the child with ADHD to perform a task, the child may assume that "no" is an acceptable response. Some parents believe that "commanding" violates proper etiquette because it lacks courtesy. When effective commands are given to children with ADHD, they are able to be more compliant. The therapist can help parents by suggesting the following specific guidelines:

1. Present the command directly and effectively, not as a question or favor.
2. Give one command at a time.
3. Follow-through is necessary. Consequences, either negative or positive, should be presented to the child.
4. Be sure to have the child's attention. There should be no distractions. Sometimes it may be necessary to gently turn the child's face toward the parent's face.
5. When comprehension is questionable, have the child repeat the command.

The parents practice giving three "easy" commands per day to the child. Each time the child completes what is required by the command, the parent replies, "I love it when you do what I ask," or "Thank you for doing what I told you to do." Some easy commands are "Pass the fork," "Hand me the napkin."

Parents are asked to name one behavior they would like to see changed, and the therapist contracts with the child to accomplish this choice. This exercise teaches the child the meaning of contracting with his or her parents and how to have successful results. However, if a parent says, "He should behave in the morning," this is not operationally definable as one behavior, but as many. Teach the parents to choose *one* behavior for contracting (e.g., brush teeth, get dressed, put clothes in hamper).

Session 5: Contracting with the Child

Read the Good Behavior Book, reemphasizing all of the pages full of the child's good behavior. This process serves as a segue to the contracting procedure. The therapist tells the child about the reward system and the potential to earn a toy. If the child is interested in earning a toy (which is almost always a "yes"), the therapist draws up the contract with the child.

> *Sample Contract*
>
> Joey will brush his teeth every morning without complaints or reminders, and [therapist's name] will give him a package of baseball cards.

Both the therapist and the child sign the contract, and each keeps a copy.

The therapist and child review special playtime. The child's perspective and feedback are very important to determine if the play has been successful. Following this review, the child picks one piece of personal "garbage" from one of the garbage bags. The therapist should be prepared to help play out (either through role play or toy miniatures) the problems in the bag. By helping the child play out the problem, solutions are explored, utilizing the child's experience. It is nonthreatening for the child to play out problems "as if" they are real. The therapist remains focused and helps the child work through solutions to these problems, using dolls or other toys.

After playing out one problem, the therapist directs the child to play Beat the Clock again for a prize. The time is now increased by 2 minutes. The directions for the game need to be reiterated at the onset (even if the child claims that he or she remembers).

Following this game, the therapist and child finish the session playing another self-control game (Rebound, Trouble, Sorry!, pick-up sticks, Connect Four, checkers). The therapist models moves, using verbal descriptions. The child is apt to listen and pay more attention to the therapist's moves than to his or her own. In addition, the child will model what the therapist has done.

Session 6: Training Parents to Focus on the Child

A review of the compliance training should be accomplished first to see if any problems exist. Working through the parental issues can help with further compliance by the parents.

The next training segment teaches parents to pay attention to their child when the child is *not* bothering them. In the case of a child with ADHD, the more attention given to the child, the more positive the behavior will be exhibited. Therefore, when the child is doing exactly what the parent wants, the parent is to reward the child with hugs, praise, a soft touch, or other positive feedback. Parents must be reminded to make the time to focus wholeheartedly on the child's independent play. As a result, parents are likely to notice longer periods of positive behavior by their child, resulting in fewer interruptions. The parents should test this new behavior while pretending to read a book or talking on the telephone. If attention is given when the child is not bothering the parents, then when the parents are not attending to the child because they are reading or paying bills, the child will be less likely to bother them.

The therapist asks for another item to add to the child's contract, thereby increasing compliance and positive feelings for the child.

Session 6: Continuing Positive Feedback with the Child

Read the Good Behavior Book first and then review the contract item. In most cases, the child has accomplished the initial task and is excited about receiving his or her prize.

The child then takes another piece of "garbage" out of the garbage bag and plays out solutions to that problem. The therapist once again directs the play, either through the use of miniatures or roleplay. In directive play therapy, the therapist remains active in the play to help the child resolve psychological problems.

By this session, the Beat the Clock game is played again with a 5-minute increase. Each week the child is able to focus more on independent work, and homework should not be the focus. Before the therapist times the child, he or she first repeats instructions. As the therapist administers praise for concentration and successful focus, the child feels successful and deserving of the prize.

In session 6, the therapist introduces the Splatz game (Kaduson, 2004). The therapist and child stand about 5 feet from a white board, and think of things they hate. The therapist goes first and gives a general statement such as, "I hate tests;" he or she then throws the *Blobz* (Play Visions, 2000) at the white board and watches it "splatz." Then it is the child's turn, and he or she does the same. This taking of turns, repeated 10 times, helps to support the child in expressing feelings of anger that he or she has had to suppress most of the week. Children with ADHD are more likely to make impulsive mistakes, get negative feedback, and feel angry. This release technique allows for the reduction of angry feelings and the venting of what is bothering the child.

The session ends with a game to teach self-control, which serves an additional purpose of "closing down" the child after all his or her feelings have been expressed.

Session 7: Parent Review and Feedback

A review of the homework assigned to the parents in the previous session is performed by the therapist while reemphasizing the lessons. The therapist must keep the parents focused on the training and not allow them to discuss every problem encountered during the week. This will allow them to practice the positive parenting approach while deemphasizing the punishment routines that have been set in motion as a regular course of business in the household. Punishments do not help a child with ADHD to stop the undesirable behavior. Punishments only engage the parent and child in negative interactions. However, it is recognized that praise and attention alone are rarely sufficient to motivate better compliance in children with ADHD. The therapist requires the parents to implement a highly effective motivational program that enlists a variety of rewards and incentives easily accomplished at home. This "token" reward system encourages compliance with commands, rules, codes of social conduct, and school regulations. For children ages 4 through 10, poker chips can be used as tokens. Older children may use a bankbook format, which utilizes debits and credits.

A sample of a token economy system is illustrated in Figure 5.5. The parents list five "easy" tasks, tasks worth 1 to 5 chips per chore; five "moderate" tasks worth 5 to 10 chips; and three "difficult" tasks worth 25 chips per successful completion. These tasks and concepts can be taken from the Good Behavior Book. The therapist guides the parents through this process by researching the repetitive behaviors (easy), the rare behaviors (moderate), and those not yet discussed (difficult). The "buy chart" allows the child to spend his or her earnings from good behavior accomplishments, but the child must now also decide whether he or she wants to spend for the activities listed, such as a half-hour of television viewing, or for 15 minutes of playing a game. Most children enjoy having control of the chips and seek to earn more and more so they can buy what they want. The aim is to have the child spend 80% of the chips earned for desired activities and save 20% of the chips for a long-term reward. The child should save for at least a week or two before earning a larger reward. Even if children never saved money before, they may hold all of their chips for a long-term (delay of gratification) reward if the reward is something they really want.

After establishing the token economy concept during the office session, allow the parents and child to finish it together at home. This creates a more effective goal-setting system because the child is involved in setting the goals.

The parents' portion of this session takes about a half-hour of the session this week. In the last 15 minutes, the child and therapist go into the playroom, where the therapist motivates the child to earn 100 or more chips to win a prize, as part of the therapist–child contract.

Good behavior chart		Buy chart	
Get up	2	Snack	5
Get dressed	3	Soda	2
Brush teeth	2	15 minutes Video games	10
Eat breakfast	1	one half hour TV	15
Put dish in sink	4	Ice cream	10
		Alone with Mom	25
		Alone with Dad	25
Put clothes in hamper	5	Rent movie	25
Take out trash	10	Go to movie	100
Make bed	10	Sleepover	100
Pack backpack	5	Dinner of choice	50
Make lunch	5	Dessert	20
		Lollipop	5
		Candy	15
		Stay up 15 minutes later	50
Nice talk			
Morning	25		
After school	25		
After dinner	25		
Go to Bed at 9	25		
Homework done	25	_____	
		Great Adventure	1,000
		Toy ($10)	1,000
		Go to	500

FIGURE 5.5. Token economy (example). © 2005 Heidi Gerard Kaduson, PhD.

Session 7 with the Child: Introduction of Token Economy

This week is the last time the Good Behavior Book is read. The therapist introduces the token economy concept using a very positive format. The child is, in most cases, very willing to participate at this time. The therapist signs another contract with the child, adding to the original contract a requirement that the child must earn 100 or more chips during the week to earn a prize.

After signing the contract, the child chooses the last piece of "garbage" from his or her bag and plays it out with the therapist. The therapist either actively helps to solve the problem or teaches coping skills during this playtime.

The Beat the Clock game is played, using real homework, for at least 10 minutes. This game is practiced at home, and the child becomes very proficient at increasing his or her attention span by the seventh week of treatment.

If a child has trouble falling asleep at night (this information is obtained during the intake), the Bubble Blowing Game (Kaduson, 2004) is introduced. This game teaches the child the art of deep breathing, using a fun format of blowing bubbles. This technique helps the body relax before bed, while doing homework, or when taking a test. The therapist uses two bottles of bubble liquid; one for the child and one for the therapist. The therapist models how to blow bubbles:

> "If I take a short breath and blow fast, there will be no bubbles; if I take a deep breath and blow fast, there are many bubbles; but if I take a deep breath and blow very slowly, then I can blow a very big bubble."

The object of the game is for the child to learn how to take deep breaths by taking in air, then slowly exhaling. When the child practices enough, the therapist and child take turns to determine who can blow the biggest bubble. The therapist encourages the child to use deep breathing to blow the biggest bubble. They practice this technique during the session, and the child takes the bubble liquid home so that the parent and child can practice the game five times before bed each night. If the therapist believes that there will be a problem in accomplishing this exercise, it can be added to the behavioral contract.

Session 8: Parent Feedback

The token economy is reviewed to determine any problems, and the therapist helps the parents modify the program to work better.

During this session, the concept of time-out is explored with the parents. This is the first week that a punishment is discussed. Time-out should be used sparingly and usually only when a child is violent or swears. If parents were to use the time-out procedure for all instances of noncompliance, the child with ADHD would spend most of the day in the time-out room. It is recommended that the time-out location be chosen by the parents, and that the same place be used every time. Many parents use the bedroom. This is sufficient as long as it does not have items or features that would be attractive to the child. A bathroom (with all movable items removed) or a utility room is more aversive and still safe. Time-out should last for 1-minute per year of life, and timing can be performed by an electronic or kitchen timer. The child needs to be quiet before coming out of the time-out. The therapist can guide parents in the proper use of this method. If the parents have been compliant and followed the weeks of parent training, most of the child's aversive behaviors have been reduced so that time-out is not overused.

Session 8: Child Feedback

The poker chips are counted, and the child reports all good behaviors. Many children remember all of the positive things they have accomplished, because the chip rewards are highly motivational. This session focuses on the child's successes, and a board game (Kaduson, 2000) about the child is created. Figure 5.6 is a sample of the board game. The child is given four happy face stickers and told to put them on the board on whichever squares he or she wants to represent "Say something good about yourself." The next stickers show an angry face, and the child puts four of them throughout the board game; these represent "Say what makes you mad." The same is done for sad face stickers. These, of course, represent "Say what makes you sad." In addition to the stickers, the child is told to put a question mark on four of the squares on the board. The question marks represent "Ask any question of any person playing the game." The rest of the game is marked by the therapist and the child, documenting all the successes the child has experienced both in the playroom and at home. The therapist guides the child to create squares, and the therapist writes inside each square what the child dictates about each success. The child then indicates how many spaces to go ahead. If there are still problem areas, they are dictated to the therapist, who writes them in every other open square, with the child noting how many spaces to go back. To play the child rolls a die and moves his or her piece along the board to the destination (roll 6, move 6 spaces) For example:

> In square two, Joey brushes his teeth without complaints—go ahead two spaces. In square five, Joey gets dressed by himself—go ahead three spaces. In square seven, Joey is late for the bus—go back two spaces, etc.

Session 9: Releasing the Child into the Parents' Care

Session 9 is used to empower the parents to take over management of the child in all respects. By this time they have attained the skills needed to manage their child with ADHD. They may feel cautious and want to stay in therapy, but it is helpful to assure them that they can manage on their own now. Several successes have been demonstrated by the parents. The therapist reiterates these in detail (keeping the Good Behavior Book, having special playtime with the child, giving better commands and following through). The parents are also ready to take over contracting with the child. Although there is no one answer to ADHD, they now have the ability to engage with school personnel because of the training and education they have received in therapy.

The therapist should also have the parents complete another Conners' Parent Rating Scale and an Achenbach Child Behavior Checklist to document posttreatment results. This can be helpful if the client returns at any time, because it measures their ratings as they change over time.

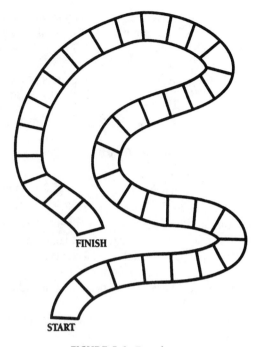

FIGURE 5.6. Board game.

Parents should be advised to examine their own behavior(s) before they call to return to treatment if the child seems to be regressing. The therapist helps the parents recall the reasons for the misbehavior and how their focus may have changed during a time of family stressor. It is important for the therapist to reemphasize the importance of positive parenting to maintain the child's compliance and self-esteem.

Session 9: Releasing the Child

The ninth session focuses on termination. A child typically feels some loss when play therapy in the office is discontinued. The therapist must empower the child by completing the board game started in Session 8. This completion serves to emphasize all of the child's accomplishments, and just notes what still has to be worked on. Any new adjustments can be managed using the same techniques the child has learned during the therapeutic relationship (staying on task; problem solving one thing at a time; self-control; stop, think, and then act; increased concentration with Beat the Clock, and so forth).

In the last portion of the session a List of Good Me is created, with the therapist's help if necessary. The therapist asks the child to list things that he or she is good at. If the child cannot think of anything, the therapist can assist by asking the child if he or she is a good swimmer; then the therapist lists "good swimmer"; if the child is a good friend, the therapist lists "good friend." This List of Good Me is typed, laminated, and given to the child during the last session.

Session 10: Termination of Parent and Child

The therapist invites the parents and child into the room together. They talk about only the good changes that have occurred in the family. Credit is given to the parents and the child for their active participation in all the changes. A Drawing Game (Kaduson, 2000) then begins; all the parties, including the therapist, sit around a table and participate in the termination drawing.

On a piece of 11" × 17" paper, the therapist starts drawing, while discussing all of the wonderful successes in the family. Then each person draws individually for 3 minutes passes the markers to the next person. For a family in which mother and father are both present, this activity requires approximately 12–15 minutes. A theme is not necessary, but the therapist may draw a picture in which a rainbow shows a transition from pretherapy to this final session. The child follows that theme while the parents draw whatever they desire. This is the last positive interaction involving the therapist. After this meeting, the family continues independently to produce successes.

The child is given the List of Good Me, and the board game created by the therapist and the child is played, with the parents included. These transitional objects are left with the child to reinforce his or her successes and accomplishments during times of doubt. The List of Good Me or the board game can be revisited at any time with the parents.

CASE ILLUSTRATION

Andrew P, a 9-year-old boy, was referred for treatment by his school and parents. They were not able to handle his hyperactivity and impulsivity. School personnel were complaining about his lack of attention and incomplete, late work.

Session 1

At the intake, several important points were brought up. Because Andrew was the youngest of two children (his brother was 3 years older), the family had known only typical behavior in school and had not spent an excessive amount of time involved in Andrew's life. To avoid Andrew's temper tantrums over daily personal hygiene routines, his parents dressed him each day. They did not want his behavior to bother their other son. This produced resentment in his older brother anyway, because all the chores were done by the older brother. To avoid tantrums, Mr. and Dr. P did not ask Andrew to do anything. All of the negative attention had encouraged and increased Andrew's negative behavior, which was constantly criticized by his older sibling. A family history showed learning and emotional problems in two cousins, and Dr. P thought that she was inattentive when she was young, but this had not interferred with her learning. She was a medical doctor, and she remembered her childhood without any problematic times. Mr. P was physically punished as a child and did not want to do the same to Andrew. Therefore, although there was a lot of arguing, there was little follow-through from either parent. Andrew had not been taking any medication for his ADHD symptoms because his parents were concerned about the side effects. Therefore, behavior at school was very difficult, as well as at home.

Both parents attended the intake session and were quite open about their problems with Andrew. Although they were angry about his behavior and thought the school was not helping, they did not blame each other. They were advised to read several books on ADHD, specifically, *Taking Charge of ADHD* by Russell A. Barkley (2000) and *The Explosive Child* by Ross Greene (2005). After they were given an explaination of the motivation for the misbehavior of children with ADHD, they seemed to understand how they had "lost control" of Andrew. They were given all of the rating scales mentioned earlier to complete before the next session. Because of the stress level seen during the intake session, Mr. and Dr. P started the Good Behavior Book immediately, before Andrew come in for his play session.

Session 2: Evaluating Andrew

Andrew's first session was very productive. He was clearly hyperactive and impulsive. He complied with all the therapist's instructions and found enjoyment in drawing his pictures and performing the Puppet Sentence Completion Task (Knell, 1993). His pictures illustrated the power he held in his home and the insecurity and anxiety he felt about it. His drawing of a person was of one wearing a military outfit, holding a gun, with fear in his eyes. He said the boy had a gun to protect himself from all of the bad stuff that was around. The family drawing illustrated that his father was very important to him, but his mother was somewhat removed. He said the family was trying to have a good time at the beach, but it kept raining on them. During his "puppet task," he said he was happiest when he got what he wanted, was afraid when it was dark, hated reading, and loved to play. Many of his answers followed the same theme. He stated that "Daddy is nice when he plays with me, and Mommy is nice when she smiles." He had trouble finishing the stems: "Mommy and/or Daddy is mean when. . . ." Such resistance is not unusual.

His ability to play Guess Who? was somewhat impaired, although he claimed to play it a lot and win most of the time. He had an impulsive style when asking and answering questions that confused him. For instance, when he asked, "Does your person have blue eyes?" and the therapist answered, "No," he looked confused and said that none of the people in his remaining pictures had blue eyes. With encouragement and direction, he was able to understand the game better, which was necessary in order to allow him to continue at all. He was so confused that it was clear that he had not played the game before and suggested that he might have auditory processing difficulties.

The game Rebound was clearly enjoyable to Andrew, but he had no ability for or awareness of self-control. He moved the pieces too fast to get them in the target area, and he did not seem to understand how to slow down. It was evident, however, that he was frustrated very easily and could probably have a tantrum without much warning.

When playing Trouble, he impulsively took his turn *and* the therapist's turn without realizing it. He quickly wanted to quit when the therapist started to win. This inability to stay on task or finish games with his family was reported at intake. Again, with encouragement, Andrew stayed with the game until the session was over.

Session 3

Dr. P attended all the sessions with Andrew. The Good Behavior Book required a few minor revisions. There was a full-time nanny who wrote in the book most of the time because Mr. and Dr. P were often at work. Mr. P did write in the book as well, but he wrote more than two words per line and included some listings that were negative. After retraining, he clearly did the job better. By the third session, Andrew performed additional positive tasks so that his parents would record them in the book. It was Dr. P's responsibility to put Andrew to bed. She read a book to him at night, and he enjoyed their time together. If Andrew had trouble settling down after that, she would lie down with him until he fell asleep.

In Andrew's first play session, he was introduced to the Feeling Word Game. During the game, it became clear that Andrew felt his parents favored his brother, that he experienced a general sense of anxiety, and that he felt school was a difficult place. Andrew did not seem to have any social problems (which is unusual for children with ADHD), but felt somewhat alienated from certain people. He loved being with his friends and found that to be a great reason to go to school. It was noted during this game that he had begun to notice that the other guys didn't find him funny when he did things that they had found funny last year.

The Beat the Clock game had a baseline time of 4 minutes. Andrew kept his eyes on his drawing without ever looking up. Toward the end of the

4-minute session, he was more fidgety and used all his energy to "win" the game. After three trials, he did pick a prize from the treasure box. He wanted to play Beat the Clock again, but the therapist insisted that they play Connect Four. He followed the therapist's suggestion without resistance.

During Connect Four, a game of self-control, Andrew was quite impulsive. The therapist began to verbalize move strategies of her own and cued Andrew to look around the board before moving. With this stopping technique, Andrew was able to slow down his responses and comment before making his moves. After that game, they played Rebound to begin the training of self-control.

Session 4: Feedback

When the therapist met with Andrew's parents in session 4, they commented on Andrew's progress with chores and accomplishments in previously difficult areas. The therapist commented on the parents' positive change of style and Andrew's responsiveness.

The Special Playtime technique was introduced next. At first, Dr. P felt that this would not be a problem, because she always liked to play with Andrew for short periods of time. The therapist then modeled the narrating behavior and playtime tracking, but Dr. P was hesitant. She thought that Mr. P would be better at it. The therapist asked that both parents share this training and that they take turns in performing these tasks every other night with Andrew.

The therapist then joined Andrew and read the Good Behavior Book to him. Andrew was excited about all that he had accomplished. He even remembered accomplishments that he had achieved that they had forgotten to record. After they played the Feeling Word Game, more positive stories were produced by Andrew. He seemed to feel more confident about "being good" and told stories reflecting this. The therapist explored the fears affecting Andrew, and once again, generalized anxiety seemed pervasive.

Andrew began the Garbage Bag technique with some resistance. He would not agree to the garbage descriptors used by the therapist. He finally related to "piles and piles of garbage" and said "You would walk around like smelling horrible and no one would want to be around you." Andrew recorded his garbage items: (1) "My brother always gets me in trouble," (2) "School is boring," and (3) "No one wants to do things my way." The three items written by the therapist included (1) "No one is ever happy with what I do," (2) "People always tell me to stop talking," and (3) "My parents are always yelling." These items were acknowledged by Andrew as he nodded his head.

After putting the "garbage" in the bag, Andrew began the Beat the Clock game. This week Andrew reached the 5-minute level and held it easily. He received all 30 chips for the three trials. For homework, he was asked to practice this at home with his mom or dad, for 5 minutes per trial, to determine his ability to cope in the "real world." He was excited to try this.

The next self-control training again consisted of playing Rebound. Andrew showed a clear preference for this game. Although he threw the pieces so fast that they jumped off the board, he was receptive to the therapist's comment, "Show more self-control now so you can get into the target." With some modeling of the game and a great deal of verbal instruction, he slowed down his moves and was able to play and gain more points at each trial. The therapist kept the game even and then won in the end to measure Andrew's ability to lose. Under the same conditions, he said he would challenge the therapist again the following week.

Session 5: More Feedback

Special playtime was hard for Dr. P, but easier for Mr. P. Dr. P felt she had no time to do it. Because Andrew still took baths, the therapist advised Dr. P to do the special play during that time. Andrew loved to play in the bath, and Dr. P could narrate then. Mr. P found this part of the training easy to do.

Compliance training was then introduced. Dr. P said that she seemed to always "ask" her children to do things, because she felt it was rude to command. With her other son, "asking" worked, but with Andrew it did not. She was willing to try this new technique, but asked if she could say "please" to make it sound less demanding. It was agreed that she would perform the commands with both children so that there would be consistency.

When the therapist asked for a contractual item, Dr. P responded immediately. She wanted Andrew to get dressed by himself by 7:30 so that she could have a portion of her morning back. This seemed like a reasonable request, inasmuch as Andrew was certainly capable of dressing himself on weekends when there was no school. The therapist commented that because he had never dressed himself on a schoolday, expectations should not be too high. Because Andrew was so playful, the therapist suggested that Dr. P set a timer and prompt Andrew with "On your mark, get set, go" for the first two times. She was then to remark on how wonderfully Andrew was doing from time to time.

Andrew's portion of the session started again with the Good Behavior Book. The therapist told Andrew that sometimes children worked for larger prizes than those in the treasure box by performing one specific behavior all week. He was excited and wanted to do that. It was agreed that he would get dressed *by himself* and finish by 7:30 A.M. each morning when there was school that day. Mom would set a timer to keep track of the time. He seemed very willing to go along with this, and a contract was signed. Andrew wanted to earn some army men as a prize.

Andrew's first piece of "garbage" pulled from the bag was "School is boring." Andrew and the therapist set up miniature people and created a small classroom. The teacher doll told the children in the class to "drop everything and read now." That meant that the children had to read to themselves. The boy doll (Andrew) had trouble sitting down and wanted to play instead. Then the boy doll said, "I can't stand reading in my head—it is so boring." The therapist went picked up on this problem and, as the teacher, instructed the boy how to pass the time even if he couldn't read silently. The teacher doll asked for his suggestions, and the boy was able to figure out different ways to pass the time without worrying that he wasn't reading, which included asking the teacher for some help or if he could help her. After coming up with a few ideas, Andrew commented, "Hey, that was easy."

The Beat the Clock game was going well at home; Andrew's baseline time was 8 minutes this week. He played twice and was able to pick a prize. (When the game is played at home, a child increases his or her attention span at a faster rate.)

This session also introduced the Splatz (Kaduson, 2004). Andrew thought it was fabulous fun to say what he hated and throw the Blobz. He was so involved in the game that he kept going without giving the therapist a turn. He said that he hated tests, doing homework, long projects, having people telling him to stop all the time, his brother telling him he is wrong, his parents' yelling, teachers calling his name, friends telling him they don't want to play. Just the release of this information clearly helped Andrew to feel better. He was smiling a lot during the game.

The session ended this week with Rebound and the Trouble game. The therapist modeled each move and talked about the process she was incorporating. Andrew focused on the therapist's moves and mimicked with his own. This week he also verbalized his own move strategies, indicating that planning capabilities were developing.

Session 6: Progress Report

Compliance training went very well for Andrew. He easily completed the tasks, and Mr. and Dr. P were amazed at Andrew's follow-through. Dr. P was congratulated for following through with Andrew as well. Previously, they had told Andrew what to do, leaving it up to him to complete the tasks independently (which rarely happened). Andrew also got dressed alone and was ready on time every day for the past week. Dr. P was truly proud of him.

Dr. P was taught how to pay attention to Andrew and his brother when they were not bothering her. She had reported that she felt they never played quietly without a fight, but with encouragement she was willing to give it a try. She chose to pretend she was reading the paper and would frequently break away to comment on the children's good behavior.

Andrew's next contractual item was to complete homework without complaints. Mr. P was practicing Beat the Clock with Andrew (coloring only). It was decided that he would motivate Andrew to do his homework in one sitting, without complaints, through use of the contract.

At the beginning of Andrew's portion of the session, he was excited about receiving his prize as a reward for completing his homework. The Good Behavior Book seemed overshadowed by his excitement. He asked if he was going to earn another prize. A contract was drawn up for him to do homework without complaints in one sitting. The therapist reminded Andrew that he was already succeeding at Beat the Clock, so this would be a simple task. Andrew was motivated to try.

The next piece of garbage chosen was "My brother always gets me in trouble." Andrew played this out with both parents and his brother, using miniatures. Andrew illustrated through his play that his brother tattled on him whenever he made a mistake or annoyed him. The "mom doll" helped Andrew practice a technique in which Andrew goes to his mom first to report any trouble, thereby thwarting his brother's efforts to make him look bad. Andrew was able to problem-solve without anger once he realized that he had some control over the situation. Andrew also showed jealousy toward his brother in play, which was understandable under the circumstances. Things came easier for his brother, and Andrew knew it. The mom doll started listing all the good things that Andrew, the younger brother, could do faster and better in order to balance those negative feelings.

Andrew's play was more involved this week, with more interventions being suggested by the therapist. It was decided that the Beat the Clock game would not be played inasmuch as Dr. P was working on it at home. Andrew had already reached 20 minutes of attending without lifting his head or becoming distracted.

At the end of the session, pick-up sticks was played in order to focus more on developing self-control. Andrew was certainly working hard on trying to control and quiet his body as he played the game. He fidgeted when the therapist took a turn, but he took a deep breath before taking his turn and said "OK," as if to prepare himself for the trial. He still had some time after the game, and he asked to play Rebound again. He was beginning to really control his actions on that game, and it was proving very reinforcing because he easily won the games.

Session 7

Interestingly, both parents attended session 7. Mr. and Dr. P were as excited as Andrew to tell the therapist that not only was Andrew dressing himelf, but he did homework without complaints for the entire week. However, Mr. P said that focusing on his children when they were not bothering him was difficult. He felt that they were actually worse this week. Although this may have been true, the therapist told him that when a change is noticed by children, their behavior tends to get worse before getting better. This information encouraged Mr. P to stay with it.

The token economy was then introduced, and both parents were informed that they no longer had to keep the Good Behavior Book. The token economy uses poker chips, and Andrew and his brother were to participate. Competition concentrates on good behaviors rather than bad. Mr. and Dr. P grasped the system quickly, and, with Andrew, they were planning to develop it together the following weekend. It would be easy for Andrew to earn 100 points, and that was added to his contract. Both parents were present, so the therapist illustrated the Bubble Blowing Game which she would introduce to Andrew. She encouraged them to play along, and to keep their pinkies up when blowing the bubbles so that they would pop their own and Andrew would win.

During Andrews session, the therapist introduced the concept of the token economy. Andrew was asked what the payment should be for the chores listed. The therapist presented the poker chips and started giving him enough to illustrate the following items:

- Get up   2
- Get dressed   5
- Brush teeth   4
- Pack backpack   5
- Take vitamin   5
- Put clothes away   10
- Set table   7
- Make bed   5
- Feed dog   5
- Walk dog   10
- Do homework without complaints   25

Andrew was excited about earning the chips and agreed in the contract that he would earn 100 chips before the next week.

Andrew played out his last piece of "garbage": "No one wants to do things my way." The play session is performed with role play this time. The therapist and Andrew dressed as different people. The play focused on friends who were very busy playing a game without Andrew. Then the therapist's character modeled asking the other guys what they were playing. Andrew's character said they were playing kick ball. The therapist's character asked if they would play his way. Then Andrew, being the other guys, said, "We will play your way after we play ours." He was able to problem-solve this more easily when he was the other guys. Taking such a stand was clearly not as threatening as it would be if he were just himself. He couldn't think of any way to solve the problem until we pretended we were at recess together. He just nodded when he felt that the problem was solved.

The Beat the Clock game was now a regular item at home, so the therapist introduced the Bubble Blowing Game. Andrew was very good at taking deep breaths, but he held them instead of slowing blowing out. After approximately 15 trials, he began to perform the activity correctly, and he was given both bottles to practice at home. He could compete with Dad five times before homework, and compete with Mom five times before bed.

Session 8

The token economy was going great with Andrew and his brother. Mr. and Dr. P felt that this was a lifesaver, because the boys were trying to do more and more (tasks and good behaviors) to get more chips. There was less hitting going on between the boys and more positive play time. They were rewarded with chips for each hour they played nicely together.

The therapist reviewed time-out procedures with both parents. They agreed to use time-out sparingly and felt that it really had not been necessary to use it in weeks. Dr. P thought the utility room would do for a time-out, because Andrew could not harm himself with anything there. The concept of taking away chips was discussed. The therapist advised the parents that after Andrew obtained a long-term reward, chips could be deducted for not accomplishing what was on the list. However, removal could not be random. They had to be consistent with the token economy and add items when necessary. The therapist suggested that they put a bonus number on the chart so that they could give extra chips for special behaviors that were performed.

Andrew showed the therapist his poker chips in the playroom and immediately wanted his prize. The prizes were given at the end of the session, so he had to control himself and did so very well. The therapist then introduced him to making his own board game. Andrew's board game was created, with all his successes listed, and he then felt that there were some things he hadn't accomplished yet. He put the stickers down in place, and the therapist wrote the key. They started listing his items for the List of Good Me (these specific items are based on Andrew's perception of himself): got dressed alone, played nicely with brother, completed homework without complaints, finished homework without getting up, called friends once per night, made bed, felt happy. He decided to use these for his board game as well. He listed the things he needed to work on before putting them on the board game; forgot to study for spelling test, left clothes on floor, watched more television than permitted, took my brother's game system without permission. He said he wanted to work on accomplishing these tasks later. The therapist and Andrew began to put the board game together, using his items for the blank spaces.

Session 9

All of Andrew's parents' successes were listed for them. They really felt that he was doing a good job. The therapist said, "I was the director, and you did all the work." It was pretty clear that they were feeling prepared to take over the contracting, especially because the token economy was the contract medium.

Both parents were again present for session 9, so they were given the rating scales to complete. They could complete the scales while Andrew had his part of the session or could fill them out at home and return them the following week. For this session, both parents were required to be present, but ever since Mr. P had started to come to the sessions, both had attended weekly. The parents were advised on managing future problems by examining their own behavior and family stressors, and determining whether Andrew was reacting to a change *before* calling the therapist. The door is always open for clients to call or come back when needed.

Andrew was then informed that there were two sessions left in therapy. He didn't want to stop, but the therapist focused on how successful he had been, and started to finish the List of Good Me. Andrew recalled many of his accomplishments, and the therapist helped him finish the list with "good son," "good brother," "wonderful student," "genuine friend."

The session ended with Andrew and therapist playing his board game, which he thoroughly enjoyed.

Session 10

Both Mr. and Dr. P joined Andrew and the therapist for the last session. Everyone was happy to report that the token economy was going well, and Andrew had earned his long-term goal of having two friends go bowling with him.

The therapist began the drawing game by drawing a bridge connecting a cloudy sky to a rainbow sky. Then it was Andrew's turn; he colored in the entire rainbow very carefully (paying attention to his work the entire time, as he was praised by both parents.) Mr. P added a golden pot at the end of the rainbow, filled with candy and prizes. Dr. P added a sun and singing birds. No one added anything to the cloudy sky side of the bridge; the transformation was complete, and the family focused on the future with new beginnings.

Andrew was given his List of Good Me and board game to take home. He asked if everyone could play it together, which they did to end the last session. Andrew was clearly more in charge of his own life, and his parents were managing to parent him very well.

SUMMARY AND CONCLUSION

ADHD is a chronic disorder that baffles many therapists and teachers alike. However, through the use of play therapy and parenting changes, families *can* function and manage the problems of ADHD so they can meet normal criteria society sets for raising children. Many families have not been able to understand the disorder well enough to know where to start. Once motivated and directed, such families often function increasingly better. There will always be setbacks, and there will always be tough days. But to see a smile on a child's face and hear how terrific the family members feel makes all the hard work worthwhile. It is eminently fulfilling to a therapist to join a family in this process.

REFERENCES

Achenbach, T. M. (1978). The child behavior profile. *Journal of Consulting and Clinical Psychology, 46*, 478–488.

American Academy of Pediatrics. (2001). Clinical practice guideline: Treatment of the school-aged child with attention-deficit hyperactivity disorder. *Pediatrics, 108*, 1033–1044.

American Psychiatric Association. (1994). *Diagnostic and Statistical Manual of Mental Disorders* (4th ed.). Washington, DC: Author.

August, G. J., Realmuto, G. M., Hektner, J. M., & Bloomquist, M. L. (2001). An integrated components preventive intervention for aggressive elementary school children: The Early Risers Program. *Journal of Consulting and Clinical Psychology, 69*, 614–626.

Barkley, R. A. (1987). *Defiant children: A clinician's manual for parent training.* New York: Guilford Press.

Barkley, R. A. (1990). *Attention-deficit hyperactivity disorder: A handbook for diagnosis and treatment.* New York: Guilford Press.

Barkley, R. A. (2000). *Attention-deficit hyperactivity disorder: A handbook for diagnosis and treatment.* New York: Guilford Press.

Barkley, R. A. (1995). *Taking charge of ADHD: The complete, authoritative guide for parents.* New York: Guilford Press.

Barkley, R. A. (2000). *Taking charge of ADHD: The complete, authoritative guide for parents* (rev. ed.) New York: Guilford Press.

Barkley, R. A., & Murphy, K. R. (1998). *Attention-deficit hyperactivity disorder: A clinical handbook* (2nd ed.). New York: Guilford Press.

Blachman, D. R., & Hinshaw, S. P. (2002). Patterns of friendship among girls with and without attention-deficit hyperactivity disorder. *Journal of Abnormal Child Psychology, 30*, 625–640.

Conners, C. K., Sitarenios, G., Parker, J. D. A., & Epstein, J. N. (1998). Revision and restandardization of the Conners Parent Rating Scale (CPRS-R): Factor structure, reliability, and criterion validity. *Journal of Abnormal Child Psychology, 26*, 257–268.

Conners, C. K., & Wells, K. C. (1986). *Hyperkinetic children: A neuropsychosocial approach.* Beverly Hills, CA: Sage.

Gioia, G. A., Isquith, P. K., Guy, S. C., & Kenworthy, L. (2000). *Behavior Rating Inventory of Executive Function.* Los Angeles, CA: Western Psychological Services.

Goldstein, S., & Goldstein, M. (1990). *Managing attention disorders in children.* New York: Wiley.

Greene, R. W. (2005). *The explosive child.* New York: HarperCollins.

Hartman, R. R., Stage, S. A., & Webster-Stratton, C. (2003). A growth curve analysis of parent training outcomes: Examining the influence of child risk factors (inattention, impulsivity, and hyperactivity problems), parental and family risk factors. *Journal of Child Psychology and Psychiatry and Allied Discipline, 44,* 388–398.

Houk, G. M., King, M. C., Tomlinson, B., Vrabel, A., & Wecks, K. (2002). Small group intervention for children with attention disorders. *Journal of School Nursing, 18,* 196–200.

Kaduson, H. G. (1993a). The feeling word game. In H. G. Kaduson & C. Schaefer (Eds.), *101 favorite play therapy techniques* (pp. 19–21). Northvale, NJ: Aronson.

Kaduson, H. G. (1993b). Play therapy for children with attention-deficit hyperactivity disorder. In H. G. Kaduson, D. Cangelosi, & C. E. Schaefer (Eds.), *The playing cure* (pp. 197–227). Northvale, NJ: Aronson.

Kaduson, H. G. (2000). Structured short-term play therapy for children with attention-deficit hyperactivity disorder. In H. G. Kaduson & C. E. Schaefer (Eds.), *Short-term play therapy for children* (pp. 105–143). New York: Guilford Press.

Kaduson, H. G. (2004). *More fun play therapy techniques.* Boiling Springs, PA: Play Therapy Press.

Knell, S. M. (1993). *Cognitive-behavioral play therapy.* Northvale, NJ: Aronson.

Loney, J. (1980). Hyperkinesis comes of age: What do we know and where should we go? *American Journal of Orthopsychiatry, 50,* 28–42.

Loney, J., Kramer, J., & Milich, M. R. (1981). The hyperkinetic child grows up: Predictors of symptoms, delinquency and achievement at follow-up. In K. D. Gadow & J. Loney (Eds.), *Psychosocial aspects of drug treatment for hyperactivity.* Boulder, CO: Westview Press.

Lord, J. (1985). *A guide to individual psychotherapy with school-age children and adolescents.* Springfield, IL: Charles C. Thomas.

Milich, R. S., & Landau, S. (1981). Socialization and peer relations in the hyperactive child. In K. D. Gadow & I. Bailer (Eds.), *Advances in learning and behavior disabilities* (Vol. 1). Greenwich, CT: JAI Press.

Mischel, W., Shoda, Y., & Rodriguez, M. L. (1989). Delay of gratification in children. *Science, 244,* 933–938.

Mrug, S., Hoza, B., & Gerdes, A. C. (2001). Children with attention-deficit hyperactivity disorder: Peer relationships and peer-oriented interventions. In D. W. Nangle & C. A. Erdley (Eds.), *The role of friendship in psychological adjustment: New directions for child and adolescent development* (pp. 51–77). San Francisco: Jossey-Bass.

Play Visions (2000). *The Blobz!* Woodinville, WA.

Routh, D. K. (1978). Hyperactivity. In P. R. Magrab (Ed.), *Psychological management of pediatric problems* (Vol. 2). Baltimore: University Park Press.

Satterfield, J. H., Satterfield, B. T., & Cantwell, D. P. (1981). Three-year multi-modality treatment study of 100 hyperactive boys. *Journal of Pediatrics, 98,* 650–655.

Van Fleet, R. (2005). *Filial therapy: Strengthening parent–child relationships through play* (2nd ed.). Sarasota, FL: Professional Resource Press.

Webster-Stratton, C., Reid, M. J., & Hammond, M. (2001). Social skills and problem solving training for children with early-onset conduct problems: Who benefits? *Journal of Child Psychology and Psychiatry, 42,* 943–952.

Webster-Stratton, C., Reid, M. J., & Hammond, M. (2004). Treating children with early-onset problems: Intervention outcomes for parent, child and teacher training. *Journal of Clinical Child and Adolescent Psychology, 33,* 105–124.

Weiss, G., & Hechtman, L. T. (1986). *Hyperactive children grown up: Empirical findings and theoretical considerations.* New York: Guilford Press.

Wender, P. H. (1987). *Minimal brain dysfunction in children.* New York: Guilford Press.

Wodrich, D. L. (2000). *Atttention-deficit hyperactivity disorder: What every parent wants to know* (2nd ed.). Baltimore: Brookes.

PART II

FAMILY PLAY THERAPY

CHAPTER 6

Short-Term Play Therapy for Adoptive Families
Facilitating Adjustment and Attachment with Filial Therapy

RISË VANFLEET

When a couple decide to adopt a child, they are embarking on a journey that is both exciting and daunting. Whereas adoption often fulfills the couple's long-time desire for a child, it also introduces significant adjustments and potential problems for the family to overcome. Older adoptive children may have longed for the adoption as much as their parents have, yet they bring years of turbulent history with them that is not so easily set aside. When an adoption is finalized by the court, it is a joyous occasion, but considerable patience, flexibility, and hard work are needed to integrate the child fully into the family's life from that point forward. Perhaps the most important developmental task of adoptive families is to create healthy, secure attachments within the family. Trusting, reliable relationships provide the base from which children and adults alike can explore and enjoy their lives fully.

This chapter describes the challenges faced by adoptive families and the importance of secure attachments for all family members. The use of Filial Therapy (FT) to assist the adjustment of adoptive children and families is discussed, including its use as a prevention/family enhancement method as well as an intervention for very difficult problems.

GENERAL DIFFICULTIES FACED BY ADOPTIVE FAMILIES

The processes by which parents decide to adopt are as varied as the reasons children become available for adoption. A "typical" adoptive family does not really exist. Although there are similarities among adoptive families, there is also tremendous diversity. A family's postadoption adjustment can be influenced by many factors. Some of the characteristics and needs of adoptive families are outlined in the following discussion.

Adoptive Children

Adoptive children vary widely in their psychosocial characteristics, as well as in their needs. Age at adoption, temperament, coping abilities, history of abuse or neglect, involvement in the foster care system, prior attachment experiences, and general life experiences all play a profound role in children's adjustment to adoption. A shared characteristic of adoptive children is the major disruption that has occurred in their normal development, including the development of attachment relationships. This disruption can interfere with children's individual development at many levels and their capacity to form satisfying, secure, intimate family relationships (Ginsberg, 1989; VanFleet, 1994, 2003).

The challenges presented by adoptive children include anxiety, behavior problems, impulsivity, attachment difficulties, unresolved reactions to past abuses, losses, or rejections, confused personal boundaries, posttraumatic stress disorder, insecurity about the family environment, and an inability to conceive of or plan for the future. Some adoptive children have lived with a long line of family members or foster families, and it may be difficult for them to believe that an adoption is "final." Sometimes they have been moved at a moment's notice, placed with a new family in a new town, and then penalized for having negative reactions to these sudden and unpredictable changes. Such experiences can intensify their feelings of rejection and helplessness and exacerbate their emotional and behavioral reactivity.

Adoptive children, especially those who come from foster placements, have sometimes been separated from the support of their siblings, and they may have many questions about their biological families. It can be difficult for them to determine their roles in the adoptive families when they have so much confusion about their biological families.

These potential problems do not appear in all adoptive children, but the disruptions in these children's lives place them at greater risk for developmental, learning, social, emotional, and behavioral difficulties.

Adoptive Parents

Adoptive parents have usually endured many stresses prior to actually adopting a child. Inability to conceive can result in feelings of loss, guilt, and anger, as well as marital stress. The adoption process can be long and frustrating, and most adoptive parents have heard horror stories of children being placed in loving adoptive homes only to be reclaimed by biological parents at the last minute. Uncertainties prevail.

When a child is placed, it is typically a happy occasion, yet it is fraught with stress. Sometimes the placement occurs suddenly and unpredictably, and the family's lifestyle is changed almost overnight. When adoptive parents are faced with the actual infant or child, self-doubt about their ability to parent him or her often arise.

Adoptive parents sometimes express concern about the role of the biological parents in the child's life. They need information about how, what, and when to tell the child about the adoption and his or her biological parents.

Adoptive parents also need as much information as possible about the child's medical and psychosocial history. For infant or toddler adoptions, parents want to know what to expect in their child's development and any potential problems to watch for. With adoptions of older children, parents may have some idea of the problems experienced by the child, yet still be at a loss as to how to handle problematic emotions, behaviors, or medical conditions. Sometimes attachment problems emerge in a totally unexpected manner. The first few months in the family home may go smoothly, followed by the sudden eruption of disturbance. Parents need to be prepared for these possibilities and how to find assistance if needed.

THE IMPORTANCE OF ATTACHMENT

One of the primary functions of a family is to provide a safe, secure environment in which all members can develop in positive ways. This is particularly important for adoptive families, in which normal developmental processes of attachment have been disrupted. Secure attachments and healthy parent–child relationships are associated with psychosocial health, whereas insecure or damaged attachments are linked with a wide range of difficulties (Belsky & Nezworski, 1988; Clark & Ladd, 2000; Humber & Moss, 2005; Ladd & Ladd, 1998; Youngblade & Belsky, 1992). Healthy attachments provide a protective shield for family members when they face and cope with life difficulties (Figley, 1989; Hart, Shaver, & Goldenberg, 2005; La Greca, Silverman, Vernberg, & Roberts, 2002; Sroufe, 1983, 1988; Sroufe & Rutter, 1984). Family psychologists, therapists, and researchers have paid increasing attention to the implications of developmental attachment processes for family relations (Bifulco & Moran, 1998; Bifulco, Moran, Ball, & Lillie, 2002; Cheung & Hong, 2005; Johnson, 2005; Marvel, Rodriguez, & Liddle, 2005). Such implications are relevant to the way in which practitioners work with adoptive families in prevention and intervention programs.

Attachment disruptions in children arise from separations from parents, temperamental factors, anxiety of parents, traumatic events, lack of physical or emotional safety, unpredictability in the child's environment, abuse, neglect, frequent changes in living conditions, and so on (VanFleet & Sniscak, 2003a). When children lack a strong connection with their parents, or worse, are abused by those entrusted with their care, they often feel insecure, frightened, helpless, and angry. When poor attachment arises from traumatic conditions in which their needs are ignored or violated, children can become mistrustful of all people. James (1994) has clearly described the dynamics through which attachment-trauma problems are created and manifested, and Terr (1990) has documented the long-term negative impact of trauma on children. Even the very system developed to protect abused children has been responsible for new abuses and victimization (Bernstein, 2001). Most child therapists can describe situations in which "the system" has failed the children in its care.

The impact of attachment disruptions on children's lives can be devastating and far-reaching. Children who have not experienced healthy attachments, or whose attachments have been weakened or broken, develop a wide range of difficult behaviors, including rage and explosiveness, numbness and detachment, dissociation, trauma reactions, unhealthy trauma bonds, depression, self-injury, intense fears, isolation, unhealthy relationships, sexualized and/or violent behaviors, and poor self-regulation (James, 1994; Ziegler, 2000). The scope and intensity of attachment problems sometimes lead to frequent changes in placement and repeated life experiences of failure and rejection. The attachment styles of caregivers can aid or exacerbate these difficulties. Because many children who are adopted have had attachment disruptions of varying degrees, it is important for parents and professionals involved with adoption to be familiar with attachment relationships and know the resources available to strengthen them.

An understanding of how healthy attachment relationships develop can inform the education and treatment of adoptive families grappling with trauma and attachment-related problems. Much has been written on the process of attachment (Ainsworth, 1982; Belsky & Nezworski, 1988; Bowlby, 1982; Brazelton & Cramer, 1990), and this can guide the interventions we employ to establish it in adoptive families. Filial therapy, the treatment approach emphasized in this chapter, aims to help adoptive children and parents develop healthy attachments, while encouraging children to work through their trauma issues in a safe, accepting environment. Furthermore, this approach is noncoercive and emphasizes the reciprocity important in healthy bonds. Although the treatment of attachment-related problems is not always short-term, it can be, and the use of the approaches defined here can substantially reduce the amount of therapy time required. Such treatment is accomplished through the involvement of adoptive parents as the primary change agents for their own children. Filial therapy, with its use of nondirective play sessions, recreates parent–child interactions similar in many ways to those that lead to healthy attachment in infancy (Ryan & Wilson, 1995).

PREVENTION AND INTERVENTION

A relatively short-term intervention that effectively strengthens attachment within adoptive families is Filial Therapy (FT). FT is a psychoeducational approach that combines family therapy and play therapy, with the goals of strengthening families and treating a wide range of child and family problems. The therapist trains the parents to conduct special child-centered play sessions with their own children. The therapist then observes the initial parent–child play sessions and provides constructive feedback to facilitate the parents' skill development. Discussions of the possible meanings of the child's play themes within the context of family and community life help the parents to understand their children better and to respond to their needs more satisfactorily. As the parents develop competence and confidence in conducting the play sessions, they eventually hold them more independently in the home setting. In the final stage of FT, the therapist helps the parents generalize and maintain the use of the skills they have learned during the play sessions. FT has been used for many years with adoptive families with considerable success.

Overview of Filial Therapy

FT, developed by Bernard and Louise Guerney (B. G. Guerney, 1964; L. F. Guerney, 1983, 2003), is a theoretically integrative and evidence-based approach that combines play therapy and family therapy. It is a highly effective intervention that can be very beneficial for adoptive families (VanFleet, 1994, 2003). In FT, the therapist trains and supervises parents as they conduct special child-centered play sessions with their own children. With appropriate training and supervision, parents usually are able to conduct these special play sessions at home without the therapist's direct supervision.

The goals of FT are to help parents create an accepting, safe environment in which their children can express their feelings fully, gain an understanding of their world, solve problems, and develop confidence in themselves and their parents. The therapy process is designed to help parents become more responsive to their children's feelings and needs, to become better at solving child- and family-related problems, and to become more skillful and confident as parents. Families who participate in FT are expected to emerge with better communication skills, problem-solving and coping skills, and stronger family relationships. FT helps the family create a network of healthy, secure attachment relationships. It is usually an enjoyable process for the entire family, and many families incorporate it into their lifestyles after formal therapy has ended (VanFleet, 1998).

Because of its educational and strengths-based nature, FT has never been a lengthy therapeutic approach. Families with mild to moderate problems typically require 15–20 1-hour sessions before discharge. It can be provided in as few as 10 sessions, however, and there are a number of relatively short-term group formats for its use as well.

Filial Play Session Skills

Parents learn four specific skills in order to conduct the special play sessions with their children. After the parents have mastered these skills during the play sessions, their use can be generalized to everyday parenting situations. The four skills, detailed in VanFleet (1999, 2000, 2005a), are briefly described here:

1. The *structuring skill* helps children understand how the play sessions work. Parents learn how to explain the sessions to their children, what to say upon entering the play session, and how to handle departure from the room and the ending of the play session. The therapist prepares parents to handle resistance from a child, particularly when the play session ends.

2. The *empathic listening skill* enhances parents' attunement to the child, helping them show greater understanding and acceptance of their child's feelings, motivations, and needs. The therapist teaches parents to rephrase aloud the child's main activities and emotions to convey interest in the child by their nonverbal behavior. Parents learn to refrain from leading, teaching, questioning, or directing the child's play.

3. The *child-centered imaginary play skill* is actually another form of attunement and empathy. The parents engage in pretend play when invited by the child, and in a manner consistent with the child's wishes. They learn to act out different roles the child might assign. Parents follow the child's ideas for the direction of the play so that themes of importance to the child can emerge.

4. The *limit-setting skill* creates safety within the play sessions as parents set and enforce the rules when needed. The number of limits is minimized, but they are important to help children understand their boundaries and how to redirect their energies if their behavior becomes unsafe or destructive. The therapist teaches parents a three-step limit-setting process: (a) state the limit clearly and specifically when it is first broken and redirect the child in a general way, (b) give the child a warning on the second infraction of the same limit, informing the child that the play session will end if he or she tries it a third time, and (c) enforcing the consequence for the third infraction of the same limit by ending the play session.

The Process of Filial Therapy

VanFleet (1999, 2005a) has detailed the methods and process of FT, as follows:

1. The therapist explains the rationale and methods of FT, answering parents' questions and engaging them as partners in the process.

2. The therapist then demonstrates the play sessions individually with the children in the family as the parents watch and record their observations and questions. The therapist fully discusses the play session demonstrations with the parents afterward.

3. The therapist trains the parents in the four basic play session skills: structuring, empathic listening, child-centered imaginary play, and limit setting. A variety of training approaches can be used, but this phase culminates in mock play sessions in which the therapist pretends to be a child and the parents practice the four basic skills. The therapist provides ongoing feedback during the mock session to help shape the parent's use of the skills, and then discusses the experience fully with the parents at the end, providing feedback on their skills and expectations of how the process will work with the children in the family. The feedback offered to parents throughout FT focuses on their strengths and offers suggestions for improvement.

4. The parents begin play sessions with their own children under the supervision of the therapist. The play sessions involve one parent and one child at a time, and the sessions can be alternated to include all family members (VanFleet, 1999, 2005). The therapist provides feedback to the parents on their play session skills, helps them understand their children's play, and discusses a variety of family dynamics issues that emerge from the play sessions.

5. After parents develop confidence and competence in conducting the play sessions, they begin to hold them independently at home. The therapist and parents meet periodically to discuss the home play sessions, problem-solve family issues that arise, and generalize the skills beyond the play sessions to daily life.

Empirical Basis of Filial Therapy

FT has been continuously researched since its inception in the early 1960s. Studies of its process and efficacy have increased steadily through the years, and research has been or is being conducted in the United States, Canada, the United Kingdom, Korea, China, South Africa, Bahrain, and elsewhere, with a variety of problem areas and in different settings and cultures. VanFleet, Ryan, and Smith (2005) have provided a critical review of the empirical basis of FT, noting its consistently positive outcomes and robustness as a therapy useful in addressing a wide range of problems. Controlled studies have demonstrated its effectiveness in (1) improving children's presenting problems and behaviors, (2) developing parental acceptance and understanding of their children, (3) strengthening parents' skills, (4) decreasing parents' stress levels, and (5) improving parents' satisfaction with outcomes. Follow-up studies have shown that family gains are maintained 3 and 5 years after therapy has ended. These quantitative outcomes are augmented by qualitative information and compelling case studies (VanFleet & Guerney, 2003), and the use of FT has grown dramatically during the past decade, largely because of its effectiveness.

The Value of Filial Therapy for Adoptive Families

FT is particularly useful for adoptive families. Because FT builds healthy attachments while simultaneously permitting children to work through problems or traumatic reactions, it provides adoptive families with the tools needed to create a satisfying home environment. It also assists adoptive parents in understanding the complex needs of their adopted child so that they are more likely to know how to address those needs in constructive ways. There are many reasons why FT is applicable, and often the treatment of choice, for adoptive families (VanFleet & Sniscak, 2003a):

1. FT creates a physically and emotionally safe environment for the child. Physical safety is ensured by the structuring and limit-setting skills, and emotional safety is demonstrated by the parent's/caregiver's empathic acceptance and child-centered imaginary play skill (another form of empathy and attunement).

2. FT offers the child acceptance of *self* by primary caregivers, and this in turn can strengthen the child's own sense of self.

3. Children in FT are free to explore their own interests, motives, struggles, wishes, and so on, and this can help strengthen identity.

4. The nondirective nature of the play sessions fosters the development of trust, as the child learns from repeated exposure during the play sessions that all of his or her feelings and expressions are accepted unconditionally.

5. Children in FT learn better emotional and behavioral regulation through the combined use of play session skills that can eventually be employed by parents in daily life. This is accomplished by providing the child with much-needed nurturance and acceptance while simultaneously and firmly limiting inappropriate behaviors.

6. The FT play session skills help build the attunement between parent and child. It helps parents to understand their children better and, consequently, to focus on and meet their needs better.

7. FT is a developmentally sensitive intervention. It uses play as the primary means of building attachment, and the child can work through clinical, developmental, and relationship issues simultaneously.

8. FT allows adoptive children to express and master their trauma issues in a nonthreatening and facilitative environment.

9. FT recognizes the reciprocity of relationships. It helps parents help their children, and parents model for their children the healthier attitudes and behaviors that they wish their children to adopt. FT encourages the interplay of parent and child as they appreciate each other, learn about each other, and have fun together.

10. FT provides parents with the empathy, encouragement, and support to use (a) the play session skills, (b) their clearer understanding of their child,

and (c) insight about their own feelings and reactions to change their own attitudes and behaviors, resulting in more satisfying relationships with their children.

11. Because the entire family is involved in the process, FT helps strengthen family identity, trust, and cohesion. As parents and children together work through their dynamic issues and develop stronger bonds, their joint sense of belongingness and attachment is forged.

12. FT involves other children already in the family, whether they are biological or previously adopted children. It helps to prevent or reduce sibling rivalries that may arise, and siblings have their own play sessions so they are less likely to resent the newly adopted child's special times with the parents. It helps the family appreciate the uniqueness of all the children and facilitates family cohesion rather than competition.

13. The FT process enables parents to "take the therapy home," often reducing the amount of office-based therapy needed.

14. FT provides parents with lifelong skills that can be used long after therapy ends and adapted as the child's developmental level changes.

15. FT is transportable and can be used in many different settings with a variety of caregivers. It can be used to facilitate difficult transitions for children, such as from foster care into adoptive placement, and to serve as a template for healthy relationships along the way.

Filial Therapy Models for Use with Adoptive Families

The needs of adoptive families are varied, and FT has the flexibility to adapt to those needs. The strength of FT lies in its training methods, its positive strengths-based focus, its use of play as a means of connecting parents and children, and its collaborative trust and involvement of parents as the primary change agents for their own children. When these essential ingredients are incorporated, the actual format for treatment can take many forms and remain effective. Descriptions of different individual and group formats are available (Caplin & Pernet, 2005; Ginsberg, 2004; Guerney, 1983; Landreth, 2002; Landreth & Bratton, 2006; VanFleet, 2005a; VanFleet & Guerney, 2003; Wright & Walker, 2003). Three general options for the use of FT with adoptive families are included in the following discussion.

Filial Therapy as a Prevention Program

Many adoptive families adjust well to the changes in their lives. Adopted infants and adopted children with less traumatic histories often adjust smoothly. Even children with backgrounds of abuse and neglect sometimes settle into life with their adoptive families rapidly and without undue strain. Even so, it is desirable for adoptive families to strengthen their attachments and to prevent at-risk children from developing difficulties at a later date. FT can help them do this. Furthermore, the filial play sessions are very enjoyable and offer a unique way for parents and children to connect, and for parents to feel confident in their parenting approach. Therefore, FT can be offered to some adoptive families simply as a prevention program to facilitate their development as a family.

In this case, FT can be offered as a very short-term program, perhaps in a 10- to 15-week individual family format, or a 10- to 15-session small group format. A session-by-session sample of such a program for individual families is outlined here. Asterisks show points in the process where sessions can be added or deleted, as needed by the family. Furthermore, sessions 1 and 2 can be combined if a full assessment of the family is deemed unnecessary.

- Session 1:   Intake with parents
                    Discussion of adoption and attachment issues
                    Explanation of the importance of play
                    Preliminary information about FT
                    Premeasures
- Session 2:   Family play observation
                    Discussion of family play observation with parents
                        only
                    Recommendation for FT
                    Overview of FT process and skills
- Session 3:   Therapist–child play session demonstration; parents
                        watch
                    Discussion of play session
                    Introductory training in the four play session skills
- Sessions 4–5:*   Training of parents in play session skills
                    Mock play sessions
- Sessions 6–10:*   Filial play sessions
                    Discussion and feedback with parents alone
- Sessions 11–15:* Home filial play sessions
                    Reports on home sessions and discussion
                    Generalization and maintenance of skills
                    Postmeasures

To accommodate a number of children and as many as two parents in this format, the filial play sessions that are directly observed by the therapist in sessions 6 through 10 are held for 20 minutes each. Each parent holds one session for 20 minutes, and the therapist uses the remaining 20 minutes for discussion and feedback. When the parents begin their home sessions, they are each asked to hold a 30-minute play session with each of their children each week, if possible.

Several short-term group adaptions are also appropriate for adoptive families as prevention programs. Landreth and Bratton (2006) have developed and researched a 10-week group filial training format that teaches parents the basic play skills and provides a small amount of direct observation of the parent–child play sessions. Descriptions of this format are also available in Landreth (2002) and in several chapters in VanFleet and Guerney (2003).

Caplin and Pernet (2005) have developed a 12-session group format for the use of FT with impoverished and at-risk families, and they have been using it in Philadelphia for more than 5 years. Their format can work very well with adoptive families. Two therapists lead a group of 10 or 12 parents. The didactic material is covered with the entire group together. When parents practice the skills and hold their filial play sessions with their children, the group divides, each half meeting with one of the therapists. This approach permits the parents to obtain considerable individualized supervision and feedback from the therapists, and it allows other children in the family to be involved in the process too. Home play sessions are reported during the final weeks of FT, with the entire group intact once more.

Wright and Walker (2003) have developed a similar approach with Head Start families that incorporates the strengths of the original Guerney FT group model (Guerney, 1983) and the Landreth/Bratton 10-week group FT training format (Landreth & Bratton, 2006). Two group leaders divide the group for the practice sessions and for observations of the actual parent–child play sessions, yet meet with the entire group jointly to cover didactic material, hold toy-making sessions, and discuss progress. They provide additional innovative interventions to ensure group attendance and involvement. The Wright and Walker (2003) format entails 12 sessions of a core program, followed by 1 or 2 "reunion sessions" held several months after the core sessions have ended. This approach, too, seems very applicable to adoptive families.

Filial Therapy for Adoptive Families Experiencing Problems

When adoptive families experience problems, often due to the child's traumatic past or the additional strains on family life, FT may be a beneficial intervention. Other play therapy and behavioral interventions may be needed as well, but because FT typically addresses emotional, social, behavioral, and parenting issues, it can often be used as a single, systemic intervention. The form of therapy offered to an adoptive family varies greatly, depending on specific child and family needs. It is not always short-term, but FT, with its involvement of the parents and entire family system, tends to reduce significantly the amount of therapy time needed.

There are instances when other interventions may be required prior to the start of FT, such as the following: (1) if the parents have exhausted their physical and emotional reserves prior to seeking therapy, (2) if the child's behaviors are so extreme that crisis intervention is needed, or (3) if the parents are unlikely to be able to accept the potentially intense emotional content of the child's play (e.g., sexualized play related to molestation or play related to other traumas). Decisions about the course of therapy, with these factors in mind, are made with full input of the parents.

For example, an adoptive mother of a child with reactive attachment disorder was exhausted after 2 years of attempts to tame the child's behavior and unsuccessfully seeking treatments that would work. She had been told that play therapy would not work for her daughter, and she and her child had been traumatized by a coercive holding method recommended and conducted by another professional. Her child had been placed in therapeutic foster care for the safety of other children in the family. The skeptical adoptive mother requested that the therapist work with the adopted girl first to see if interventions would be successful, and if so, she would become involved in FT at a later date. The therapist conducted child-centered play therapy and more directive trauma interventions with the child, while working with the foster mother and the adoptive mother on consistent behavior management approaches. During 35 play sessions, the child worked on intense trauma and attachment issues and showed behavioral improvements in her daily life with her foster parents and on weekend visits with her adoptive family. The adoptive mother then learned to conduct the filial play sessions, and after 10 such sessions, the child returned home. The adoptive mother had been given a much needed respite and the daughter's intensity had diminished. The filial play sessions continued at home while the child participated in a small play-based social skills group. FT, combined with a variety of play therapy and parenting interventions, was successful in helping the adoptive family establish more secure attachment relationships that have continued for several years posttreatment (VanFleet & Sniscak, 2003a).

Other child-oriented therapies that may be considered as an adjunct to FT with adoptive families include cognitive-behavioral play therapy (Kaduson, 1994; Knell, 1993); release play therapy for trauma (Kaduson, 1994; Schaefer, 1994), identity activities, sandtray interventions, thematic play therapy (Benedict & Mongoven, 2000), dramatic play therapy (Gallo-Lopez & Schaefer, 2005), bibliotherapy (e.g., *Brave Bart* by Sheppard, 1998) and the use of educational workbooks (e.g., *When Something Terrible Happens* by Heegaard, 1991), developmental play therapy (Brody, 1993), and animal assisted therapies (Becker, 2002; Chandler, 2005; Crawford & Pomerinke, 2003; Davis, 1992; Fine, 2000; Levinson & Mallon, 1997). These interventions can help children address the legacy of their prior traumas and develop a clearer understanding of themselves; they can also reduce levels of emotional arousal and anxiety and enhance social skills and adjustment. Of course, children should also be referred for appropriate physical/biological interventions as needed, such as medical treatment, physical therapy, occupational therapy/sensory integration, and speech/hearing services.

Other family-oriented therapies can be useful as well. These include training in behavior management and parenting skills (although these are also built into the FT process), Theraplay (Booth & Lindaman, 2000; Jernberg & Booth, 1999; Munns, 2000), the Circle of Security program (Marvin, Cooper, Hoffman, & Powell, 2002), the Watch, Wait and Wonder program for infants (Cohen et al., 1999; Muir, Lojkasek, & Cohen, 1999), parental involvement in therapist-directed activities (as in Hughes, 1997), and other family collaborative play activities.

Whether FT is used alone or in conjunction with other therapeutic interventions, some adjustments may be needed to assist adoptive families. Possible adaptations of the FT method are described in detail elsewhere for trauma issues (VanFleet & Sniscak, 2003b) and attachment-related problems (VanFleet & Sniscak, 2003a), both areas that intersect with adoptive families. Adaptations of the method are briefly discussed in the following paragraphs.

First, where relevant to the child's history, adoptive families need to understand the impact of attachment/trauma problems on the child. Internet chat rooms are full of dire predictions and punitive "solutions" that can exacerbate tensions at home. Therapists need to educate parents about trauma, attachment, affective, and relationship issues, how their child's behavior is related to such issues, and how they and their children discharge distress (Jackins, 1994; James, 1994; Ziegler, 2000).

Second, when the adoptive family comes to treatment in crisis mode, parenting skills and behavior management interventions may be required immediately to reduce the level of emotional arousal in the family. Guerney's (1995) parenting skills program is useful here, and it is consistent with FT.

Third, adoptive parents sometimes need a bit more time spent in the training phase of FT. This is true when the child exhibits extreme conduct problems or intense posttrauma reactions. After parents learn the basic play session skills during the normal FT process, they may benefit from additional observations of therapist-conducted play sessions with their child and/or a third mock play session during which the therapist prepares them for the more difficult child behaviors that may emerge during play sessions.

Fourth, adoptive parents may need extra encouragement and support as they conduct filial play sessions with their children. Although always an integral part of the FT process, therapists may need to provide considerable empathy, patience, and practical guidance for parents as they conduct the play sessions, discuss the play themes, and decide how to handle problematic situations at home. Sometimes, with severely distressed children, the therapist and adoptive parents may decide to continue play sessions under the therapist's supervision for a longer-than-usual time before starting the home filial play sessions.

Additional child and family interventions and adaptations to the FT method are not always needed for adoptive families. The systemic FT process is powerfully effective as a short-term intervention, and it often ameliorates adoptive family problems readily. An advantage of the systemic nature of FT is that it reduces the amount of therapy that an adoptive family needs. Additions and adaptations are made only a case-by-case basis.

Filial Therapy Model for Successful Transition from Foster Care to Adoption

Children who have been involved in the foster care system sometimes have difficulty in making the transition from home to home, and the move into adoption is no exception. Although most of these children desperately want to be part of a family, the abuse or neglect they suffered in their biological families, coupled with frequent and unexpected moves from placement to placement, leave them wary and unbelieving that the adoptive placement is "for real." FT can help stabilize foster placements and provide an excellent transition tool to ease the move into adoption. In this model, the therapist trains and supervises foster parents or kinship carers as they hold filial play sessions with the child. When adoptive parents are identified, the therapist trains them as well, and through a series of alternating filial play sessions with caregivers and adoptive parents, helps the child move from an emotionally safe placement to a secure adoptive home.

FT has been used successfully with foster parents (Sweeney, 2003), kinship caregivers (Malon, 2003), and adoptive families (Ginsberg, 1989; VanFleet, 1994, 2003). This FT transition model combines these approaches in a continuous, but relatively short-term intervention across the systems in which the child lives.

Mental health professionals sometimes worry about a child forming an attachment to foster parents or temporary kinship caregivers, fearing that it will be damaging to the child to have that attachment broken when the child moves into adoption. This FT transition model encourages healthy attachments with foster or kinship caregivers for several reasons.

First, many children in the care system have little or no experience with healthy attachments. Their only experiences are with insecure attachments and hurtful relationships. If they can experience a healthy relationship with their caregivers, then it adds a "template" of secure attachment to the child's frame of reference. This can help increase the child's eventual ability to discern healthy from unhealthy relationships. Even for parents, the experience of connection during their own life histories can provide this template for future relationships. An adoptive mother reported, during FT, "When I was growing up myself, I wasn't very close to my parents. They were always too busy or very critical. But my grandmother saved the day. I could talk with her about *anything*, and she really listened and understood. That's the kind of mother I want to be for Brad."

Second, filial play sessions provide foster children with perhaps their first experience of empathy from another person. It is difficult for a person to have empathy for another person if he or she has not experienced it first.

Third, foster children develop bonds with their caregivers by virtue of living with them. Using FT can help ensure that the bonds are healthy ones. It is not unusual for foster children to begin immediately calling new foster parents "Mom" and "Dad" and saying, "I love you" to them. This demonstrates their need and desire for engagement. Foster children can also behave in provocative ways that result in relationships that mimic the abusive relationships of their past. FT can prevent this from happening, and it can deepen the relationship so that the child's needs for security and attachment are better met. This, in turn, can reduce problematic behaviors of the child, which in turn can reduce or eliminate changes in the child's placement.

Fourth, children sometimes remain in foster placement or kinship care for extended periods of time. Because healthy relationships are so critical to children's well-being, it may be a disservice to children to "wait" until they are adopted before facilitating their healthy attachment with caregivers. To counteract feelings of rejection, isolation, and self-esteem, these children also need to feel valued. FT helps foster or kinship caregivers *show* children how valued they are by their acceptance during the play sessions.

Fifth, most people's lives are populated with a variety of relationships, of varying degrees of connection and health. In all lives, some of the attachments (i.e., friendships, family relationships, intimate relationships) are broken or left behind. When the relationship of best friends is disrupted by one child's move to another city, their friendship may endure through e-mails and visits, or it may dissolve, but the experience of that friendship stays with the children throughout their lives. Moreover, most people have a number of attachment relationships at any given time, with some closer than others. Therefore, it is a relatively normal experience to have multiple attachments, some of which change or end, and it is a developmental task to adjust to such changes. The transition model that follows helps children engage in healthy relationships and then adjust to changes in those relationships.

For many children awaiting adoption, the transition from the foster home to the adoptive home is relatively abrupt. The child meets the preadoptive parents, has several visits with them, including some overnight visits, and then moves in with them permanently. This entire process is sometimes completed in 1–2 months. Although the visits help alleviate the anxieties the adoptive child and parents are likely to feel, this process does not always permit true relationships to develop. A 16-year-old adoptive boy commented on his adoption at age 12: "I met them a few times and liked them, but we were all on our best behavior. I didn't really know them. I liked my foster family and knew them pretty well, so it was pretty scary to just leave and move in with my adoption parents, knowing that it was supposed to be forever, and I hardly knew them!"

Some placement agencies have espoused the view that children should leave their foster homes and "move on with their lives." A prevalent belief is that the fostering relationship must end in order for the adoptive relationship to start. For the reasons stated earlier, this belief seems misguided. It is difficult for children to leave a predictable, safe relationship with a foster family to enter the unknown world of an adoptive family. Instead, it can be much easier for children to make a transition from the foster family when they are moving toward another family with whom they have already forged some very positive bonds.

FT has been used successfully to help adoptive families establish meaningful relationships *during* the visitation process, thereby reducing transition anxieties. The adoptive child is moving from one healthy attachment relationship to another. This process provides adoptive families with specific activities to get their new relationships off on the right foot.

The FT transition model (VanFleet, 2005b) includes training both foster parents/kinship caregivers and preadoptive parents to hold filial play sessions with the children involved. The process weans children from the play sessions in the foster home to regular play sessions in the adoptive home. FT serves as a core intervention that follows the child through all transitions until the need for treatment has ended.

While the child is in foster or kinship placement, the therapist employs FT to stabilize the placement and to create healthy relationship patterns for the entire family. The children often use these play sessions to work on a variety of issues, including their trauma experiences, anxieties, past and current relationships, hopes for the future, and so on. The foster parents learn a set of skills they can use with other foster children in the future, although a filial therapist should monitor that use when it occurs. Overall, the placement can be stabilized and the child has an opportunity to work through a variety of issues with weekly filial play sessions. The foster parents are supported and supervised on a weekly or biweekly basis by the filial therapist. Other interventions, such as therapist-conducted play therapy, behavior management, or other family/parent consultations are added as needed.

Immediately after a match has been found for the adoptive family, the therapist meets with the preadoptive parents to provide them with (1) an overview of what to expect, good and bad, from the child's behavior, (2) education about trauma, its impact on emotions and behaviors, and the importance of healthy attachments, (3) tips on interacting with the child, including some basic positive parenting and behavior management skills, if needed, and (4) training in the filial play session skills. This takes approximately three or four sessions. During this training phase, the preadoptive parents observe a play session conducted by one of the foster parents or the therapist, with the child's advance knowledge and agreement.

Next, a series of day visits and overnight visits are accompanied by filial play sessions with the already-trained adoptive parents. Initially, these take place at the therapist's office, in coordination with the visits, and then shift to home play sessions when the adoptive family is ready. During this visitation period, the play sessions continue in the foster home as well.

After the child has moved permanently to the adoptive home, there are several visits with the foster parents, during which play sessions are held, terminating in a final visit, play session, and "farewell" activity. The filial play sessions continue in the adoptive home as long as they are needed, and parents hold play sessions with any siblings as well. The filial therapist monitors and supports these play sessions until a satisfactory adjustment and attachment have been made, helping the adoptive parents to generalize the use of the play session skills to daily life. The filial play sessions can be augmented with other family interventions, such as family storytelling for sharing histories and creating a new combined history, special family rituals including enjoyable times, the creation of a special scrapbook and/or photo album for the child and family, and the like.

The FT transition model has been used in transitions from foster care to adoption with more than 40 families to date, where appropriate funding could be secured. In all cases where the foster and adoptive parents and the child placement and adoption agencies cooperated fully with the therapy plan, successful, smooth adoptions took place. Although some of the adoptive children exhibited serious trauma and attachment problems while in care, their adjustment to adoption was facilitated by the use of FT. One adoptive father put it this way: "We knew we wanted to add this boy to our family, and we liked him. What we didn't expect was how traumatized he was. Filial therapy gave us the tools we needed to help him adjust to us and for us to understand what was going on for him. The foster mom helped him settle down to a point where he was ready for us, and then when we took over the play sessions, he just seemed to hit his stride and keep on going. It was great for us, and we still do the play sessions 2 years later!"

Although FT has a strong empirical history, this specific model of transitioning children from foster care to adoption using FT as a bridge has not yet been researched fully. Initial results from in-depth case studies and small pre- and postmeasurement evaluations are promising, leading to a major international research project that is now under way.

CASE ILLUSTRATION

Identifying information about the following case has been disguised in order to protect the privacy of the children and families. The case illustration reflects a composite of several families, but it accurately represents the course of treatment using FT.

Jake's History

Jake had a long history of physical abuse at the hands of his mother's boyfriends and neglect by his mother, resulting in his placement in foster care when he was 9 years old. His initial adjustment to foster care was satisfactory, but he had to be moved after 6 months when the foster mother's teenage daughter became pregnant and the mother no longer wished to be a foster mother. No one informed Jake of this move until the day it happened. He reacted badly to the abrupt change in his life, and his subsequent adjustment with the next foster family was poor. There were several more changes in his foster placement, all of them without warning. He was further abused by an older foster child in one of the homes, and again it was he who was moved. Two families expressed interest in adopting him, but when he was placed with them, they were ill prepared for his intense emotional outbursts and defiant behaviors. Both adoptions failed.

The Start of Play Therapy

Jake was in his seventh placement when he and his foster parents were referred for therapy. The foster parents were minimally cooperative with therapy, so the therapist began a course of child-centered play therapy with him and basic positive parenting and behavior management with the foster parents, with the hope of including FT in the near future. Jake, now 11, immediately began playing out themes relevant to his trauma history and the unpredictable nature of his life. His play was aggressive, and he always cast himself in powerful roles, effectively communicating and counteracting the vulnerability he felt in everyday life. He rarely broke the limits, however, and he clearly loved the play sessions. Although the foster parents immediately noticed some positive changes at home, they had quickly "burned out" with his poor behavior, and after just 10 sessions, they requested that he be moved from their home. The therapist continued to conduct child-centered play sessions with Jake while another home was sought, and she added trauma education, using bibliotherapy, some art and expressive work, and cognitive-behavioral play therapy methods designed to improve his emotional and behavioral regulation, his impulse control, and his social skills and interpersonal problem solving. The directive methods were held in a room separate from the nondirective playroom.

Filial Therapy with Jake's Foster Mother

At play session 15, Jake was living in yet another placement, this time with a single foster mother. She eagerly took part in therapy sessions. Because she needed immediate assistance with his behavioral challenges, the therapist spent time covering some basic child management approaches and then began preparing her for FT. The FT training was coupled with education about the impact of trauma. The foster mother, Carly, quickly learned the play session skills and was eager to begin play sessions. The therapist alternated her own individual play therapy sessions with Carly's initial filial play sessions with Jake. Carly quickly mastered the skills, and as she held her third play session with Jake, the therapist began phasing out her own sessions with him.

Jake responded quickly to the play sessions with Carly. Her acceptance of him seemed to relax him, and her firm limit-setting added a sense of security he had not felt before. His play involved themes of family relationships, authority figures, unexpected "tricks" played on people, and aggression. He often pretended he was a police officer chasing down drug lords or burglars or other "bad guys." In the course of his duties, he was sometimes shot down, and he fell to the floor in dramatic near-death scenes. Carly, in her assigned imaginary role as his wife, was expected to bandage his wounds, whereupon he always recovered from his injuries and then disposed of the bad guys. These scenes also involved times when the police officer came home to dinner with his wife, during which he fed and carried the baby dolls around the playroom, giving them nurturance and care until he was called back to his police work. At times, he asked Carly to play the burglars, and he pretended to apprehend her with aggressive play fighting, yet whenever he touched her, he did so very gently and took great care not to actually harm her. Both the therapist and Carly found his themes of vulnerability, power, resilience, and nurturance quite poignant.

Within just five play sessions, Jake was noticeably happier at home, and he and Carly developed a satisfactory relationship. He still had episodes of problematic impulsive behaviors and making emotionally hurtful remarks to Carly. Carly discussed these with the therapist, and she understood that they stemmed from his history. She continued steadfastly to manage his daily behaviors with the nurturance and consistent firmness that he needed. The filial play sessions were enjoyable for them both, and with the therapist's help, Carly quickly learned how to use the play session skills in day-to-day situations.

Progress continued steadily, but an adoptive family was not found for more than a year. Carly and Jake continued their weekly play sessions with the biweekly support of the therapist.

Filial Therapy during Jake's Preadoptive Transition

Eventually a couple was approved to adopt Jake. The therapist met with the couple, Charlie and Betti, prior to their meeting Jake. She provided a synopsis of his history and treatment, explained what they might expect from him during the transition phase, and recommended that they start trauma education and FT right away. They agreed.

Charlie and Betti first met Jake and Carly at a local restaurant for dinner. The meeting went well, after which Jake agreed to let them watch one of his filial play sessions with Carly. Two weeks later, the foster family and the preadoptive family met for dinner, then came together to the therapist's office for the play session. Charlie and Betti stayed afterward to discuss the play session with the therapist and to begin their training. After three training sessions with the therapist, they began holding play sessions with Jake; they came to the therapist's office, held a play session, and then had their visit. During this time, Jake continued play sessions with Carly as well.

Jake was soon playing out significant themes during his play sessions with Charlie and Betti. He played with Betti in ways similar to the way he played with Carly. With Charlie, he chose to play with cars and trucks, with dragons and dinosaurs. His play themes still reflected the vulnerability he felt, his need for control, and his desire for connection and a family. Two meetings at the therapist's office for Charlie, Betti, and Carly helped all involved to share their strategies for managing Jake's difficult behaviors, and Charlie and Betti understood the need to maintain a consistent approach, especially because it had worked so well for Carly and Jake.

After a number of successful overnight visits, the date for Jake to move in with Charlie and Betti was set. He moved 3 months after the match had been made. The therapist held a final session for Jake and Carly, during which they had a play session and created sandtrays representing what they had meant to each other and what they hoped for Jake's future. Arrangements were made for a short visit with Carly after Jake had moved. Jake was part of all of this planning.

Jake's move was without incident, and Charlie and Betti each held a play session with him during the first 4 days he was in their home. After 2 weeks, Jake had a brief visit and short play session with Carly. Carly continued to have contact with Jake for months afterward, mostly by phone. Charlie and Betti continued to have weekly play sessions with Jake, and he made a good adjustment. The therapist continued to monitor the play sessions and to assist with other parenting dilemmas that arose periodically.

The new adoptive family worked with the therapist for a total of 20 hourly sessions. Jake had made a smooth transition, and he attached well to Charlie and Betti, as they did with him. They all reported that things were continuing to go well for them during 1-month, 6-month, and 12-month follow-up phone calls by the therapist.

SUMMARY

Adoption poses many challenges for children and parents alike. The primary task is to provide healthy, strong relationships within the family that meet everyone's needs. This can be challenging, especially when the adopted children have histories of attachment disruption. FT is a relatively short-term evidence-based family play intervention that simultaneously allows children to work through salient psychosocial issues while establishing secure attachments with adoptive parents. It can be used as a prevention program to provide an avenue for secure attachment, or it can be used to intervene in significant problems of the child and family. Finally, it holds great promise as a mechanism through which the transition from foster care to adoption can be facilitated, allowing the child to have several experiences of genuine, healthy engagement along the way and culminating in strong, satisfying adoptive relationships for everyone involved.

REFERENCES

Ainsworth, M. D. S. (1982). Attachment: Retrospect and prospect. In C. M. Parkes & J. Stevenson-Hinde (Eds.), *The place of attachment in human behavior.* New York: Basic Books.

Becker, M. (2002). *The healing power of pets.* New York: Hyperion.

Belsky, J., & Nezworski, T. (Eds.). (1988). *Clinical implications of attachment.* Hillsdale, NJ: Erlbaum.

Benedict, H. E., & Mongoven, L. B. (2000). Thematic play therapy: An approach to treatment of attachment disorders in young children. In H. Kaduson, D. Cangelosi, & C. E. Schaefer (Eds.), *The playing cure* (pp. 277–315) Northvale, NJ: Aronson.

Bernstein, N. (2001). *The lost children of Wilder: The epic struggle to change foster care.* New York: Pantheon Books.

Bifulco, A., & Moran, P. (1998). *Wednesday's child.* London: Taylor & Francis.

Bifulco, A., Moran, P. M., Ball, C., & Lillie, A. (2002). Adult attachment style: Its relationship to psychosocial depressive-vulnerability. *Social Psychiatry and Psychiatric Epidemiology, 37,* 60–67.

Booth, P. B., & Lindaman, S. L. (2000). Theraplay for enhancing attachment in adopted children. In H. G. Kaduson & C. G. Schaefer (Eds.), *Short-term play therapy for children* (pp. 194–227). New York: Guilford Press.

Bowlby, J. (1982). *Attachment* (2nd ed.). New York: Basic Books

Brazelton, T. B., & Cramer, B. G. (1990). *The earliest relationship: Parents, infants, and the drama of early attachment.* Cambridge, MA: Perseus Books.

Brody, V. (1993). *The dialogue of touch: Developmental play therapy.* Treasure Island, FL: Developmental Play Training Associates.

Caplin, W., & Pernet, K. (2005). *A 12-session group model of filial therapy.* Boiling Springs, PA: Play Therapy Press.

Chandler, C. K. (2005). *Animal assisted therapy in counseling.* New York: Routledge.

Cheung, S., & Hong, G. K. (2005). Clinical application of attachment theory: Cultural implications. *Family Psychologist, 21*(2), 15–16.

Clark, K. E., & Ladd, G. W. (2000). Connectedness and autonomy support in parent–child relationships: Links to children's socioemotional orientation and peer relationships. *Developmental Psychology, 36*(4), 485–498.

Cohen, N. J., Muir, E., Lojkasek, M., Muir, R., Parker, C. J., Barwick, M., et al. (1999). Watch, Wait, and Wonder: Testing the effectiveness of a new approach to mother–infant psychotherapy. *Infant Mental Health Journal, 20*(4), 429–451.

Crawford, J. J., & Pomerinke, K. A. (2003). *Therapy pets.* Amherst, NY: Prometheus Books.

Davis, K. D. (1992). *Therapy dogs.* New York: Howell Book House.

Figley, C. R. (1989). *Helping traumatized families.* San Francisco, CA: Jossey-Bass.

Fine, A. (Ed.). (2000). *Animal-assisted therapy: Theoretical foundations and guidelines for practice.* San Diego, CA: Academic Press.

Gallo-Lopez, L., & Schaefer, C. E. (2005). *Play therapy with adolescents.* New York: Aronson.

Ginsberg, B. G. (1989). Training parents as therapeutic agents with foster/adoptive children using the filial approach. In C. E. Schaefer & J. M. Briesmeister (Eds.), *Handbook of parent training* (pp. 442–478). New York: Wiley.

Ginsberg, B. G. (2004). *Relationship Enhancement family therapy* (2nd ed.). Doylestown, PA: Relationship Enhancement Press.

Guerney, B. G. (1964). Filial therapy: Description and rationale. *Journal of Consulting Psychology, 28,* 303–310.

Guerney, L. F. (1983). Introduction to filial therapy: Training parents as therapists. In P. A. Keller & L. G. Ritt (Eds.), *Innovations in clinical practice: A source book* (Vol. 2, pp. 26–39). Sarasota, FL: Professional Resource Exchange.

Guerney, L. F. (1995). *Parenting: A skills training manual* (5th ed.). North Bethesda, MD: Institute for the Development of Emotional and Life Skills.

Guerney, L. (2003). The history, principles, and empirical basis of filial therapy. In R. VanFleet & L. Guerney (Eds.), *Casebook of Filial Therapy* (pp. 1–20). Boiling Springs, PA: Play Therapy Press.

Hart, J., Shaver, P. R., & Goldenberg, J. L. (2005). Attachment, self-esteem, worldviews, and terror management: Evidence for a tripartite security system. *Journal of Personality and Social Psychology, 88*(6), 999–1013.

Heegaard, M. (1991). *When something terrible happens.* Minneapolis, MN: Woodland Press.

Hughes, D. A. (1997). *Facilitating developmental attachment.* Northvale, NJ: Aronson.

Humber, N., & Moss, E. (2005). The relationship of preschool and early school age attachment to mother–child interaction. *American Journal of Orthopsychiatry, 75*(1), 128–141.

Jackins, H. (1994). *The human side of human beings: The theory of re-evaluation counseling* (3rd ed.). Seattle, WA: Rational Island.

James, B. (1994). *Handbook for treatment of attachment-trauma problems in children.* New York: Free Press.

Jernberg, A. M., & Booth, P. B. (1999). *Theraplay* (2nd ed.). San Francisco: Jossey-Bass.

Johnson, S. (2005). So now we know what love is—It's all about attachment. *Family Psychologist, 21*(2), 13–14.

Kaduson, H. G. (1994). Play therapy for children with attention-deficit hyperactivity disorder. In H. G. Kaduson, D. Cangelosi, & C. Schaefer (Eds.), *The playing cure* (pp. 197–227). New York: Rowan & Littlefield.

Knell, S. M. (1993*). Cognitive-behavioral play therapy.* Northvale, NJ: Aronson.

Ladd, G. W., & Ladd, B. K. (1998). Parenting behaviors and parent–child relationships: Correlates of peer victimization in kindergarten? *Developmental Psychology, 34*(6), 1450–1458.

La Greca, A. M., Silverman, W. K., Vernberg, E. M., & Roberts, M. C. (Eds.). (2002). *Helping children cope with disasters and terrorism.* Washington, DC: American Psychological Association.

Landreth, G. L. 2002. *Play therapy: The art of the relationship* (2nd ed.). Philadelphia: Brunner-Routledge.

Landreth, G. L., & Bratton, S. C. (2006). *Child parent relationship therapy: A 10-session filial therapy model.* New York: Taylor & Francis.

Levinson, B. M., & Mallon, G. P. (1997). *Pet-oriented child psychotherapy* (2nd ed.). Springfield, IL: Charles C. Thomas.

Malon, S. (2003). The efficacy of Filial Therapy with kinship care. In R. VanFleet & L. Guerney (Eds.), *Casebook of Filial Therapy* (pp. 209–234). Boiling Springs, PA: Play Therapy Press.

Marvel, F. A., Rodriguez, R. A., & Liddle, H. A. (2005). Attachment and family therapy: Theory informing practice. *Family Psychologist, 21*(2), 10–12.

Marvin, R., Cooper, G., Hoffman, K., & Powell, B. (2002). The Circle of Security project: Attachment-based intervention with caregiver–pre-school child dyads. *Attachment and Human Development, 4*(1), 107–124.

Muir, E., Lojkasek, M., & Cohen, N.J. (1999). *Watch, Wait, and Wonder.* Toronto: Hincks-Dellcrest Institute.

Munns, E. (Ed.). (2000). *Theraplay: Innovations in attachment-enhancing play therapy.* Northvale, NJ: Aronson.

Ryan, V., & Wilson, K. (1995). Non-directive play therapy as a means of recreating optimal infant socialization patterns. *Early Development and Parenting, 4*(1), 29–38.

Schaefer, C. E. (1994). Play therapy for psychic trauma in children. In K. J. O'Connor & C. E. Schaefer (Eds.), *Handbook of play therapy* (Vol. 2, pp. 297–318). New York: Wiley.

Sheppard, C. H. (1998). *Brave Bart: A story for traumatized and grieving children.* Grosse Pointe Woods, MI: Institute for Trauma and Loss in Children.

Sroufe, L. A. (1983). Infant–caregiver attachment and patterns of adaptation in the preschool: The roots of competence and maladaptation. In M. Perlmutter (Ed.), *Minnesota symposia in child psychology* (Vol. 16, pp. 41–83). Hillsdale, NJ: Erlbaum.

Sroufe, L. A. (1988). The role of infant–caregiver attachment in development. In J. Belsky & T. Nezworski (Eds.), *Clinical implications of attachment.* Hillsdale, NJ: Erlbaum.

Sroufe, L. A., & Rutter, M. (1984). The domain of developmental psychopathology. *Child Development, 55,* 17–29.

Sweeney, D. S. (2003). Filial Therapy in foster care. In R. VanFleet & L. Guerney (Eds.), *Casebook of Filial Therapy* (pp. 235–258). Boiling Springs, PA: Play Therapy Press.

Terr, L. (1990). *Too scared to cry: How trauma affects children . . . and ultimately us all.* New York: Basic Books.

VanFleet, R. (1994). Filial therapy for adoptive children and parents. In K. O'Connor

& C. Schaefer (Eds.), *Handbook of play therapy* (Vol. II, pp. 371–385). New York: Wiley.

VanFleet, R. (1998). A parent's guide to filial therapy. In L. VandeCreek, S. Knapp, & T. Jackson (Eds.), *Innovations in clinical practice: A source book* (Vol. 16, pp. 457–463). Sarasota, FL: Professional Resource Press.

VanFleet, R. (1999). *Introduction to filial play therapy: A video workshop.* Boiling Springs, PA: Play Therapy Press.

VanFleet, R. (2000). *A parent's handbook of filial play therapy.* Boiling Springs, PA: Play Therapy Press.

VanFleet, R. (2003). Filial Therapy with adoptive children and parents. In R. Van Fleet & L. Guerney (Eds.), *Casebook of Filial Therapy* (pp. 259–278). Boiling Springs, PA: Play Therapy Press. (Adapted and reprinted from VanFleet, 1994.)

VanFleet, R. (2005a). *Filial Therapy: Strengthening parent–child relationships through play* (2nd ed.). Sarasota, FL: Professional Resource Press.

VanFleet, R. (2005b). *Filial Therapy transition model for foster children.* (Working Paper and Report No. 05-7STC-R). Boiling Springs, PA: Author.

VanFleet, R., & Guerney, L. (Eds.). (2003). *Casebook of Filial Therapy.* Boiling Springs, PA: Play Therapy Press.

VanFleet, R., Ryan, S. D., & Smith, S. (2005). Filial Therapy: A critical review. In L. Reddy, T. Files-Hall, & C.E. Schaefer (Eds.), *Empirically based play interventions for children* (pp. 241–264). Washington, DC: American Psychological Association.

VanFleet, R., & Sniscak, C. C. (2003a). Filial Therapy for attachment-disrupted and disordered children. In R. Van Fleet & L. Guerney (Eds.), *Casebook of Filial Therapy* (pp. 279–308). Boiling Springs, PA: Play Therapy Press.

VanFleet, R., & Sniscak, C. C. (2003b). Filial Therapy for children exposed to traumatic events. In R. VanFleet & L. Guerney (Eds.), *Casebook of Filial Therapy* (pp. 113–138). Boiling Springs, PA: Play Therapy Press.

Wright, C., & Walker, J. (2003). Using Filial Therapy with Head Start families. In R. VanFleet & L. Guerney (Eds.), *Casebook of Filial Therapy* (pp. 309–325). Boiling Springs, PA: Play Therapy Press.

Youngblade, L. M., & Belsky, J. (1992). Parent–child antecedents of 5-year-olds' close friendships: A longitudinal analysis. *Developmental Psychology, 28*(4), 700–713.

Ziegler, D. (2000). *Raising children who refuse to be raised: Parenting skills and therapy interventions for the most difficult children.* Phoenix, AZ: Acacia Press.

CHAPTER 7

Involving and Empowering Parents in Short-Term Play Therapy for Disruptive Children

CHERYL B. McNEIL
ALISA B. BAHL
AMY D. HERSCHELL

In this chapter, we discuss a 12-session model for conducting play therapy with disruptive children (McNeil, Hembree-Kigin, & Eyberg, 1996, 1998). Sessions 1 through 7 focus on individual therapy with the child, and sessions 8 through 12 focus on teaching play therapy to parents. We believe that parents are the key to accomplishing goals in a short time because they can support our efforts outside the therapy hour. Parents are incorporated into this model in three ways: (1) by structuring time so that we check in and check out with them in each session, (2) by giving them weekly homework assignments to support the therapy goals, and (3) by coaching them to use play therapy skills at home to accomplish such goals as enhancing the parent–child relationship and improving child self-esteem (McNeil et al., 1996). In addition to featuring parental involvement, this 12-session model is unique in that it focuses on productivity. Treatment goals are carefully articulated, and weekly objectives are established prior to the sessions so that they build on each other. These session objectives are met by structuring each session so that there is a therapist-directed, task-oriented portion that precedes the child-directed play. In addition, behavior management strategies are used to help prevent disruptive behavior from interfering with session objectives (McNeil et al., 1996).

PARENT–CHILD INTERACTION THERAPY: THE EMPIRICAL
AND THEORETICAL FOUNDATION FOR THIS APPROACH

The approach described in this chapter is based, in part, on parent–child interaction therapy (PCIT), which is an evidence-based, parent training program (Eyberg & Calzada, 1998; Hembree-Kigin & McNeil, 1995). PCIT, developed in the 1970s by Sheila Eyberg, PhD, is designed for children ages 2–7 years who are exhibiting disruptive behavior and early-onset conduct problems. The focus of the approach is on teaching parents to work more effectively with their behaviorally challenged children. PCIT is based on the two-stage Hanf (1969) model of parent training.

The two stages of PCIT are (1) child-directed interaction, and (2) parent-directed interaction. During child-directed interaction, parents are taught to follow their child's lead by using behavioral play therapy skills (Capage, Foote, McNeil, & Eyberg, 1998; Herschell, Calzada, Eyberg, & McNeil, 2002a). These skills, sometimes referred to as the "PRIDE" skills, are designed to strengthen the parent–child relationship by increasing parents' use of (1) Praise, (2) Reflection, (3) Imitation, (4) Description, and (5) Enthusiasm. Parents are taught to praise positive behavior and attributes in a very specific way, called "labeled praise." They also learn to listen actively to their children using reflection, a verbal statement that repeats back or paraphrases what the child says. The essence of play therapy involves following the child's lead; therefore, parents are taught how to imitate the child's play. They also learn to describe the child's activities. These descriptions become like a running commentary of behavior. By being enthusiastic in the use of these skills, parents increase the likelihood that the child will remain interested and behave appropriately during play. In addition to the PRIDE skills, parents are taught to use selective attention and ignoring to manage minor disruptive behaviors. For example, if a child is playing roughly with toys, the father is instructed to turn his back to the child and play enthusiastically by himself. When the child begins behaving again in an appropriate manner, the father returns his attention to the child and praises prosocial behaviors.

During the parent-directed interaction stage of PCIT, sometimes referred to as the discipline stage, parents are taught to be consistent in dealing with noncompliant and aggressive behaviors. Parents learn to give effective instructions to their child, to praise compliance, and to provide choices when the child does not comply. For example, a parent may provide a two-choice warning for noncompliance such as, "You have two choices: you can either pick up the toy or you can go to time-out." Parents are taught step-by-step how to implement an effective time-out as a consequence for noncompliance.

Instead of relying only on didactic training, PCIT employs a coaching model of teaching. That is, the therapist actively directs the parent's interactions with the child. (In two-parent families, each parent is coached separately while interacting with the child). Many clinics that use PCIT are equipped with a one-way mirror and a bug-in-ear microphone system. This allows the therapist to unobtrusively observe the parent–child interaction and communicate directly with the parent during this interaction. In this way, parents can benefit from frequent, immediate, and specific feedback, and children learn to respond to their parents rather than to the therapist. When the one-way mirror and bug-in-ear system are unavailable, the therapist can coach the parent discretely within the room.

Empirical Support for PCIT

Through numerous empirical investigations, PCIT has been demonstrated to decrease child behavior problems, increase parent skill, and decrease parent stress. Parents also report improvements on measures of parent and child psychopathology, as well as high satisfaction with the treatment's content and process (see Gallagher, 2003; Herschell, Calzada, Eyberg, & McNeil, 2002b, for reviews). Follow-up studies have reported treatment gains maintained up to 6 years after completion of treatment (Eyberg et al., 2001; Hood & Eyberg, 2003; Schumann, Foote, Eyberg, Boggs, & Algina, 1998).

Though originally developed and most often used to treat disruptive behavior problems, PCIT also has been used to treat separation anxiety disorder (Choate, Pincus, Eyberg, & Barlow, 2005; Pincus, Eyberg, & Choate, 2005), disruptive behaviors comorbid with bladder cancer (Bagner, Fernandez, & Eyberg, 2004), developmental disorders (Eyberg & Matarazzo, 1980), and in cases of general child maltreatment (Fricker-Elhai, Ruggiero, & Smith, 2005), child physical abuse (Chaffin et al., 2004; Timmer, Urquiza, Zebell, & McGrath, 2005), and foster parents caring for disruptive children (McNeil, Herschell, Gurwitch, & Clemens-Mowrer, 2005). Recently, adaptations have been made to conduct PCIT in a group format (Niec, Hemme, Yopp, & Brestan, 2005) and with toddlers (ages 12–30 months; Dombrowski, Timmer, Blacker, & Urquiza, 2005).

PCIT Applied to Child Physical Abuse

An alarming number of children are the victims of maltreatment. The most recent statistics indicate that in 2001, 903,000 children in the United States were victims of abuse or neglect (U.S. Department of Health and Human Services, 2003). Younger children (birth through age 7 years) have the highest victimization rates, suffer the most severe injuries, and are the most likely to experience a recurrence of maltreatment (U.S. Department of Health and Human Services, 2003). Further compounding this problem is that, for specific types of abuse (e.g., physical abuse), biological mothers are the most likely to be the perpetrators.

Children who have been abused suffer many short- and long-term difficulties. In comparison to nonabused peers, children with histories of physical abuse demonstrate poor school performance, difficulty in achieving secure attachments (Crittenden & Ainsworth, 1989), problems with peer relationships (Hoffman-Plotkin & Twentyman, 1984), social withdrawal (Azar & Wolfe, 1989), and an increased number of suicide attempts and self-mutilations (Green, 1978). These negative outcomes continue across the lifespan. Child physical abuse is strongly correlated with committing juvenile and adult crime (Luntz & Widom, 1994; McCord, 1983; Widom, 1989). In light of these concerns, several expert groups have highlighted the importance of developing better treatments for children who have been abused (Kauffman Foundation, 2004; Satcher, 2000). PCIT has been recommended as a "best practice" approach for treatment of child physical abuse, which is related to the empirical support of its effectiveness with that population.

In addition to theoretical justifications (Herschell & McNeil, 2005; Urquiza & McNeil, 1996), case examples (e.g., Filcheck, McNeil, & Herschell, 2005; Herschell et al., 2002a), and single-subject design studies (e.g., Fricker-Elhai et al., 2005), two treatment outcome studies have been completed (Chaffin et al., 2004; Timmer et al., 2005) that support the use of PCIT with physically abusive parents and their abused children. Chaffin and colleagues (2004) completed a treatment outcome study that included 110 physically abusive parent–child dyads. To test the impact of PCIT in preventing re-reports of physical abuse, parent–child dyads referred by child welfare were randomized to one of three treatment groups: (1) PCIT, (2) PCIT with individualized, enhanced services, and (3) treatment as usual via standard community-based parenting groups. Findings supported the efficacy of PCIT for reducing rates of re-abuse. At a median follow-up time of 850 days, 19% of participants in the PCIT condition had a re-abuse report, whereas 36% of participants in the PCIT with individualized, enhanced services condition had a re-abuse report and 49% of participants in the community group had a re-abuse report. All conditions were helpful in increasing positive parent behaviors; however, only the groups that included PCIT were associated with reductions in negative parent behaviors. Surprisingly, additional services did not improve the efficacy of PCIT. Instead, adding in-home and individualized treatment services for other parental mental health needs tended to attenuate treatment outcome.

Timmer and colleagues (2005) completed a quasi-experimental study of 126 biological parents and their children who completed PCIT. The effectiveness of PCIT was evaluated for parent–child dyads with high versus low risks of abuse on measures of child behavior, parent functioning (e.g., stress, psychopathology, abuse potential), and parent satisfaction before and after treatment. Results indicated decreases in child and parent problems (e.g., behavior problems, child psychopathology, parent stress) from pre- to posttreatment.

However, participants with histories of physical abuse showed smaller reductions in problems than those with no history of physical abuse (e.g., child behavior problems, parent psychopathology).

PCIT and Cultural Diversity

Most psychosocial treatments for children have been developed on the basis of Western theories, studied with predominantly Caucasian samples, and have largely underappreciated the influence of cultural issues. However, there are data that indicate that PCIT is effective with diverse groups, including African American and Hispanic families. When the effects of socioeconomic status are controlled for, PCIT has been found to be equally effective with African American and Caucasian families (Capage, Bennett, & McNeil, 2001). Similarly, Boggs et al. (2004) found that ethnicity did not predict treatment response or attrition in PCIT. Calzada and Eyberg (2002) examined specific parenting practices among Dominican and Puerto Rican mothers living in the United States. Their results indicated that the parenting values of these Hispanic groups are similar to those of U.S. Caucasian mothers, which may mean that PCIT can be applied effectively with such families. Additional research is under way to understand how culture affects treatment with Mexican American parent–child dyads (e.g., McCabe, Yeh, Garland, Lau, & Chavez, 2005; McCabe, Yeh, Lau, Garland, & Hough, 2003).

RELATIONSHIP BETWEEN PCIT AND THIS SHORT-TERM PLAY THERAPY MODEL

The 12-session model described in this chapter is based in part on PCIT. For example, a portion of the first seven sessions is devoted to the therapist using the child-directed interaction (or PRIDE) skills from PCIT. Among other benefits, these skills are helpful in establishing rapport, making the session fun for the child, and improving child self-esteem. In sessions 8 through 12, parents are taught these nondirective play skills through the use of the coaching model derived from PCIT. Again, this model assumes that parents are the key to success in short-term treatment. Thus, parents are taught child-directed play skills, which they use to (1) enhance their relationship with their child, (2) help their child deal with anger and frustration, (3) manage disruptive behaviors, and (4) improve child self-esteem. The principal difference between this 12-session model and PCIT is that this is primarily a play therapy model, whereas PCIT is a parent training model. In PCIT the therapist does not typically work individually with the child.

SHORT-TERM PLAY THERAPY APPROACH

Structure of the Play Therapy Session

In order to use time efficiently and minimize disruptive behavior, a great deal of structure (e.g., predictable routines, clear limits, and transition rituals) is incorporated into the short-term play therapy approach. In fact, each of the sessions has a predictable four-part structure: (1) check-in with the caregiver—approximately 10 minutes, (2) child's work (therapist-directed activities)—approximately 20 minutes, (3) child's play (child-directed activities)—approximately 20 minutes, and (4) check-out with the caregiver—approximately 10 minutes. In contrast to the typical stimulating play therapy rooms that have many toys in the open (e.g., sandtrays, pretend kitchens, dollhouses), the playroom used in this type of therapy contains only those toys and materials that the therapist brings in for a particular part of the session. The purpose of structuring the room is to prevent children with disruptive behavior from becoming overactive and overstimulated. With only 12 sessions to achieve treatment goals, every attempt is made to minimize disruptive behavior and keep the child on task.

Check-In

Each session begins with a 10-minute check-in period with the child's caregivers. In most cases, the child is present during this time so that he or she (1) does not become concerned that the therapist is revealing confidential information, (2) can participate, and (3) can be adequately supervised. The purpose of check-in is to provide parents and children with an opportunity to share information that may contribute to the therapeutic process. They are asked about progress on weekly homework assignments and problems that have occurred during the week, as well as family stressors and significant events. This check-in time is also a valuable opportunity for the therapist to build rapport with parents and help them feel like powerful contributors to their child's progress in treatment.

Child's Work

Child's work is the therapist-directed portion of each session, which incorporates planned activities to address preestablished therapeutic goals. Examples of activities conducted during child's work include therapeutic games, role plays, presentation of educational materials, and thematic drawings. Child's work always precedes child's play, for several practical and therapeutic reasons. The first is that disruptive children are typically more cooperative with planned activities if they know a "free play" will follow. In contrast, such children are likely to be less cooperative if they are required to transition from a free play activity to a structured activity chosen by the therapist. In terms of therapeutic benefits, beginning with thematic activities allows conflictual issues and emotional responses to be triggered early in the session. The child is then likely to carry these issues and responses into the child's play portion of the session, providing rich therapeutic material for nondirective play therapy. Placing child's work before child's play also allows ample time for the child to work through strong reactions before leaving the session.

Child's Play

In child's play, the therapist follows the child's lead and provides a supportive atmosphere in which the child can work through difficult issues. A primary goal of this portion of play therapy is to build a strong relationship between the therapist and the child. Other goals, such as building self-esteem, improving communication skills, and improving social skills, are also part of child's play. Through careful use of some very specific skills, the therapist works toward these goals.

These specific skills are used throughout the hour session, but are more concentrated during child's play. In addition to the PRIDE skills discussed earlier (i.e., *P*raise, *R*eflection, *I*mitation, *D*escription, and *E*nthusiasm), the therapist uses questions and interpretations to make child's play a richly, therapeutic time. Questions make an explicit demand on the child to provide specific information and are therefore used in moderation. Examples of such questions include "When does your daddy come to visit you?" and "How do you feel about visiting your dad?" In the beginning sessions of therapy, questions are often arouse anxiety in a child and yield little information; however, questions tend to become more productive with time. Questions are also more productive when they are open-ended, used sparingly, and interspersed with pauses long enough to let the child respond.

Interpretations are therapist statements that make a link between the child's behavior and his or her motivations or feelings. Interpretations are used to make the child more aware of this link. Because interpretations are "educated guesses" or hypotheses, they should be stated hesitantly so that the child may agree or disagree. Interpretations are often stated with tentative beginnings such as "I wonder," "Perhaps," "Maybe," or "Sometimes." An example of an interpretation in response to a child's statement, "I hate my dad's girlfriend because she's always talking to him," is "Maybe you're feeling angry at her because she gets so much of your dad's attention."

Check-Out

Similar to check-in, check-out is a time when the therapist meets with the child and his or her parents. During these 10 minutes, the therapist informs the

parents of the therapeutic nature of the play therapy work. This helps to facilitate communication between the parents and the therapist and to keep the parents invested in their child's therapy. An important consideration is the child's
right to confidentiality. This right must always be balanced with the parents' need
to know about the content of therapy. Thus, at the end of child's play, the therapist and child should have a discussion about what material should be shared
with the parents. Typically, sensitive material regarding the child's feelings and
thoughts is not shared with the parents. Another important goal of check-out is
to promote generalization of treatment gains. Through homework assignments,
parents can prompt and reinforce skills acquired during child's work. Homework assignments are given each week and are specific to the session's content. If child's work involved helping the child express anger though acceptable channels, the homework assignment might be for the parent to prompt
and reinforce appropriate ways of expressing anger, such as scribbling on a piece
of paper really hard or writing an angry letter and tearing it up. Similarly, if
child's work involved prompting the child to recognize accomplishments, the
homework assignment might include having the child keep a chart of things
he or she did well each day.

Managing Disruptive Behavior during Sessions

Although some play therapies view disruptive behavior as rich therapeutic
material from which valuable information can be gleaned and interpreted, the
sort-term play therapy approach views disruptive behavior as an impediment
to treatment progress. Little energy can be focused on therapeutic goals when
a child is engaged in off-task and oppositional behaviors. Therefore, throughout all four portions of the session, managing disruptive behavior is a priority.
This management is accomplished though proactive structuring that inhibits
disruptive behavior, as well as controlled responses to disruptive behavior when
it occurs. Proactive structuring of each session includes established rules, consistent routines for transitions, careful attention to precedents, choosing appealing child's work activities, and requiring work before play. Even with these
preventive features in place, strategies such as the use of praise, tangible reinforcers, rules for being a good listener, contingent attention, effective directions, the "when–then" strategy, special game rules, and the "turtle technique"
are used for managing disruptive behavior during play therapy. A summary of
these procedures is provided in Table 7.1.

A 12-Session Model for Short-Term Play Therapy

This play therapy approach follows a 12-session model in which the first 7 sessions are mainly conducted with the therapist working individually with the
child. The remaining 5 sessions emphasize joint therapy with the child and

TABLE 7.1. Skills for Managing Disruptive Behaviors

Management skill	Explanation and example
Establish rules	Establishing rules clearly indicates to the child what is acceptable versus unacceptable behavior. Before the child's work portion of a session begins, the child is told that he or she must stay in the playroom, play gently with the toys and materials, and not do anything that would endanger him- or herself or the therapist. Rules are typically reviewed at the beginning of each session as a reminder to the child.
Develop transition routines	Transitions are often times when a disruptive child becomes overactive and distracted. One way to minimize misbehavior is to provide the child with a warning that the transition is about to occur. Approximately 5 minutes before the end of child's play, the child should be given a transitional statement such as "In just a few minutes, it will be time to stop playing and clean up. Singing special songs can also make transitions easier.
Pay careful attention to precedents	If the child is allowed to engage in any minor problematic behaviors during the first sessions (e.g., running from the waiting room to the playroom, demanding choice of toys, running out of the session to visit parents), these behaviors will continue throughout the sessions and become larger issues. It is best to establish clear, strict boundaries early on.
Use unlabeled and labeled praise	Unlabeled praise is a general comment indicating approval (e.g., "Good job"), whereas labeled praise is a specific statement that tells the child exactly what he or she did that the therapist liked (e.g., "Good job using your words to tell me how you feel.") To manage disruptive behavior using praise, the therapist should identify a problem behavior, identify behaviors that are incompatible with the problem behavior, and then praise the incompatible behavior. For example, the problem behavior may be screaming. A behavior incompatible with screaming is talking in an indoor voice. So the therapist would give a labeled praise for talking in an indoor voice.
Incorporate tangible reinforcers	The best systems for tangible reinforcers involve immediate rewards for specific behaviors. For example, a hand stamp can be used for good listening. Also, a star chart can be used so that the child earns a reward once a certain number of stars has been acquired.

continued

TABLE 7.1. *continued*

Develop rules for being a good listener	Because one of the greatest challenges in doing play therapy with disruptive children is maintaining their attention, children are taught three "good listening rules" early in treatment: (1) Look in my eyes when you talk, (2) Hold your body very, very still, and (3) Think hard about what I am saying (McGinnis & Goldstein, 2003).
Use strategic ignoring and contingent attention	Many disruptive behaviors are a child's attempt to gain attention, and therefore can be managed by ignoring. The therapist explains and models in advance that he or she will turn and ignore disruptive behavior (e.g., aggressive play, hiding from the therapist). For example, if the child is playing roughly with toy farm animals, the therapist can ignore the rough play, model appropriate play, and then praise the child for playing gently.
Give good directions	Directions are defined as specific instructions the child is told (rather than asked) to follow. When it is important for the child to comply, the direction should be positively stated, polite, and specific. For example if a child begins to run ahead during a transition time, the therapist can say, "Please come back and walk with me."
Use the "When–then" strategy	Children are told that a pleasant, rewarding activity will be provided once they engage in specified behaviors. For example, "When you practice your breathing one more time, then we can use our colored markers."
Create special game rules	The therapist assigns special rules to nonthreatening, typical board games (e.g., checkers). Most often, the special rule is that the child must produce a small amount of work in exchange for a turn at the game. The therapist may introduce this as follows: "Today we get to play checkers, but this is a special kind of checkers. The rule is that before we can take a turn, we each have to tell about a time when we felt mad."
Use the turtle technique	Developed by Robin (1976), this technique helps disruptive children to regain self-control by teaching them to react to aggressive impulses by imagining that they are turtles (e.g., pulling their heads into their shells).

parents. Throughout the course of therapy, increasing parental involvement is encouraged. During joint therapy, this idea is extended as parents are taught to be "cotherapists." Teaching parents valuable "therapist" skills helps to improve their relationship with their child, empowers them to become more independent of the therapist, and enhances generalization of treatment gains. Essentially, there is a transfer of dependence and responsibility from the therapist–child relationship to the longer-term and more primary parent–child relationship.

The first two sessions of this play model establish precedents and routines for all sessions to follow. During these sessions, procedures are explained to the parents as well as to the child. The structure of the sessions follows the general four-part outline. During check-in, consent and confidentiality are reviewed, parents are educated regarding play therapy, the treatment plan and goals are discussed, and a therapy contract is devised. Child's work involves explaining and modeling the play therapy structure for the child. Child's play is spent in child-directed activities, and check-out includes a review of the session's content and assignment of homework.

The content for sessions 3 through 7 is more flexible, considering that children are referred for short-term play therapy for a variety of reasons. However, these middle sessions should adhere to the same established structure (i.e., check-in, child's work, child's play, and check-out) and incorporate the same behavior management (e.g., establishing rules, giving good directions) and process skills (e.g., praise, reflection). In terms of content, the therapist should develop a flexible but detailed treatment plan prior to the beginning of session 3 and progress toward identified goals. The contents of the sessions should be well planned and build on one another so that skills learned in earlier sessions form a foundation for more advanced skills to be acquired in later sessions. An additional consideration is that the treatment plan should incorporate homework. Assigning meaningful weekly homework enhances progress and facilitates parental involvement. Termination themes are introduced at the end of session 7, because this session immediately precedes a major shift in treatment. Sessions 1 through 7 are mainly conducted by the therapist working individually with the child and involving the parents in the beginning and end of each session. However, beginning with session 8, the focus of the therapist is on working with the parents and child together.

Essentially, session 8 begins the transfer of the child's dependence on the therapist to the parents. Decreasing amounts of time are spent individually with the child, as the parents are coached in play therapy skills. Parents are asked to attend session 8 without their child and are taught play therapy skills. In sessions 9 thorough 11 parents are directly coached in the use of these play therapy skills. Their skills are monitored each week by the therapist's observing the parent–child interaction for 5 minutes and coding specific behaviors using the Dyadic Parent–Child Interaction Coding System (Eyberg & Robinson, 1983).

This careful monitoring provides the therapist with a more objective measure of the parents' skill acquisition and therefore provides the therapist with a valuable piece of information to aid in treatment decisions. After sessions 9 through 11, homework is assigned that requires parents to provide daily play therapy sessions at home.

Session 12 includes conducting termination rituals with the parents, such as reviewing the treatment plan, examining pre- to posttreatment changes with assessment measures, and praising the parents' accomplishments. Termination rituals with the child include a review of the course of treatment and a posttreatment party. Typically, one or two "booster sessions" are scheduled to address a few unresolved issues and gradually reduce dependence on the therapist. Parents are also invited to call if they feel it is necessary and are given appropriate resources and referrals.

Teaching Play Therapy Skills to Parents

Parents attend session 8 without their child and are taught play therapy skills. (For a detailed description of teaching play therapy to parents, see Hembree-Kigin & McNeil, 1995). This session is structured so that 10 minutes are devoted to check-in, 40 minutes are allotted to instruction, and 10 minutes are spent on check-out. During check-in, the previous week's homework and life events are reviewed. The 40 minutes of instruction time are very active for the parents, as well as the therapist. Because most people learn best by being involved in the material and by repetition, the therapist strives to incorporate examples relevant to the family—role playing, humor, opportunities for parents to ask questions, and frequent summaries of information during the instruction period. Check-out consists of a brief review and homework assignment. The assignment given is for parents to spend 5–10 minutes of special playtime with their child each day.

Parents are told that they will be taught a set of play therapy skills to use with their child in the daily 5- to 10-minute play sessions. To help them understand the purpose of this "special playtime," they are told that they can assist treatment progress by serving as "cotherapists." The emphasis is on how the parents can help their child accomplish more in a shorter amount of time by actively participating in their child's treatment. Special playtime goals are established and individualized for the family. These goals may include increasing the child's self-esteem, decreasing anger, improving social skills, developing constructive play skills, strengthening family relationships, and using words to communicate feelings.

In conducting special playtime, parents are asked to avoid using commands, criticisms, and questions. Instead, they are encouraged to use skills such as praise, reflection, imitation, description, and enthusiasm (i.e., PRIDE skills).

Parents are taught that a key component for managing behavior and making special playtime a high-quality, positive time is the use of attention. Parents are instructed to provide a lot of positive attention (e.g., labeled praise, descriptions, and enthusiasm) to the child when he or she is engaging in appropriate behaviors and to ignore the child when he or she is engaging in inappropriate behaviors during play therapy. This skill is commonly referred to as selective attention/strategic ignoring, or contingent attention.

Parents are also instructed on how to handle misbehavior during play therapy. The therapist explains that misbehavior can fall into one of two categories: (1) dangerous/destructive, or (2) annoying/obnoxious. Dangerous/destructive behaviors can cause physical harm to people or property. Examples include hitting, biting, scratching, throwing toys, and writing on walls. Annoying/obnoxious behaviors are inappropriate, but do not result in harm. Examples of these behaviors are bossiness, whining, spitting, teasing, and using foul language. Parents are taught different strategies for handling the two types of misbehavior. They are encouraged to stop special playtime if the child engages in any dangerous/destructive behaviors and provide an additional consequence if they feel it is appropriate. In contrast, parents are instructed to use strategic ignoring if the child engages in any annoying/obnoxious behaviors during special playtime.

Just as structure is important in the clinical setting, it is recommended that parents add structure to the special playtime by establishing a routine. Parents are instructed to try to hold play therapy at the same time every day so that it is predictable. This makes the child less likely to beg or nag for special playtime and makes the parent more likely to remember it. Parents are also instructed that the best materials for special playtime are construction-oriented toys that encourage creativity and imagination, such as blocks, garage and car sets, tea sets, toy farms, dollhouses, and crayons and paper. Toys to avoid include those that have set rules (e.g., board games), encourage aggressive play (e.g., superhero figures, punching bags), require limit setting (e.g., scissors) or discourage real conversations (e.g., audiotapes, books, puppets). To start special playtime, parents select three or four acceptable toys or activities and place them in a space free of distractions. The ideal setting is a quiet area where the parent and child will not be interrupted (e.g., the parents' bedroom, a dining room). After the toys have been selected, the parent tells the child that it is time for special playtime and explains the rules as follows:

> It is time for our special playtime. You can play with any of the toys in front of us and I'll play along with you, but there are two rules you must follow. First, you have to stay right here with me. And second, you have to play gently with the toys. If you wander around the room or play roughly with

the toys, I will turn around like this and play by myself. Then, when you come back or play nicely again, I'll turn back around like this and play with you again. Thanks for listening to the rules. We can play with anything you want to play with now. (McNeil et al., 1996, p. 68)

The skills taught to parents are very similar to those used by the therapist; however, there are some important differences. Because parents do not have extensive training or objectivity, they are not instructed or encouraged to use interpretations. They are also not prepared to formulate treatment plans or utilize specialized therapeutic techniques, like those used in the child's work part of a session.

Coaching Play Therapy Skills

The direct coaching component of this approach helps to increase time-effectiveness. In more traditional, didactic approaches parents would be taught a skill and sent home to practice it with their child throughout the week. The parents would return the following week and report failed attempts to implement the skill. The therapist would then help the parents make modifications and send the parents home again to practice. In contrast, a direct coaching approach involves teaching parents skills in session and asking them to practice the skills with their child in session. The therapist observes this interaction and provides immediate, specific feedback to the parents regarding their use of the skills. This feedback or coaching can occur with the therapist outside the room (which requires the use of a one-way mirror, intercom speaker system, and a bug-in-the-ear auditory transmission system) or inside the room. When the therapist is coaching in the room, children are told to pretend that the therapist is not there. It also is explained to a child that the therapist will not talk or play with the child until the coaching is over. Direct coaching is one of the most expedient ways of acquiring new skills because it involves the use of two powerful learning strategies: rehearsal and immediate feedback.

Coaching is most effective when feedback is provided consistently after each parent verbalization. Essentially, the parent makes a comment, the therapist responds, the parent makes another comment, the therapist responds, and so on. This rhythm helps the parent to learn to pause and listen after each comment so that the therapist and parent avoid talking over one another and instead communicate effectively. Coaching at each parent verbalization also allows skills to be shaped in a time-efficient manner. The parent receives a large amount of specific, immediate feedback. It is this continuous and active coaching that leads to quick and meaningful improvements in play therapy skills.

Coaches should also emphasize the positives (Harwood & Eyberg, 2004). Parents are very sensitive about their parenting skills, and little is learned from criticism. Rather than telling parents what they are doing wrong, the therapist should instruct parents as to what to do instead. Another way to emphasize the positives is to frequently provide labeled praise to parents when they are using skills correctly or are engaging in other therapeutic behaviors such as being warm, genuine, or playful. Similarly, coaches should be selective when correcting mistakes. Providing frequent, corrective suggestions may make the session tense, the parent feel unduly criticized, and ultimately hurt rapport. Instead, it is better to ignore some minor mistakes even though it may break the coaching rhythm.

Feedback should be brief and specific. Although an occasional lengthy observation may be provided to parents, most of the coaching should consist of brief, specific phrases. Examples might include "Good description," "Great labeled praise," "I like the way you ignored that inappropriate behavior," and "Go ahead and describe that." It is also helpful to coach qualitative aspects of the parent–child interaction such as eye contact, physical closeness, expression of feelings, patience, playfulness, and creativity. Finally, it is important to be decisive and quick when coaching, particularly in coaching ignoring. When a child engages in a negative attention-seeking behavior, the therapist has only seconds to coach the parent through the situation.

CASE ILLUSTRATION

This case example illustrates the use of the short-term model for behavioral play therapy with Luis Palomo (a pseudonym). A 13-session treatment is presented, briefly discussing the session objectives, the use of child's work, the use of child's play, and the use of homework activities to further address the goals of treatment. Issues related to Luis's mother's harboring of resentment toward the child are addressed as treatment progresses.

Background Information

Luis was a 5½-year-old mixed-race boy whose parents recently ended a bitter divorce in which there were allegations of abuse against each parent. Luis's mother, Ms. Palomo, was Mexican American and his father was African American. Luis's parents were granted joint custody, in which Luis would live with his mother, Ms. Palomo, during the school year and with his father during the summer. In addition to the custody ruling, the court ordered both of Luis's parents to attend parent training. The court also recommended that Luis attend therapy, to address issues surrounding the divorce and his new living arrangements. Attempts were made to involve Luis's father in parent training with the therapists (on a different day than when Ms. Palomo attended) to promote consistency in parenting approaches; however, he chose to seek his own therapist.

Session 1

Session Objectives

1. Obtain parental consent and child assent for treatment.
2. Agree on attendance contract.
3. Introduce the parent and child to basic concepts of play therapy.
4. Establish playroom rules and behavioral expectations.
5. Build rapport.

Check-In

During the check-in, the structure of the play therapy sessions was explained to Luis and his mother. Both agreed to the format of therapy and to attending for at least 12 sessions.

In the first session, Ms. Palomo stated that she had been raised in a strict Hispanic home in which children were taught to respect their elders. She said that she was concerned that she would not be allowed to punish Luis and that his disrespect for adults would worsen. In addition, Ms. Palomo confessed that she was very angry with Luis. She said that Luis's "awful" behavior was the reason that his father ran out on them. She said that she loved Luis, but she did not like his personality. Moreover, she stated that she harbored resentment toward Luis because he looked like his father, with dark skin and similar hair, and because he acted like his father, with a "short temper" and "bossy personality." Although she stated that she would like to enjoy Luis again and get him to be "sweet like he used to be," she said that she did not have fun being around him any more. Furthermore, she was skeptical about parent training being helpful for improving Luis's disrespectful and bossy personality.

Before beginning the child's work portion of the session with Luis, the therapist asked Ms. Palomo if she would complete the Eyberg Child Behavior Inventory (ECBI; Eyberg & Pincus, 1999), a parent-completed behavior rating form.

Child's Work

The therapist walked to the playroom with Luis and explained the rules of that room. The therapist then told Luis that they would read a book together that would explain a little more about what he and the therapist might do together during the next couple of months. When reading *A Child's First Book about Play Therapy* (Nemiroff & Annunziata, 1990), the therapist asked Luis what problems he had that could be worked on in play therapy. Interestingly, Luis identified with one of the characters in the book and stated that he sometimes got into fights too, but it was the other person's fault. The therapist said that fighting might be one thing they would talk about in play therapy, but that they would also talk about other things, such as his feelings about his parents' divorce and what it would be like to have two homes.

Child's Play

During the child's play part of the session, Luis played with the construction straws. The therapist, to gain rapport, played alongside Luis and described what he was constructing. When Luis looked at what the therapist was constructing, he said that the therapist wasn't building the right way and that he didn't think the therapist's work was any good. The therapist continued to focus on describing Luis's constructions and ignored his negative statements. In response to the therapist's positive attention to his construction, Luis returned his focus to what he had been building and did not make any more negative comments.

Check-Out

Ms. Palomo joined the therapist and Luis for the check-out. During this time, the therapist briefly explained Luis's child's work session. The therapist provided an inexpensive paperback copy of the book *A Child's First Book about Play Therapy* (Nemiroff & Annunziata, 1990) for Ms. Palomo and asked that she read it at home with Luis.

Session 2

Session Objectives

1. Continue establishing rapport.
2. Begin to discuss divorce.

Check-In

Ms. Palomo reported that she had completed the homework assignment from the previous week. To emphasize the importance of completing homework, the therapist praised Ms. Palomo and explained that beginning that day, therapy would be more focused on the presenting problems.

Child's Work

The child's work portion of the session began with the therapist introducing two identical dollhouses. The therapist said, "Remember the play therapy book that we read last week together? It's the same one that you read with your mother at home. Well, today we are going to play together and start talking about what it is like to have two homes. Here are two houses that look the same on the outside, but different people live on the inside." When asked, Luis stated that he thought that his mother lived in one house and his father lived in the second house. The therapist and Luis placed the appropriate figures in each house. Then the therapist picked up a boy doll and asked where Luis would live. The therapist and Luis continued to role-play with the dolls and the houses, talking about what things might be the same in Luis's two homes and what things might be different.

Child's Play

Luis chose to continue playing with the two homes during child's play. His play consisted of pretending that the adult dolls met together outside and argued. Then Luis pretended that the boy doll was getting into trouble with both of the parent dolls. After the boy doll was scolded, the father doll went away to his home.

Check-Out

During check-out, Ms. Palomo was encouraged to avoid having any arguments with Luis's father while Luis was watching. The importance of modeling respectful, nonargumentative behavior for Luis was discussed, in addition to discussing that children who witness lower levels of conflict in divorce tend to have better long-term outcomes.

Session 3

Session Objectives

1. Convey the idea that divorce is not Luis's fault.
2. Assign homework book about divorce.

Check-In

Ms. Palomo reported that she had argued with Luis's father on the telephone when she thought that Luis was outside playing, but it so happened that Luis had been listening from another room in the house. She said that Luis "was so mean" to her for the next 2 days. The therapist suggested that Luis was still learning to understand divorce and that he acted "mean" because he had not yet learned a better way to express his feelings about divorce. The therapist showed Ms. Palomo the book *Was It the Chocolate Pudding?: A Story for Little Kids about Divorce* (Levins, 2005) to be used for that day's therapy session.

Child's Work

The book, *Was It the Chocolate Pudding?: A Story for Little Kids about Divorce* was read to Luis during child's work. Luis appeared sullen during the story and did not speak after the story was completed. The therapist talked about the children in the book feeling that the divorce was their fault and asked Luis if he felt that the divorce was his fault. Luis said that his "Mommy and Daddy got a divorce because I was so bad." The therapist summarized the story by saying, "Sometimes children think that divorce is their fault, but that's not true. Divorce is something that is decided by a mommy and a daddy. It happens for adult reasons."

Child's Play

During Child's Play, Luis chose to play with the construction straws. He did not say anything about the book that the therapist had read. However, his mood became more animated when he led the play.

Check-Out

The therapist spent some time with Ms. Palomo discussing the reasons for her divorce from Luis's father. Ms. Palomo stated that there were relationship issues, but that these issues were exacerbated by Luis's difficult behavior. Ms. Palomo was told that it was important to convey to Luis that the divorce was not his fault, and that divorce is a decision that adults make for adult reasons. The therapist asked Ms. Palomo to read the book *Was It the Chocolate Pudding? A Story for Little Kids about Divorce* (Levins, 2005) at home with Luis to foster further conversation about blame and divorce.

Session 4

Session Objectives

Express feelings.

Check-In

The homework assignment was reviewed with Luis and his mother during check-in. Ms. Palomo reported that Luis seemed to be more reserved since reading *Was It the Chocolate Pudding?* However, he had asked to reread it on several occasions. The therapist said that his reaction would be a good lead-in for the work to be done in today's session focusing on expressing feelings.

Child's Work

The therapist already had the Talking, Feeling, and Doing Game (Gardner, 1973) set up in the play therapy room when Luis came in. The therapist explained that today they were going to play a game in which they would pick certain situations and use words to express how these situations would make each of them feel. The therapist selected the Divorce Card Game (Shapiro & Shore, 2004), which is used with the original Talking, Feeling, and Doing Game, so that the situations would be especially relevant for Luis. During the game, Luis referred to the book that he had been reading at home. He stated that he knew that the children in the book had feelings of sadness because of the divorce, because that was how he felt too. The therapist validated Luis's experience by saying that it was normal and OK to have sad feelings about a divorce.

Child's Play

Luis chose to play with the Legos during the child-led play therapy portion of the session. At first Luis took one of the Lego people and aggressively acted out, kicking down a Lego house. The therapist turned and ignored this aggressive play. Then Luis independently took another Lego person and started a dialogue between the Legos, using the feeling words from the game he had just played with the therapist (e.g., he made one Lego person say, "I'm so mad at you"). The therapist praised Luis for using the words, and stated that they could keep playing together when words were used to express feelings.

Check-Out

During check-out, the therapist explained the Divorce Card Game that was used with the Talking, Feeling and Doing Game during the therapy session and discussed how Luis had independently used feeling words when playing with the Legos. Ms. Palomo was encouraged to model the use of "I feel . . ." statements at home and to try to recognize when Luis's use of feeling words at home.

Session 5

Session Objectives

1. Discuss the play therapy (PRIDE) skills with Ms. Palomo.
2. Role-play the skills.
3. Assign the first home practice of special playtime skills.

Check-In

The therapist had asked Ms. Palomo to attend this session alone so that she could be taught the skills for the child-directed play interaction. The therapist explained to Ms. Palomo that the PRIDE skills would be useful for increasing her focus on Luis's appropriate behaviors and decreasing her attention to his inappropriate behaviors, such as his talking back and bossiness.

Ms. Palomo stated that Luis needed more one-on-one time with the therapist because his disrespectful and bossy behavior had not improved, especially when family members were visiting. She said that she was worried that because she was taking up his therapy time, Luis would never get better. The therapist assured Ms. Palomo that the time she spent in therapy with Luis would prove to be very valuable, inasmuch as Ms. Palomo would be able to use the new skills to help Luis every day of the week. In addition, the special playtime would address the issues that Ms. Palomo discussed in the first session regarding her wish to enjoy time with Luis again and would help her get over her anger and resentment toward him.

During the session, the therapist explained the child-directed interaction skills and allowed Ms. Palomo to ask questions. Ms. Palomo was encouraged to use the PRIDE (i.e., *P*raise, *R*eflect, *I*mitate, *D*escribe, *E*nthusiasm) skills when conducting play therapy with Luis. The PRIDE skills include the following: labeled praise for specific things that Luis does well, reflection of Luis's appropriate talk, imitation of his play, and description of his activities, all using an enthusiastic tone of voice. She was encouraged to avoid using commands and asking questions, because this would take the lead away from Luis during his play therapy time. The therapist also asked Ms. Palomo to avoid criticizing Luis during special playtime by not using the words "no," "don't," "stop," "not," and "quit." Finally, Ms. Palomo was taught to turn away from Luis to ignore his bossy and disrespectful comments during play therapy, and to respond only to his appropriate behaviors and comments.

After the skills were taught, Ms. Palomo role-played the play therapy with the therapist. The therapist made some contrived rude comments, similar to those that Luis had made in the past. This gave Ms. Palomo are opportunity to practice turning her back to ignore the disrespectful comments and returning to play when the behaviors were appropriate.

Check-Out

Ms. Palomo was given a handout on the play therapy (i.e., child-directed interaction) skills. Her homework assignment was to begin practicing these skills in a daily 5-minute special playtime with Luis. Ms. Palomo was also asked to record her special playtimes with checkmarks on a homework sheet.

Session 6

Session Objectives

1. Coach Ms. Palomo in child-directed play skills.
2. Begin decreasing the amount of time spent in child's play with the therapist and transferring the playtime to Luis's mother.

Check-In

Ms. Palomo said that she tried the special playtime with Luis only on the first 3 days after last week's appointment. She said that when she played with Luis, he always started telling her what to do and that it was not enjoyable for her to spend the time with him. The therapist reminded Ms. Palomo that the goal of this special playtime was to improve her relationship with Luis overall, and that his bossiness would be addressed once a solid positive ground for their relationship was developed and as therapy progressed. Finally, the therapist asked Ms. Palomo if she would mind if the first 5 minutes of playtime were videotaped to be used for comparison later in therapy, and Ms. Palomo agreed that she would not mind and signed a consent form.

The therapist explained the new structure for the remaining sessions of play therapy to Luis and asked if he would mind if they videotaped some of the playtime. He said he did not mind. The therapist said to Luis, "Today, I am going to coach your mom while she plays with you. I won't talk to you during this time. But after your special playtime is over, you and I will have some time to spend alone together. During the playtime, just pretend that you can't see me or hear me."

Coding

The first 5 minutes of the playtime were used to record Ms. Palomo's use of the play therapy skills. The therapist observed that Ms. Palomo played with Luis, but that she did not make many verbalizations.

Coaching

The therapist began the coaching portion by identifying Ms. Palomo's strengths (i.e., her imitation skills, her play interactions with Luis). Next, the therapist chose to focus on increasing Ms. Palomo's verbalizations by emphasizing the use of reflections and descriptions. Luis began telling his mother that she was "stupid" and did not "know how to build right," and he began to knock down and pull apart her Lego structure. At first, Ms. Palomo criticized Luis when he began making negative comments and directing her play. She scolded, "That's not the way to speak to your mother," and "What you're saying is rude," and pushed his hands away from her Legos. The therapist quickly jumped in and reminded Ms. Palomo to ignore Luis' disrespectful comments by turning her back and describing her own play. Ms. Palomo turned away from Luis and the therapist coached her to say, "I'm building a tall tower with my Legos, and now I'm going to put a light on the very top of it. And now I'm going to add some people walking around." At first Luis's negative comments increased (e.g., "That's a dumb tower," "You used the wrong colors"). But when his mother did not respond, he became quiet and continued playing with his own Legos. When this occurred, the therapist coached Ms. Palomo to turn back toward Luis and begin describing what he was building.

Child's Work/Child's Play

Because most of this session was spent in coaching, Luis's individual time was reduced to approximately 15 minutes. Luis said that he had liked playing with his mother because she "used to never play like that" with him at home. The therapist praised Luis for using words to express his feelings. Luis then asked if they could use the rest of the session to play with the two homes.

Check-Out

Ms. Palomo stated that she was surprised by how quickly Luis's behavior changed, even when she did not reprimand him for his "rude" comments. She said that although she felt awkward playing with Luis in front of the therapist, she really liked having someone tell her exactly what to do and say in her interactions with her son. She stated that it helped her remain calm, even when his behavior worsened, because she had someone else to rely on for ways to handle the behavior. The therapist encouraged Ms. Palomo to concentrate on either praising or describing Luis's appropriate behavior during her playtime with him at home. Again, Ms. Palomo was asked to record her special playtimes with checkmarks on a homework sheet.

Sessions 7 and 8

Session Objectives

1. Continue coaching Ms. Palomo in child-directed play skills.
2. Spend less time in child's play in anticipation of termination.

Check-In

The therapist reviewed Ms. Palomo's homework sheet recording her playtimes with Luis. Ms. Palomo indicated that she and Luis had had the special playtime every day, except for one when her family had come to visit in the evening. Ms. Palomo also stated that Luis' behavior was the worst it had been in a while on the day her family had visited. The therapist suggested the importance of doing the playtime at home, particularly on days when attention to Luis was less than usual. Ms. Palomo stated, however, that despite these few bad days, she had noticed that Luis looked forward to the special playtime at home, and that she believed she was starting to see the "sweet kid underneath the bossy one" again. She also stated that as she was making progress with Luis and as the divorce rulings were now 2 months in the past, she was beginning to feel less resentment toward Luis.

Coding

During the 5-minute coding period, Luis chose to play with the two homes. Luis's mother used many descriptions, but asked a number of leading questions about who was in the home and his feelings about living in two homes.

Coaching

Based on the information derived from the coding period, the therapist chose to emphasize the use of labeled praise, with the idea that focusing positively on skills to increase (such as praise) would result in a decrease in the use of questions. The therapist reminded Ms. Palomo that the more she used labeled praise, the greater influence she could have on maintaining Luis's appropriate behaviors during the playtime. Ms. Palomo independently used labeled praise regarding Luis's play. The therapist helped Ms. Palomo identify and use labeled praise for desirable target behaviors that Luis exhibited (e.g., sitting at the table, playing nicely with his mom, using kind words, sharing with his mom). At one point, Luis said that he "hated the stupid homes," "hated his stupid aunt," and that he wished "that she would get sick, disappear, and never come again." He acted this out aggressively with the dolls by throwing one doll out the window. At first, Ms. Palomo froze, but then continued with describing her play. When Luis was quiet, the therapist coached Ms. Palomo to return her attention to Luis and say, "Thanks for playing nicely with the dolls. It sounds like you're really angry about your aunt coming over." Luis said, "She makes me really angry." The therapist coached Ms. Palomo to respond by saying, "I am so proud of you for using your feelings words. You are a big boy for saying how you feel." The therapist then coached Ms. Palomo to continue playing with Luis while focusing on praising his appropriate behaviors. Luis continued to play with the homes, acting out the family's coming to visit, but using appropriate play and language to describe the actions.

Child's Work/Child's Play

Luis's individual time was reduced to approximately 10 minutes this week. Luis asked if the therapist would read the *Was It the Chocolate Pudding?* book again with him. Throughout the book, Luis independently identified feelings that the characters might be having, and the therapist praised Luis for using words to express feelings.

Check-Out

The therapist praised Ms. Palomo for her progress in the child-directed play skills and for her ability to use strategic attention and selective ignoring effectively. She was asked to continue using the special playtime at home, and to be sure to keep a time designated for it on Luis's "tough" days, because this is when he could benefit from it even more than on his "good" days.

Session 9

Session Objectives

1. Discuss the discipline skills with Ms. Palomo.
2. Role-play the skills.

Check-In

Ms. Palomo was asked to attend this therapy session without Luis so that the therapist could introduce the discipline skills (i.e., parent-directed skills). The therapist explained that these skills would be useful in addressing Ms. Palomo's lingering concerns about Luis's "disrespectful" behavior toward her and other adults.

The parent-directed skills were explained to Ms. Palomo, followed by examples and role plays. The first of these skills is giving effective commands. This includes multiple techniques, such as giving commands that are simple, direct, positively stated, clearly worded, and at an appropriate developmental level. Then the application of consequences for following directions (e.g., labeled praise for compliance) and not following directions (e.g., time-out) were discussed. Ms. Palomo was taught to use a two-choice statement. A two-choice statement specifies two options for Luis; he may either (1) comply with the initial command or (2) go to time-out. She then was taught a consistent, effective procedure for implementing time-out in a calm and consistent manner.

Ms. Palomo stated that she had tried time-out before and that it did not work for Luis. The therapist discussed the changes that Ms. Palomo had made in her relationship with Luis through the use of the special playtime and the child-directed play therapy skills. These changes, which already had resulted in a better relationship, would make Luis more motivated to please her by complying with her requests.

Check-Out

Ms. Palomo stated that she was surprised that play therapy included methods of handling Luis's more difficult behaviors. She said that she was pleased that she was being taught a way to teach important values, such as respect for elders, to her son, in a way that was less strict and more positive and nurturing than what she had learned to do as a parent.

Ms. Palomo was given a handout on the discipline (i.e., parent-directed interaction) skills. However, her homework assignment was to continue using only the play therapy skills in the upcoming week.

Sessions 10–12

Session Objectives

1. Coach Ms. Palomo in using the discipline skills with Luis.
2. Teach Luis to comply with directions.
3. Teach Luis to respect his mother and other adults.

Check-In

Ms. Palomo reported that she and Luis were continuing to enjoy the time spent during the special playtime, but that she was looking forward to having a more active discipline strategy in place. She stated that Luis still became bossy with her, especially when close friends or family members were around.

Coaching

The therapist coached Ms. Palomo to explain the new rules for their special playtime. Luis was told the following:

> "Today, special playtime is going to be a little different. While we are playing, I am going to tell you to do things, like 'hand me that block' or 'put the doll in the house.' If you listen, then we will get to keep playing. But if you choose not to listen, then you will have to go to time-out. And time-out is no fun. When you go to time-out, you walk on your own to the chair like this, and then you sit in the chair as quiet as a mouse until I tell you that you can get up."

Ms. Palomo walked Luis through the time-out procedure and rewarded him with stickers for practicing going to time-out independently and sitting in the time-out chair quietly.

Coding

The first 5 minutes of the playtime were used to record Ms. Palomo's use of only the child-directed play therapy skills. Ms. Palomo was observed to meet the mastery criteria for play therapy. She used 23 behavioral descriptions, 12 reflections, and 17 praises (mostly labeled praises) during the coding period. In addition, her interactions with Luis were rich and enthusiastic, and Luis appeared to really enjoy the interactive play. In session 12, the therapist again asked Ms. Palomo and Luis if they would mind if the first 5 minutes were videotaped. Both said that they did not mind.

Coaching

Ms. Palomo continued to use the child-directed interaction play skills for another few minutes. Then the therapist began working with Ms. Palomo to develop the first direct instruction. Ms. Palomo chose to tell Luis to give her a car that he had been driving around the dollhouse. The therapist coached Luis's mother to say, "Luis, we are going to practice listening now. Please put the car in my hand," while she pointed from the car to her hand. The therapist then said to Ms. Palomo, "That was a good direct command. Now just gesture from the car to your hand, but stay quiet. We're counting in our heads to see if Luis starts to comply. Good, there he goes. When he puts the car in your hand, praise his compliance by saying, 'Thanks for listening,' and remind him that when he listens, he doesn't have to go to time-out and you can continue to play together." Ms. Palomo looked relieved that Luis had complied with her first instruction. The therapist coached Luis's mother to continue using the child-directed interaction play skills for a few more minutes before issuing a new command.

After a few minutes of enthusiastic play, the therapist coached Ms. Palomo to develop another, more difficult instruction. By now, Luis was engaged in play with the construction straws, a favorite toy. The therapist told Ms. Palomo that she wanted her to tell Luis to put the straws away. The therapist coached Ms. Palomo to say, "Luis, we're going to practice listening again. Please put all of the construction straws back into the box." Luis started to take apart his construction, but then began waving the straws in front of his mother's face in a taunting manner. The therapist said to Ms. Palomo:

> "This is OK. He's just testing to see what you are going to do. Keep your face neutral and say, 'You have two choices. You can either put all of the straws in the box or you can go to time-out,' and just point to the box and then to the time-out chair."

Ms. Palomo said what the therapist had coached her to say, but appeared to be getting frustrated with Luis. The therapist said:

"You're doing fine. Remember to stay calm. If Luis knows that he is getting to you, he is more likely to continue taunting. Just point again to the construction straws and to the box, but don't say anything else. There, that's good. He's trying to get a rise out of you. OK, it looks as though he's not going to listen, so what I want you to say is, 'You chose not to listen, so you'll have to go to time-out,' and gently take Luis by the hand and walk with him to the time-out chair. Now step back a little and say, 'Stay here until I tell you to get up,' and walk back to the play table."

The therapist asked Ms. Palomo to move distractions away so that the construction straws and the box were at the front of the table by Luis's chair. Then the therapist asked Ms. Palomo to describe her own play with another toy while she was at the table. Luis was intently watching Ms. Palomo play with the toys, and was remaining quiet and in the chair, so the therapist coached Ms. Palomo to walk back to Luis and say, "Are you ready to put the construction straws in the box?" Rather than waiting for a verbal answer, Ms. Palomo put her hand out toward Luis. Luis did not take her hand, but did get up and walk over to the play therapy table and start putting away the straws. When they were all put away, the therapist coached Ms. Palomo to say, "OK. Now please put the dollhouse people back in the house." Luis quickly put the dolls in the house and then looked up at his mother. The therapist coached Ms. Palomo to use a very emphatic, enthusiastic labeled praise by saying, "Fantastic job of listening, Luis! When you listen, you don't have to go to time-out, and now we can keep on playing." The rest of the session was devoted to the use of the child-directed interaction skills to help diffuse Luis's frustration and regain the positive momentum of the play therapy time.

Over the course of the next few discipline-focused sessions, the therapist gradually shifted the use of direct commands about tangible items to the application of using direct instructions for redirecting inappropriate behavior. For example, when Luis began to destroy a picture that his mother had drawn, the therapist coached Ms. Palomo to instruct Luis to draw scribbles on his own paper (an instruction that could be followed up in the same, structured manner as any other direct command). In this way, the therapist was able to problem solve with Ms. Palomo how to address Luis's "disrespectful" behaviors exhibited at home and with other familiar adults.

Child's Work/Child's Play

The therapist asked Ms. Palomo to complete the ECBI while Luis had his individual time with the therapist during the session 12. Because of the duration and intensity of the discipline coaching sessions, this portion of Luis's therapy was shortened to just 5–10 minutes. Typically, Luis chose to continue playing with the toys he had used with his mother, and often he described to the therapist what he and his mother had done together. The therapist encouraged Luis to continue expressing his feelings about his time with his mother, using the feeling words that he had learned earlier in therapy.

Check-Out

The therapist praised Ms. Palomo for her ability to stay calm during the direct commands and time-out steps that she had implemented. Ms. Palomo discussed how good she felt as a parent because she was teaching Luis important lessons about respecting adults and following directions, but she was doing it in a way that did not put him down, harm him, or model physical aggression as a way to solve problems.

Session 13

1. Have an end of therapy celebration.
2. Evaluate pre- to posttreatment changes.
3. Praise Luis's accomplishments.
4. Praise Luis's mother's accomplishments.

Check-In

The therapist provided a copy of Luis's treatment plan to Ms. Palomo. The gains that both she and Luis had made throughout treatment were discussed, and future needs were identified (e.g., issues that may arise regarding transitioning to Luis's father's home in the summer, possibility of remarriage and stepsiblings).

Next, the therapist focused on the gains that Ms. Palomo had made throughout treatment. A portion of a videotape showing Ms. Palomo's interaction with Luis in session 6 was shown, followed by a portion of a videotape from session 12. Ms. Palomo was surprised at how different her interactions with Luis had been just 2½ months earlier, as compared with their interactions today. In addition, gains that were evident in the ratings provided by Ms. Palomo on the ECBI were highlighted. Ms. Palomo was praised for (1) attending the sessions regularly (and attending one more session than originally planned), (2) keeping an open mind and attempting the therapist's suggestions, (3) following through on homework assignments, (4) improving her interaction skills with Luis, (5) keeping her "adult" comments about Luis's father to herself, and (6) reducing Luis's feelings of blame for the divorce.

Child's Work

The therapist briefly reviewed the course of treatment with Luis, reminding him about the work they had done early on about feelings, talking about divorce, and all the other exercises and activities of therapy. Luis was praised for the hard work he had done in play therapy, both alone with the therapist and with his mother. He also was praised for becoming such a polite, respectful boy.

Child's Play

The therapist, Luis, and Ms. Palomo had a termination party together. The therapist noted to Ms. Palomo that she used the PRIDE skills naturally now, even during an unstructured time such as the party. Ms. Palomo stated that it was easy to use the skills now, and that she was so happy that she really enjoyed her son again.

Check-Out

During check-out, Ms. Palomo was reminded about the importance of continuing to practice her skills during special playtime with Luis. She was told to continue praising Luis for his respectful interactions with adults, and was encouraged to contact the therapist in the future should she have any concerns.

REFERENCES

Azar, S. T., & Wolfe, D. A. (1989). Child abuse and neglect. In E. J. Marsh & R. A. Barkley (Eds.), *Treatment of childhood disorders* (pp. 451–493). New York: Guilford Press.

Bagner, D. M., Fernandez, M. A., & Eyberg, S. M. (2004). Parent–child interaction therapy and chronic illness: A case study. *Journal of Clinical Psychology in Medical Settings, 11*, 1–6.

Boggs, S. R., Eyberg, S. M., Edwards, D. L., Rayfield, A., Jacobs, J., Bagner, D., & Hood, K. K. (2004). Outcomes of Parent–Child Interaction Therapy: A Comparison of treatment completes and study dropouts one to three years later. *Child and Family Behavior Therapy, 26*(4), 1–22.

Capage, L. C., Bennett, G. M., & McNeil, C. B. (2001). A comparison between African American and Caucasian children referred for treatment of behavior problems. *Child and Family Behavior Therapy, 23*(1), 1–14.

Capage, L. C., Foote, R., McNeil, C. B., & Eyberg, S. M. (1998). Parent–child interaction therapy: An effective treatment for young children with conduct problems. *Behavior Therapist, 21*, 137–138.

Calzada, E. J., & Eyberg, S. M. (2002). Self-reported parenting practices in Dominican and Puerto Rican mothers of young children. *Journal of Clinical Child and Adolescent Psychology, 3*, 354–363.

Chaffin, M., Silovsky, J. F., Funderburk, B., Valle, L. A., Brestan, E. V., Balachova, T., et al. (2004). Parent–child interaction therapy with physically abusive parents: Efficacy for reducing future abuse reports. *Journal of Consulting and Clinical Psychology, 72*(3), 500–510.

Choate, M. L., Pincus, D. B., Eyberg, S. M., & Barlow, D. H. (2005). Parent–child interaction therapy for treatment of separation anxiety disorder in young children: A pilot study. *Cognitive and Behavioral Practice, 12,* 126–135.

Crittenden, P. M., & Ainsworth, M. S. (1989). *Child maltreatment and attachment theory.* In D. Cicchetti & V. Carlson (Eds.), *Child maltreatment: Theory and research on the causes and consequences of child abuse and neglect.* New York: Cambridge University Press.

Dombrowski, S. C., Timmer, S. G., Blacker, D. M., & Urquiza, A. J. (2005). A positive behavioural intervention for toddlers: Parent–child attunement therapy. *Child Abuse Review, 14,* 132–151.

Eyberg, S. M., & Calzada, E. J. (1998). *Parent–child interaction therapy: Procedures manual.* Unpublished manuscript, University of Florida.

Eyberg, S. M., Funderburk, B. W., Hembree-Kigin, T. L., McNeil, C. B., Querido, J. G., & Hood, K. K. (2001). Parent–child interaction therapy with behavior problem children: One and two year maintenance of treatment effects in the family. *Child and Family Behavior Therapy, 23,* 1–20.

Eyberg, S. M., & Matarazzo, R. G. (1980). Training parents as therapists: A comparison between individual parent–child interaction training and parent group didactic training. *Journal of Clinical Psychology, 36,* 492–499.

Eyberg, S. M., & Pincus, D. (1999). *Eyberg Child Behavior Inventory and Sutter-Eyberg Behavior Inventory—Revised: Professional manual.* Odessa, FL: Psychological Assessment Resources.

Eyberg, S. M., & Robinson, E. A. (1983). Dyadic parent–child interaction coding system: A manual. *Psychological Documents, 13,* MS. No. 2582.

Filcheck, H. A., McNeil, C. B., & Herschell, A. D. (2005). Parent interventions with physically abused children. In P. Forrest Talley (Ed.), *Handbook for the treatment of abused and neglected children.* Binghamton, NY: Haworth Press.

Fricker-Elhai, A. E., Ruggiero, K. J., & Smith, D. W. (2005). Parent–child interaction therapy with two maltreated siblings in foster care. *Clinical Case Studies, 4,* 13–39.

Gallagher, N. (2003). Effects of parent–child interaction therapy on young children with disruptive behavior disorders. *Bridges Practice-Based Research Syntheses, 1,* 1–17.

Gardner, R. A. (1973). *The talking, feeling, and doing game.* Cresskill, NJ: Creative Therapeutics.

Green, A. H. (1978). Self-destructive behavior in battered children. *American Journal of Child Psychiatry, 135,* 579–582.

Hanf, C. (1969). *A two-stage program for modifying maternal controlling during mother–child interaction.* Paper presented at the meeting of the Western Psychological Association, Vancouver, BC.

Harwood, M. D., & Eyberg, S. M. (2004). Therapist verbal behavior early in treatment: Relation to successful completion of parent–child interaction therapy. *Journal of Clinical Child and Adolescent Psychiatry, 33,* 601–612.

Hembree-Kigin, T., & McNeil, C. B. (1995). *Parent–child interaction therapy.* New York: Plenum Press.

Herschell, A. D., Calzada, E. J., Eyberg, S. M., & McNeil, C. B. (2002a). Clinical issues in parent–child interaction therapy. *Cognitive and Behavioral Practice, 9,* 16–27.

Herschell, A. D., Calzada, E. J., Eyberg, S. M., & McNeil, C. B. (2002b). Parent–child interaction therapy: New directions in research. *Cognitive and Behavioral Practice, 9,* 9–16.

Herschell, A. D., & McNeil, C. B. (2005). Theoretical and empirical underpinnings for use of parent–child interaction therapy with child physical abuse populations. *Education and Treatment of Children, 28*(2), 142–162.

Hoffman-Plotkin, D., & Twentyman, C. T. (1984). A multimodal assessment of behavioral and cognitive deficits in abused and neglected preschoolers. *Child Development, 55,* 794–802.

Hood, K. K., & Eyberg, S. M. (2003). Outcomes of parent–child interaction therapy: Mothers' reports of maintenance three to six years after treatment. *Journal of Clinical Child and Adolescent Psychology, 32,* 419–429.

Kauffman Foundation. (2004). *Closing the quality chasm in child abuse treatment: Identifying and disseminating best practices. The findings of the Kauffman Best Practices Project to help children heal from child abuse.* San Diego, CA: Author.

Levins, S. (2005). *Was it the chocolate pudding? A story for little kids about divorce.* Washington, DC: American Psychological Association.

Luntz, B., & Widom, C. S. (1994). Antisocial personality disorder in abused and neglected children grown up. *American Journal of Psychiatry, 151,* 670–674.

McCabe, K. M., Yeh, M., Garland, A. F., Lau, A. S., & Chavez, G. (2005). The GANA program: A tailoring approach to adapting parent–child interaction therapy for Mexican Americans. *Education and Treatment of Children, 28*(2), 111–129.

McCabe, K. M., Yeh, M., Lau, A., Garland, A., & Hough, R. (2003). Racial/ethnic differences in caregiver strain and perceived social support among parents of youth with emotional and behavioral problems. *Mental Health Services Research, 5*(3), 137–147.

McCord, J. (1983). A forty year perspective on effects of child abuse and neglect. *Child Abuse and Neglect, 7,* 265–270.

McGinnis, E., & Goldstein, A. P. (2003). *Skillstreaming in early childhood: New strategies and perspectives for teaching prosocial skills.* Champaign, IL: Research Press.

McNeil, C. B., Hembree-Kigin, T., & Eyberg, S. M. (1996). *Short-term play therapy for disruptive children.* King of Prussia, PA: Center for Applied Psychology.

McNeil, C. B., Hembree-Kigin, T., & Eyberg, S. M. (1998). *Working with oppositional defiant disorder in children: An audio and video training program.* Secaucus, NJ: Childswork/Childsplay of Genesis Direct.

McNeil, C. B., Herschell, A. D., Gurwitch, R. H., & Clemens-Mowrer, L. (2005). Training foster parents in parent–child interaction therapy. *Education and Treatment of Children, 28*(2), 182–196.

Neic, L. N., Hemme, J. M., Yopp, J. M., & Brestan, E. V. (2005). Parent–child interaction therapy: The rewards and challenges of a group format. *Cognitive and Behavioral Practice, 12,* 113–125.

Nemiroff, M. A., & Annunziata, J. (1990). *A child's first book about play therapy.* Washington, DC: American Psychological Association.

Pincus, D. B., Eyberg, S. M., & Choate, M. L. (2005). Adapting parent–child interaction therapy for young children with separation anxiety disorder. *Education and Treatment of Children, 28*(2), 163–181.

Robin, A. (1976). The turtle technique: An extended case study of self-control in the classroom. *Psychology in the Schools, 13,* 449–453.

Satcher, D. (2000). Mental health: A report of the surgeon general: Executive summary. *Professional Psychology: Research and Practice, 31*(1), 5–13.

Schumann, E., Foote, R., Eyberg, S. M., Boggs, S., & Algina, J. (1998). Parent–child interaction therapy: Interim report of a randomized trial with short-term maintenance. *Journal of Clinical Child Psychology, 27,* 34–45.

Shapiro, L. E., & Shore, H. (2004). *The talking, feeling, and doing divorce card game.* Plainview, NY: Child's Work/Child's Play.

Timmer, S. G., Urquiza, A. J., Zebell, N. M., & McGrath, J. M. (2005). Parent–child interaction therapy: Application to physically abusive and high-risk parent–child dyads. *Child Abuse and Neglect, 29,* 825–842.

Urquiza, A. J., & McNeil, C. B. (1996). Parent–child interaction therapy: An intensive dyadic intervention for physically abusive families. *Child Maltreatment, 1,* 134–144.

U.S. Department of Health and Human Services Administration on Children, Youth, and Families. (2003). *Child Maltreatment 2001.* Washington, DC: U.S. Government Printing Office.

Widom, C. S. (1989). Child abuse, neglect, and adult behavior: Design and findings on criminality, violence and child abuse. *American Journal of Orthopsychiatry, 59,* 355–367.

CHAPTER 8

Short-Term Family
Sandplay Therapy

LOIS CAREY

The major focus of managed care companies today is on "short-term" therapies. Most therapists, myself included, were trained in a psychodynamic format that was pretty much open-ended. We were not trained to do short-term
work, and insurance companies did not play such an important role in treatment decisions. In order to keep up with current trends, it behooves all of us
to find productive methods that address this need and still allow us to maintain our integrity as therapists and to resolve the problems that are presented
to us.

The book *Short-Term Play Therapy for Children* (Kaduson & Schaefer,
2000) illustrated to professionals and students just how valuable and time saving
this method can be. Short-term therapy enables us to treat more children in
less time so that we can meet the demands of managed care and allows us to
see an additional number of patients in any given year.

My earlier paper, "Family Sandplay Therapy" (Carey, 1991) demonstrated
the effectiveness of combining sandplay and family therapy. In that article, I
showed how sand can be an effective healing milieu with families and stressed
the differences of approach when one uses sand with an individual or with a
family. In this chapter, I demonstrate the application of a "short-term" approach to family sandplay therapy. The reader is advised that this milieu requires training in sandplay, play therapy, and family therapy.

A BRIEF INTRODUCTION TO FAMILY SANDPLAY THERAPY

The use of sandplay, as a Jungian technique, was spread primarily through the work of Dora Kalff, a Swiss Jungian analyst. The focus in Kalff's work was with the individual child and his or her "journey to wholeness" (see Kalff, 1980, and Appendix 8.1).

When a child is presented as the identified patient, perhaps showing symptoms after a breakup or death in the family, or for other causes, however, an increasing number of therapists are finding that it is beneficial to include the family in the child's treatment and so use a family therapy approach.

Family therapy views the family as the patient and is designed to improve communication and respect among the family members in order for them to reach a more optimal level of functioning.

The sandplay therapist can quickly assess some of the family dynamics just by watching how family members pursue the task of making a sand scene together.

- Are they cooperative or argumentative?
- Does one person overrule the others?
- Do they talk, or do they work silently?
- Do they all participate, or does someone stay in the background?

The answers to some of these questions can be apparent to the family members as well as to the therapist. Some families can see almost immediately what needs to change in order for their relationships to be strengthened. In other families, the needs are not as apparent, and the therapist, by keeping his or her remarks within the metaphor of the sand tray, can influence the family to move in a positive direction. The major problem for play therapists is that they are not always comfortable with the families of their young patients and, conversely, family therapists are not always comfortable with either play or young children.

It is widely believed that for some patients, sandplay therapy can be more quickly effective than verbal therapy just by virtue of the tactile nature of the medium.[1] This brings to mind the adage "A picture is worth a thousand words." Recent brain studies by van der Kolk (2003), Siegel (1999), and others have demonstrated that many nonverbal therapies such as art, drama, and neurolinguistic Programming (Shapiro & Maxfield, 2003), can tap into the area of the right brain, where symbol formation is located, and thus reach a deeper level more quickly than verbal therapies alone. This finding can extend to sandplay therapy as well, because positive results are much more attainable in less time with this nonverbal therapy than when words and reasoning are used as the primary method. Much of this research has been with trauma victims, for whom words cannot do justice to their feelings.

THE PROCESS OF FAMILY SANDPLAY THERAPY

Introductory Session

Family members are first shown the playroom, with an explanation that they are free to use one or both boxes to construct a scene in the tray, using whatever miniatures they prefer. They are told that at the end of the session they will be given time to share what they have observed, or tell a story about what they have done, or what the entire scene might represent to each one of them. They can agree to use one sandbox, or they can divide into teams and use both. The choice is the family's to make. The therapist can set a limit on the number of items used, but in the first session I usually do not do this, as I prefer letting the family members try to set their own limits. I instruct them that they will know when the scene feels complete and that 10 or 15 minutes will be allowed for discussion near the end of the time. My role during the initial session is primarily one of observer (as well as timekeeper). I take note of the process as it evolves, particularly:

- Where do I see alliances?
- Where do I see conflict?
- Does one or another assume a leadership role?
- Is there cooperation or conflict?
- Does everyone participate?
- If not, why not?
- What affect is shown by each member?

Subsequent Sessions

The therapist becomes more of a "director" during the following sessions. If the family in treatment is one that uses verbalization as a defense, the therapist can direct its members to work silently. If it is a noncommunicative family, he or she she can direct them to discuss what they want to do and how to do it. The therapist can choose those who should work together and in which tray. If the family members originally elected to use two trays, they may continue to do so, or they may all use one box if that was the original choice. One of the important aspects of family sandplay therapy is that the therapist can elect (in subsequent sessions) to pair certain family members together if there are particular issues to be addressed between them (for example, if there is conflict evident between a father and son). Some of these decisions are based on the size of the family. I have found that if there are more than three or four persons, it is often best to use two trays.

Postscene Discussion

The postscene discussion is incorporated into each therapy session. This is the culminating point of each session in which the family dynamics that have been observed during the process can be verbally elicited. Each member is given an opportunity to tell a story about what he or she has contributed, but any discussion should always be kept within the metaphor of the tray. An example of this is shown in the case of Martin (to follow), in Clarice's explanation of the girl in the yellow dress.

Another example might be, "What is the sheep feeling with that lion in the background?" This is the portion of the session in which the intuition and empathy of the therapist allows him or her to begin to summarize what has been observed and to put it all into perspective. This is not an easy task, but one that becomes easier as one has more experience with this technique.

Termination

A short-term contract has allowed termination to begin almost from the first session. This means that there is very little in the way of transference material that needs to be addressed, because it is the family members who need to assess and correct their problematic relationships. The therapist sets the stage for this to occur. There are definite feelings involved, as illustrated in the case of Martin (to follow), in which his passive–aggressive behavior evoked my countertransference reaction. With a careful consideration of all of the dynamics in any case, termination is usually effected without incident. In the final session, all of the family members are told that they can return in the future if that proves to be necessary.

AN EXAMPLE OF SHORT-TERM FAMILY SANDPLAY THERAPY

The various time limits on what is considered "short-term" therapy can range from 4 to 20 sessions. I believe that family sandplay therapy, as a technique, is quite conducive to a short-term model of roughly 12–16 sessions. This model is vastly different from other sandplay approaches by virtue of being more directive and more highly structured. For example, the format I use is this:

1. The first two or three sessions are devoted to relationship building.
2. The next eight or nine sessions are given to working through the problem.
3. The final three or four sessions are devoted to termination issues.

This model relies more heavily on the medium and the family's instinctual understanding and striving toward health, rather than on the strength of the bond between therapist and client.

A Case of School Refusal

This is the case of a 9½-year-old boy whom I will call Martin. Martin had been resisting school since the term began and, for the 2 weeks prior to the referral, had not wanted to attend at all. Mrs. K, his mother, had not been very insistent on his attendance because his special education teacher had told her not to be unduly concerned. She took the teacher at her word, but decided she needed to pursue treatment for Martin to try to change this pattern. The decision was made at the suggestion of Mrs. K's individual therapist, from whom she was receiving treatment at a local agency (in addition to regular attendance at Al-Anon).

At age 3, Martin had been evaluated for developmental delays and speech problems and had attended a therapeutic nursery where these problems were addressed. He once told his mother that he had been "screaming inside for 2 years," a comment that was of major concern to her. Martin was also prone to temper tantrums and would shut himself in his room when angry. He had a history of separation anxiety that began when he started nursery school and had apparently continued intermittently.

Martin had one sister, Clarice, a 10½-year-old. Martin was a very heavy child, whereas Clarice was a slight, pale, and shy girl. Clarice's history was nonremarkable. She was a bright student and, unfortunately, her mother's confidante. Her major issues were lack of friends and unwillingness to be involved in after-school activities. Both children were seen to have severe socialization problems, preferring to stay at home with their mother whenever possible. Their mother, at the beginning of family therapy, was happy with this arrangement, as the children provided her with her only outlet for socialization aside from work. Clarice had attended Project Rainbow (for children of alcoholic parents) for about a year.

The K's had been separated for 2 years because of Mr. K's alcoholism. The children had witnessed numerous parental arguments and some instances of domestic violence when Dad was drinking. One year prior to Martin's coming to treatment, the maternal grandmother had died. Mrs. K felt that this double loss (father and grandmother) may have affected both children badly, but was most concerned about Martin, as she perceived him to be quite depressed. Martin accompanied his sister to Project Rainbow once, then refused to go back because, he said, "Everyone there is so happy." He had a pattern of going to an activity or program once, after which he refused to return.

Both children had frequent contact with their father. He helped out, when needed, with child care and financial support; however, finances were an ongoing concern for both parents. I had one session with Mr. K and found him quite limited in psychological understanding. He was, however, interested in maintaining a close relationship with his children.

One of the biggest problems observed at the outset was that both children slept with their mother every single night. It took a great effort to change that pattern, but it was eventually resolved. Because of the numerous issues confronting the family members (divorce, loss of a parent and a grandparent, financial concerns, etc.), a short-term contract was set up, with the goals being to get Martin to return to school; to normalize the sleeping patterns; for both children to begin to move toward more independence; and for Mrs. K to "let go."

Clarice seemed to be doing all right. However, as noted earlier, she had no peer relationships and was not involved in any extracurricular school activities. She was at risk of becoming overattached to her mother; indeed, that appeared to have already occurred.

Mrs. K reported in the beginning of treatment that when she was able to get Martin into his own bed, she would lie down with him and, subsequently, she would often fall asleep. If she moved to her own bed, it was not long before he joined her, and being too sleepy to fight with him, she allowed him to stay with her. Clarice more readily accepted sleeping in her own bed. There was an overdependence on mother in this case, and I had to more or less insist that Mrs. K deal with the sleeping arrangements. Gentle reminders in the early stages of treatment did not produce the desired results, so I had to be quite direct and let her know that this pattern of sleeping together was much too seductive for any 9-year-old male. This finally made an impression. Mrs. K had, herself, grown up in a home where alcoholism was present and had great difficulty with boundary issues.

Martin was a reluctant participant in therapy and, like his father, had limited psychological understanding. Nevertheless, he began to make some changes. There was no more school refusal after the second family session, so Martin believed that because he was now attending school there was no need to continue with family therapy. I reminded all of the participants that we had made a contract for 16 sessions, and the mother was able to persuade the children to continue. However, in many of the sessions, Martin refused to participate, remaining mute throughout the entire time. In some sessions, he made some limited attempts to take part, as long as it was on his terms. Nothing seemed to make any difference—he resisted my attempts, and those of his mother and sister, to include him.

During the fifth session, the mother reported that Clarice had been sick one day and stayed home from school. Martin had tried to manipulate his mother to allow him to stay home too. When she insisted, however, that he go to school, he did not put up much of a fuss. Mrs. K was definitely learning.

For most sessions, we all met in the playroom; Martin would stand with his back to us, staring out a door. He said that it was "boring," "there's nothing to do" (in spite of the fact that the room was filled with sandplay toys and art materials). We talked around and about him while he stayed in the same mute position. During one session, he sat and manipulated his upper torso in such a way that it seemed to me as if he were trying to form a breast out of the fat. I made a comment about this, and he stopped immediately. Mrs. K called me later to find out why I had said anything, as he was sensitive about being "fat." I told her I was hoping to find a way to elicit some anger from him, but even that didn't work. I believed that if he could get good and angry, we might be able to proceed in a positive direction. I was certainly aware of his anger, but it came across in a very passive–aggressive style that did not help him in his expression of feelings. (My countertransference allowed me to truly feel his anger.)

In the middle of the course of therapy, I began to allow Martin and Clarice to go to the playroom while I met with Mrs. K to explore parenting issues. This seemed to contribute to Martin's being somewhat more cooperative. A session began with all of them together; then, after about 15 minutes, the children were sent off to the playroom. Mrs. K and I joined them for the last 10 minutes, and they told us about their scenes.

This was one of the more difficult families I have treated, and I tried to be as flexible as possible while keeping the children's issues in the forefront. The obvious problems were Martin's, but Clarice was of concern as well, because she was the parentified, almost forgotten child. Because the focus had been on Martin from an early age, she had not had a chance to find out who she was. Her recent report card, however, was excellent, as opposed to earlier ones showing that she had just "squeaked through." This was her first year in middle school, with all the adjustments that go along with it, and she was truly making good progress. Martin was mainstreamed into a regular class and did satisfactorily. However, he resisted doing homework, using resistance as an excuse to continue demanding his mother's attention.

Mrs. K was a teacher in a religious high school and was attending college to get her master's degree as a reading specialist. This degree would enable her to get a job in a public school, where the pay was about double the amount she was earning.

Creating the Sandplay Scene

To begin sandplay therapy with a family, I first introduce its members to the medium by leading them into the playroom, where everything is set up. I point out the two sandboxes and invite them to feel the sand in each, to determine which one they prefer—the one that contains wet sand or the box with dry sand. In some families, one or two members may prefer wet sand and the others prefer dry. In these cases, those who prefer wet sand can use it, and those who prefer dry sand can use dry. The miniatures (see Appendix 8.1 for a list of suggested items), arranged on shelves, are visible. I make a simple statement to the effect that they can choose as many miniatures as they want and then construct a scene with them in the sand. They are told that when the scene feels complete to them, each person will have an opportunity to comment on what they have made.

The K family all preferred the dry sand and used that throughout most of the session. Four pictures were taken, at different stages of the therapy, and are described below.

The first scene (Figure 8.1) was made during our second session by Martin and Clarice working together. Mrs. K and I were the observers. It is very difficult to know who did what in this picture; there are many aggressive figures, and at least two or three are eating small objects. One dinosaur on the right-hand side, just above the Beast, is swallowing a small girl. In the center on the left, a crocodile is eating a very large marble. The dinosaur in the upper right is likewise chewing up Aladdin. Scenes such as this, which show animals eating people, often represent a deep-seated rage. There are also soldiers, tanks, and a cannon. Most of the aggressive images were put in by Martin. Of note in the lower left is a family of cows and calves, all eating food. This was Clarice's contribution.

I asked each one for comments. Martin was quite sarcastic as he asked, "Can't you see what is going on?" Clarice, however, said that the cows eating their food made her feel good. Mrs. K said that she found the whole thing quite

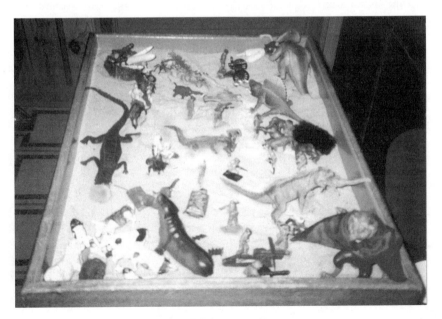

FIGURE 8.1 Anger erupts.

upsetting. I agreed that a lot was going on, but pointed out that there was hopeful imagery, such as the cows being fed.[2] This comment was made to support Clarice as well as to help Mrs. K recognize that not everything was a total disaster. I thought about the anger Martin displayed and about the role in which Clarice saw herself—family peacemaker and nurturer. I did not share that thought; the therapist's response to scenes like this are not always verbalized, especially in the beginning stage of treatment.

The next scene (Figure 8.2) was done by Clarice and Martin at the sixth session when they were in the sandplay room by themselves. It was made just 4 weeks after the first scene and is much more cohesive and less aggressive than that in Figure 8.1. Now we have an Indian village with the Indians all engaged in various pursuits. Some are warriors on horseback, two are paddling a canoe, some of the women are cooking, and some are tending babies. There is a treasure chest in the lower left and a girl at the center right, who is wearing a yellow dress; she is the only one who seems out of place. When a figure seems incongruous with the rest of the scene, the therapist makes a mental note to see if anyone comments on it. If the family members do not say anything, the therapist may interject his or her own questions.

When Mrs. K and I joined them, both children were in a very happy frame of mind. Martin was eager to tell the story of the Indians who had had a fight with their enemies and had captured one of them.[3] He was almost gleeful as he told this story. Clarice said that the girl in the yellow dress[4] came to visit the Indians, as she was curious about them. I asked what she was curious about,

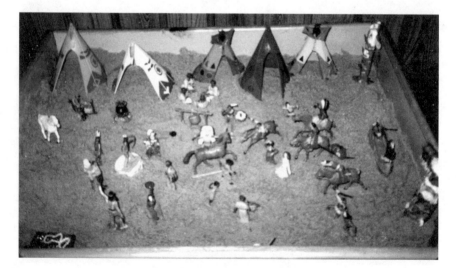

FIGURE 8.2 Indian village.

and she said that she didn't understand what the war was about. She went on to say that the Indians were trying to protect their land. Mrs. K asked about the treasure chest, and Clarice responded that it was there so that the Indians would have money to spend (this was possibly Clarice's allusion to the family's financial struggles). Mrs. K felt much calmer with this Indian scene than with the one that was discussed earlier. Parental reactions are always important, and these two scenes provided examples of Mrs. K's feeling responses to what they exhibited. She commented that the aggression displayed in the first scene (Figure 8.1) frightened her, but she felt much calmer when she saw the second (Figure 8.2). I explored these reactions with her, and she expressed the thought that "something positive was occurring." She could not verbalize what the positives were, just that she felt better. The reader is reminded that these two scenes were 4 weeks apart and others, not discussed, were produced. Space does not permit inclusion of all of the pictures.

The scene depicted in Figure 8.3 was produced 3 weeks later, during a time when Martin was again refusing to participate in the session. He seemed be feeling that there was too much focus on him during that time and responded by becoming more aggressive again. During session 7, I suggested that Mrs. K, Clarice, and I work together to make a scene to help demonstrate what we thought Martin might be feeling. Clarice put in the large and small dinosaurs with the wizard and a witch nearby, which that seemed to replicate the family constellation—the huge dinosaur perhaps being Mom; the small one, Martin (or herself). I also believed that the figures of the wizard and the witch might

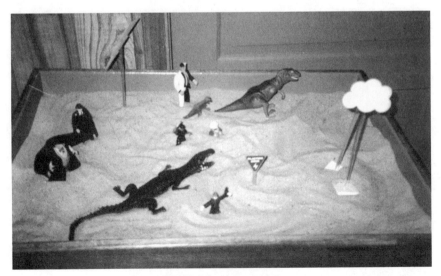

FIGURE 8.3 About Martin.

represent her parents. Mrs. K put in the scarecrow, the sign that read "Blasting Zone," and the sun hidden behind a cloud—possibly an expression of her concerns about her son. Clarice then added the lightning on the opposite side. I added the large crocodile and the two-sided man. I intended this to illustrate Martin's two sides and the strong aggression that he seemed to project. Martin had his back to us while we were making the scene. When Martin turned toward us to look at it, he was visibly upset—I assume because of how we viewed him. He quickly added the Penguin (from "Batman") and the man in the black cloak, two quite aggressive figures, then turned his back to us once again and said absolutely nothing while I tried to find some way to get him involved with the rest of us. I talked to his back as he stared out the window, telling him that the crocodile, although very scary, could also serve as a protector by keeping other, more aggressive figures away. He appeared to like this idea but continued to be resistant and mute. Martin displayed his anger in two ways: in the scenes he contributed to in sandplay as well as in his nonverbal behavior. At those times when I felt anger well up in me, I had to consciously (but nonverbally) recognize that I was, in fact, internalizing Martin's projected anger. Being attendant to my own inner process helped me to avoid expressing the anger I was feeling, because I understood that the anger was really Martin's, and not mine.

The scene depicted in Figure 8.4 was produced in the next to last session, with Mother, Martin, and Clarice all present. By now it was reported that both

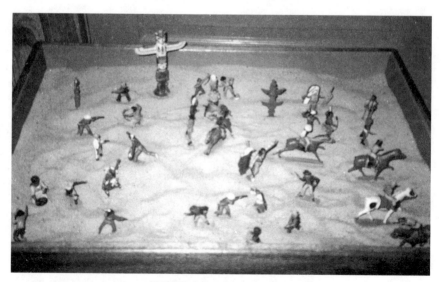

FIGURE 8.4. War and peace.

children were beginning to make friends, each one was sleeping in his or her own bed, and Mom was working on her own boundary issues in her individual therapy.

Another Indian scene is depicted here, similar to the earlier one, but the horses are moving toward the right[5]—as though they are leaving the scene—while an Indian chief is waving goodbye. The battles continue, but are far less intense. The short-term contract concluded with the stated goals having been fulfilled:

- Martin had returned to school.
- Sleeping patterns had been altered; each child now slept in his or her own bed.
- Both children had begun to move toward more independence.
- Mrs. K. had begun to "let go."

Conclusion of Case

This was a case of a very troubled family that came to treatment with issues of loss and grief, learning disabilities, and poor socialization skills. In a follow-up telephone call 3 years later, Mrs. K reported remarkable progress with both children. Martin, then 12, had become involved in football and baseball and had important positions in both sports. He had been mainstreamed out of special education and was then in a regular class achieving satisfactory marks. He was well liked by peers and teachers and no longer demonstrated clinging behavior.

Clarice, then almost 14, was involved in numerous clubs and activities. In fact, Mrs. K had to limit the number of her after-school activities. She had gone to a sleep-away camp for an entire month the previous summer and had made several new friends.

Mrs. K had completed her master's program and was working in a public school at a job in which she really seemed to excel. She said that she was happier than she had ever been, never regretted her decision to separate, but still maintained a positive working relationship with her ex-husband. Financial struggles continued to be a problem, but she was slowly getting her debts paid and had a strong sense of improved self-esteem.

This case presented compelling evidence of the effectiveness of short-term family sandplay therapy in locating the strengths in a family that had been troubled by several issues, and in helping the family then move to a healthier adaptation. The issues included parental divorce, death of a favored grandparent, poor socialization skills, overdependence on the mother, and poor parenting skills. Martin, by refusing school, was the one most responsible for getting his family into therapy. Although reticent to take part in verbal communication, he provided the stimulus for all the family members, including himself, to make significant progress, which continued until the time of follow-up 3 years later. This is not meant to imply that all of this family's problems were solved, but that the family members found the tools to support each other in difficult times and to meet obstacles that might befall them in the future. Helping this family to set appropriate boundaries seemed to be the key to a positive resolution of the major issues, enabling Mrs. K to more effectively parent each child.

I believe that this short-term model can be applied to a number of different problems, in addition to those addressed in this case. It can be effective with adjustment disorders, anxiety, depression, and bereavement and loss, to name just a few. One does not expect to "cure" all of a family's ills in a short span of time, but this is a form of treatment that can help a family address its problem situations and begin to function in a healthier way in a relatively short period of time. Needless to say, short-term therapy should be used selectively. When used judiciously, it can be a positive experience for a family.

APPENDIX 8.1. MATERIALS AND RESOURCES

Materials Needed

1. Two sandboxes, each one 19½" × 28½" × 4"; Inside bottoms are painted blue. One box contains damp sand. One box contains dry sand.
2. Miniatures of various types. The following are suggestions for miniature figures, which can be added to or subtracted from, depending on each therapist's choice; however, the categories are general.
   a. Animals: wild, domestic, prehistoric, sea creatures, birds, fish, butterflies.
   b. Living people: men, women, children; varied races; various occupations; royalty; historic; farm; soldiers; knights; cowboys; Indians.
   c. Fantasy figures: superheroes, Disney, fairies, mermaids, gnomes, etc.
   d. Transportation: Land, Sea, and air items (cars, trucks, fire trucks, police cars, ambulance; tanks, boats, ships; planes, helicopters, military).
   e. Scenery: buildings (all types), vegetation (trees, flowers), bridges, fences.
   f. Equipment: implements to make roads; farm equipment; signs, fences, children's playground, items; hospital beds, doctor kits.
   g. Miscellaneous: wishing well, coffin, rocks, shells, beads.

Sources and Resources

Sources and resources for sandplay therapy are constantly being added to. Some of my favorites are Oak Hill Specialties (wooden equipment and sandboxes; 800-615-4155); Bijou Archetypes (510-939-3111); Playrooms (800-667–2470); Self-Esteem Shop (800-251-8336); and Anna's Toy Depot (888-227-9169). Other sources can be found in the *APT NewsLetter*.

Sandplay therapists have always depended on garage sales, flea markets, dollar stores, and toystores, as well as after-Christmas ornament and crèche sales for items needed to appeal to the eyes, hearts, and unconscious processes of clients.

NOTES

1. Personal notes, D. Kalff workshop.
2. Cows often represent the positive mother archetype as they tend to their young.
3. Man who is tied to a post, center left.
4. Items that seem out of place can be explored for clarification and to focus family members on them. I believe that Clarice's use of this figure was intended to bring some attention to her needs.
5. This is a typical scene of termination. The horses are moving to the right, which can signify going into the future.

REFERENCES

Carey, L. (1991). Family sandplay therapy. *The Arts in Psychotherapy, 18*, 231–239.
Kaduson, H. G., & Schaefer, C. E. (Eds.). (2000). *Short-term play therapy for children.* New York: Guilford Press.
Kalff, D. (1980). *Sandplay: A psychotherapeutic approach to the psyche.* Santa Monica, CA: Sigo Press.
Shapiro, F., & Maxfield, L. (2003). EMDR and information processing in psychotherapy treatment: Personal development and global Implications. In M. Solomon & D. Siegel (Eds.), *Healing trauma: Attachment, mind, body, and brain.* New York: Norton.
Siegel, D. J. (1999). *The developing mind: How relationships and the brain interact to shape who we are.* New York: Guilford Press.
van der Kolk, B. A. (2003). In *terror's grip: Healing the ravages of trauma.* Printed handout from Trauma Conference, Fishkill, NY.

CHAPTER 9

Enhancing Play Therapy with Parent Consultation
A Behavioral/Solution-Focused Approach

HOLLY E. SHAW
SANDY MAGNUSON

Therapy is often a matter of tipping the first domino.
—Erickson (1948/1980)

What is important in every treatment is encouragement.
—Dreikurs (1964/1990)

One of our tasks as counselors is to assist in the process of restoring patterns of hope.
—Littrell (1998)

Parents are not always available to be fully involved in the process of play therapy. This may be for a wide variety of reasons, including problems with work, lack of commitment, or discomfort with therapy in general. Parents may be accessible for face-to-face contact only during the times they are dropping off or picking up their children.

It is beneficial for both parents and children when parents are involved in the play therapy process. This chapter presents a model of working with parents each week to use the limited amount of contact time all therapists have with parents. This is a short-term model, characterized by the play therapist working with parents briefly in consultation prior to facilitating traditional play therapy with the child. Although the parent consultation model was originally based on child-centered play therapy, this model can be used with various forms of play therapy.

Working with parents in play therapy is not a new concept. There are many well-established modes of involving parents in play therapy, including child-centered Filial Therapy (Guerney, 1964, 1991, 1997; Kraft & Landreth, 1998; Van Fleet, 1994), Theraplay (Jernberg, 1973, 1979), Parent–Child Interaction Therapy (Hembree-Kigin & McNeil, 1995), and the Adlerian model of play therapy (Kottman, 1994, 1995). Many of these modes are intensive and involve the parents as much as the child. A meta-analysis of 94 existing play therapy studies demonstrated that involving parents in the play therapy process has greater treatment effects than play therapy alone (Ray, Bratton, Rhine, & Jones, 2001) and that the effects are greatest in models of Filial Therapy in which parents are highly involved (Ray et al., 2001). Results of these inquiries strongly endorse intensive approaches as highly desirable.

But when parents are available for only brief periods, enhancing play therapy with parent consultation is an option for parents who cannot be involved in more intensive approaches, for whatever reason. This model is not equivalent to more intensive models of working with parents. Rather, it provides a way for parents to still be involved to some degree. When parents are initially included in the therapy and relationships are developed, they tend to remain involved as time goes on.

This model was developed in the context of a play therapy training clinic at a university. The target audience was master's level students needing a simple, consistent approach for working with parents. There were two positive outcomes to this approach: (1) students could begin to feel more confident in their approach toward parents, and (2) all parents could receive at least brief training and consultation.

This model would be appropriate for any play therapy clinical setting in which parents can be seen prior to or immediately after play therapy sessions. This may involve having a second person who can watch the child while the therapist and parent meet. An alternate approach is for a second therapist to provide consultation to parents while the child is in the play therapy session. In either case, it is recommended that the parents and therapist have opportunities for consultation without the child present, because the consultation time

Brief Consultation with Parents	→	Traditional Individual Play Therapy with Child and Therapist
10 minutes		40–45 minutes

FIGURE 9.1. Enhancing play therapy with parent consultation: two separate components to the therapy process.

should be considered a separate component of the process (see Figure 9.1 for the two separate components of this model, enhancing play therapy with parent consultation).

INVOLVING PARENTS IN PLAY THERAPY

Before a discussion of the model, an outline is presented of the basic beliefs about the need to involve parents, regardless of circumstances. Parents are inextricably involved in play therapy, for many reasons.

1. Parents bring their children to play therapy because they are concerned about a problem behavior. It is essential for therapists to communicate that they too are concerned about the behavior, and to communicate how play therapy may reduce it.

2. Parents who bring their children to play therapy are significantly more "depressed, upset by stress, anxious . . . and worried" (Landreth, 2002, p. 157) about their children's problems than other parents and are usually greatly relieved when help is offered.

3. Parents who bring their children to play therapy are discouraged. They may be embarrassed or afraid that they have poor parenting skills. They need positive reinforcement for their willingness to bring their children to play therapy, and for what they have done that *has worked*.

4. Even though they may not realize it at the beginning of treatment because of their frustration or discouragement, parents have the most influential and powerful relationship with their children. More than anything, children want their parents to give them attention, acceptance, and love.

5. Parents are essential allies in the play therapy process. Therapists can effect great change by working with parents, even if for only a few minutes a week. The aim is for the benefits of play therapy to extend beyond the time the child is in therapy, and strengthening the parent–child bond can greatly improve the chances of that happening.

6. Parents *will* be affected by their children's experiences in therapy. As a child changes, so will his or her relationships and the dynamics within the family.

CREATING A SHIFT IN THE FAMILY

In addition to expressing feelings and gaining self-confidence in play therapy (Landreth, 2002), children also learn how to have a connected relationship with an adult. Children learn to be in a relationship in which they are completely accepted for *who* they are—and *as* they are (Axline, 1969; Landreth, 2002). As children learn to feel safe with the play therapist, they learn that they can truly *be* with others (Axline, 1964).

Virginia Axline (1964) beautifully describes this shift in her work with a young boy in *Dibs in Search of Self*. In the beginning of Axline's story, Dibs's confidence and self-awareness are so restricted that he rarely talks to others. He is depressed and discouraged. His mother seems to be a cold person who keeps Dibs at an emotional and physical distance. From a practical viewpoint, it *appears* they will never be able to connect in a mother–son relationship and that Dibs will grow up feeling emotionally isolated and alone.

In play therapy, Dibs experiences unconditional positive regard, empathic understanding, and acceptance. As he spends time with Virginia Axline, whom he calls "Miss A" (p. 45), he learns how to engage in a relationship with an adult. As Miss A explains play therapy to Dibs, "It's a time when you can be the way you want to be . . . a time when you can be *you*" (p. 120).

After many weeks of play therapy, Dibs begins to understand what she means. Dibs reflects his comfort with play therapy when he says, "I'm in no hurry. For now, I'll just be" (p. 118). Later he says, "I think I will sing. . . . And if I want to be quiet, I'll be quiet. And if I want to think, I just think. . . . And if I want to play, I play. Like that, hmm?" (p. 127).

And so, slowly, through the process of play therapy, Dibs learns to accept and have more trust in himself. He also learns how to have a relationship with Miss A. As children learn to have a relationship with the play therapist, they also learn to have better relationships with the important people in their lives.

At one point, Miss A says it is nearly time to leave the playroom. Dibs turns the clock toward himself so that he can see it and says, "I'll have three minutes of just this. I'm being happy" (p. 149). At the end of a session Dibs says, "Soon it'll be time to go home. And when I go, I'll be all happy inside. . . . I'll be back next Thursday and fill up again with happiness" (p. 162). When he sees his mother after this session, he first looks at Miss A, then races down the hall to greet his surprised mother. He hugs her and cries out, "Oh Mother, I love you!" (p. 162). Dibs and his mother leave the office hand in hand.

After the experience of being in play therapy, it appeared that Dibs had so much happiness and so much to give that he could strengthen his relationship with his mother—even though he was a child. Dibs's relationship with his mother continued to improve after the initial play therapy sessions, and he also learned to connect to many more friends and members of his family. He was no longer depressed or discouraged.

And so within Dibs's story, the elements of family systems theory are illuminated: if change happens in one family member, the whole family will be affected. Even a small change has an enormous ripple effect throughout the family, with the whole family becoming more functional when the parent–child bond is strengthened (Kerr & Bowen, 1988; Kraft & Landreth, 1998; Minuchin, 1974; VanFleet, 1994).

The model of enhancing play therapy with consultation model rests on these assumptions and their related goals. The therapist works briefly with parents each week in order to create a small shift in the whole system.

INVOLVING PARENTS IN THE PLAY THERAPY PROCESS

As discussed earlier, the degree to which parents are involved in the play therapy process varies according to theoretical models. For example, in Gestalt therapy, Oaklander (Oaklander, 1978; Carroll, 1997) included regular consultation with parents to orient them to the therapy process and to ask about the child's environment. In Adlerian therapy, parents are deeply involved throughout the connection, exploration, assessment, and application phases (Kottman, 1995, 1999). In Theraplay, parents are actively involved in all aspects of the therapy as they can learn to encourage and nurture their children (Jernberg, 1973, 1979). In Filial Therapy, parents learn essential play therapy skills so that they can provide weekly play sessions for their children (Guerney, 1964, 1991, 1997; VanFleet, 1994). In Parent–Child Interaction Therapy, parents learn basic play therapy responding skills, which are employed during daily special playtimes of 5 minutes. In addition, they learn behavioral tools to redirect children's misbehavior (Hembree-Kigin & McNeil, 1995). In all of these models, the parents are as involved in the process as the children.

In the model of enhancing play therapy with parent consultation, parents are less involved in the process of therapy than their children. If one were to visualize a continuum of parents' involvement in play therapy, the enhancing play therapy with parent consultation model falls along the lower end of the continuum, with the models mentioned in the previous paragraph along the higher end (see Figure 9.2 for a continuum of parent involvement in play therapy).

In enhancing play therapy with parent consultation, the therapist has two concurrent roles (see Figure 9.1 for the two separate components of the model). During the initial 10 minutes of each session, the therapist adopts a consult-

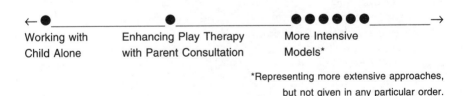

FIGURE 9.2. A continuum of parent involvement in play therapy: no involvement to intensive involvement.

ant role and meets with the parents. During the remaining time (approximately 40–45 minutes), the therapist provides individual play therapy for the child. The foundation of this model relies on a number of theories. These include consultation theories (e.g., Brown, Pryzwansky, & Schulte, 1991; Dinkmeyer & Carlson, 1973; Dougherty, 2005), behavioral theory (Bandura, 1977; Pavlov, 1910, 1927; Skinner, 1953), behavioral consultation theories (Bergan, 1977; Bergan & Kratochwill, 1990; Carlson & Dinkmeyer, 2001; Guerney, 1995), solution-focused brief therapy theory (Berg, 1990; Davis & Osborn, 2000; de Shazer, 1985; O'Hanlon & Weiner-Davis, 1989; Presbury, Echterling, & McKee, 2002; Sklare, 1997; Walter & Peller, 1992; Watts & Piertzak, 2000), and Adlerian theory (Adler, 1957, 1963; Dreikurs, 1948/1958, 1964/1990; Kottman, 1999; Lew & Bettner, 1996/2000).

The next section discusses the specific principles, derived from these theoretical approaches, that are utilized in this model. Then in the subsequent section, enhancing play therapy with parent consultation is introduced, along with the five main tasks for implementing this model with parents.

THEORY BASIS FOR OUR MODEL: ENHANCING PLAY THERAPY WITH PARENT CONSULTATION

Enhancing play therapy with parent consultation is based primarily on three theoretical approaches to therapy: (1) behavioral theory (e.g., Bergan, 1977; Bergan & Kratchwill, 1990; Pavlov, 1910, 1927; Skinner, 1953), (2) solution-focused brief therapy (de Shazer, 1985; O'Hanlon & Weiner-Davis, 1989), and (3) Adlerian theory (Adler, 1957, 1963; Dreikurs, 1948/1958, 1964/1990). The essential elements of these theories are explored in the following discussion.

Principles from Behavioral Theory

Behavioral theories are greatly influenced by the seminal work of three key scientists in the field: Ivan Pavlov (1910, 1927), B. F. Skinner (1953), and Albert Bandura (1977). In Pavlov's research related to classical conditioning, he established that each behavior has a stimulus that precedes the behavior. By identifying this *antecedent* stimulus, one can identify the most primary causal links for the behavior.

Pavlov stressed that *all behaviors are learned*, and that behaviors can also be unlearned. He further discovered that if one feared stimulus (the unconditioned stimulus) is paired frequently and regularly with a neutral stimulus, eventually that second stimulus (then called the conditioned stimulus) alone will result in the same initial behavior. For example, if a child is fearful every time he or she sees a frightening, large dog being walked by its owner, eventually the child will become fearful of the dog's owner whether or not the dog is present.

Rather than focus on the stimulus that precedes behavior, Skinner focused on what occurs immediately following the behavior, or the *consequences* of the behavior. Skinner theorized that one could predict whether *any human behavior* would be repeated or abandoned, based on whether the behavior was reinforced or punished. According to Skinner, then, *any behavior that increases has been reinforced in some manner.* Any behavior that decreases has not been reinforced, or has resulted in a punishment of some kind. Skinner also hypothesized that the more closely the reinforcement or punishment follows a behavior, the more powerful an impact it will have (Skinner, 1953).

Attention, praise, and any consequence experienced as positive are reinforcements. Positive reinforcement is highly personal; things that one person experiences as positive may not be seen as desirable by another. For example, a child who acts out in class and then gets attention from the teacher may find the attention to be extremely reinforcing, whereas another child would be horrified by it. Removing something aversive can also be seen as a reinforcement—note the classic example of learning to put on a car seat belt to turn off the annoying buzzer.

Punishment can be applied by administering something unpleasant, such as giving a time-out. A behavior can also be punished by removing something pleasant, such as removing a privilege for a child.

Bandura (1977) also stressed that reinforcement and punishment can occur vicariously when a person sees the consequences of another's behavior. In other words, if a child sees another child receiving recognition or a reward for a certain behavior, he or she may imitate that behavior expecting to also be rewarded.

Principles from Solution-Focused Brief Therapy

Brief therapy was traditionally used in the field of family counseling. It is now used widely in a variety of sectors, including individual counseling and school counseling. Contemporary solution-focused approaches were greatly influenced by the work of Milton Erickson, Steve de Shazer, Insoo Kim Berg, Michelle Weiner-Davis, and Bill O'Hanlon.

Some underpinnings of solution-focused brief therapy models differ dramatically from traditional therapy orientations. For example, acquisition of an extensive history and examination of the etiology of problems are not emphasized. Rather, the focus is on current behavioral patterns and interactions. Yet, many aspects of the solution-focused approach are complementary to other common approaches to therapy, such as (1) the centrality of the relationship, (2) the belief that reality is subjective, (3) a nonpathological focus, and (4) an emphasis on facilitating change.

Solution-focused therapists use language that is positive. They *focus on what is working* for clients. Solution-focused approaches are based on the assumptions that *the situation will be resolved, the client has the resources to find a workable solution,* and *change is inevitable* (de Shazer, 1985; O'Hanlon & Weiner-Davis, 1989.)The precise use of language in solution-focused approaches is critical. By consistently focusing on resolution, solution-focused therapists set up expectations for change (de Shazer, 1985). Essential components of solution-focused approaches include (1) joining with the client, (2) identifying the problem, (3) identifying exceptions to the problem, (4) articulating goals, (5) giving compliments, and (6) assigning tasks.

Even within this brief therapy model, the facilitation of rapport and a working alliance is critical. This is the crucial task of *joining* with clients. Adopting clients' language patterns contributes to rapport, therefore therapists refrain from using jargon. As therapists reflect and respond with similar or related phrases and terminology, clients feel that they are understood (O'Hanlon & Weiner-Davis, 1989).

When helping clients identify primary concerns, it is important to fully understand how a problem is experienced. Thus, the therapist might ask, "What about Luke's behavior is most problematic for you?" (Carlson & Dinkmeyer, 2001). When identifying the problem, it is also critical to begin to use language that is focused on solutions. The therapist might ask, "How do you think starting this therapy process will be most helpful to you and Luke?" This helps clients imagine desired outcomes, rather than focus only on problems.

In addition, much attention is given to identification of exceptions, solutions, and strengths. For example, the therapist might say to the client, "Tell me about a time last week when Jill *did* complete a task on her own." This prompts the to client begin recognizing exceptions when the child is behaving well.

The articulation of goals begins to surface as clients consider exceptions and strengths. With careful selection of terminology, therapists create mental images of resolutions to difficulties previously discussed. They use questions such as "What will David *do differently* during mealtimes when he stops fighting with his brother?"

The use of compliments is another fundamental aspect of solution-focused approaches. Compliments focus the family members' attention on existing strengths that will contribute to achieving the desired outcomes. Such compliments may include "I can tell that you have a very deep concern about Jose" or "You saw that Nick needed your help way before the situation got out of hand." These compliments are resources for clients to overcome their challenges; in addition, clients may be energized to invest in working with the therapist.

Finally, with a solution-focused approach, therapists typically end a session by assigning a task (de Shazer, 1985). De Shazer typically gives this first-session task: "Pay attention to what happens during the week at times when things are going well. I'd like to hear about those times next week." Again, the language and the task help clients focus on what is working, and on potential solutions.

Principles from Adlerian Theory

Alfred Adler (1957, 1963) developed individual psychology as a reaction to psychoanalysis and as a reflection of his humanistic beliefs. Adler suggested that human beings are primarily social, goal-directed, and creative beings (Dinkmeyer, Dinkmeyer, & Sperry, 1987; Kottman, 1999). These three aspects of the Adlerian philosophy fit well with solution-focused approaches, particularly the assumptions that clients have the resources they need and that they will be able to find solutions for their problems.

In addition, the concept of phenomenology is central to Adlerian theory. Each human being's experience is unique and must be understood from his or her point of view. Accordingly, even in a family that has had a shared history, each person in that family has had a different experience of the events. This belief is consistent with the solution-focused premise that reality is subjective and that the client's reality is important.

Adler and his followers provided a rich, detailed model for working with clients, which includes extensive assessment in a number of different areas. For the purposes of this chapter, the focus is on three essential aspects of an Adlerian approach to working with clients. In addition to that drawn from Adler, work is also drawn from Adler's former student, Rudolph Dreikurs. Dreikurs popularized many of Adler's ideas in the United States upon the publication of his book *Children the Challenge*, first published in 1964 (1964/1990).

When Dreikurs wrote about encouragement, he wrote that encouragement "is more important than any other aspect of child-raising . . . [and] the lack of it can be considered the basic cause for misbehavior" (Dreikurs, 1964/ 1990, p. 36). Children need to be given an opportunity to try things on their own and must be given encouragement to do so. A child who is misbehaving is a child who is not receiving encouragement (Dreikurs, 1964/1990).

From a behavioral point of view, the lack of encouragement is analogous to a lack of positive reinforcements. The child who is not receiving positive reinforcements, or positive attention for good behaviors, will eventually stop repeating those behaviors. The child will seek attention in some other way, usually as negative attention. If negative attention is all that is available, then the child will focus on negative attention. Pure behaviorists believe that a lack of positive reinforcement also has another consequence: the onset of depression.

Parents also need encouragement. When they feel that their parenting methods are not working and that they are receiving little positive attention for their efforts, they too become discouraged. When parents bring their children to play therapy, they are often suffering from both (1) feelings of discouragement and (2) a lack of positive reinforcement about what they are doing right as parents. The aspect of giving parents compliments in a solution-focused approach is also compatible with this theory of providing more positive reinforcement.

Feeling connected is also a strategic aspect of Adlerian theory. Adler believed that social interest is crucial to being psychologically healthy (Adler, 1957, 1963). Children need to feel connected to their families and to feel that they are unique, important individuals in the families. Lew and Bettner (1996/2000) described this in children as the need to feel connected, the need to feel capable, the need to count and feel special, and the need to have courage to try new behaviors. Lew and Bettner called these the "Crucial Cs" (Lew & Bettner, 1996/2000, p.3).

Adler and Dreikurs also wrote about *the four main reasons that children misbehave* (Adler, 1957, 1963; Dreikurs, 1964/1990). In addition to the general tenet that children who misbehave are not receiving adequate encouragement, there is a conviction that children who have repeated patterns of misbehavior have specific goals. Children who are misbehaving as a pattern are acting to (1) get attention, (2) achieve more power, (3) get revenge, or (4) avoid new or difficult tasks (Dreikurs, 1964/1990). Adler and Dreikurs called these *mistaken goals*, inasmuch as what such children really need is to feel connected. Both Lew and Bettner (1996/2000) and Terry Kottman (1995, 1999) write a great deal about the connection between children's misbehaviors and the Crucial Cs.

ENHANCING PLAY THERAPY WITH PARENT CONSULTATION: THE FIVE KEY TASKS

The theory base for the model having been established, the focus now shifts to a thorough description of implementing the model with parents. This implementation of the model is illustrated by a description of the five key tasks (see Table 9.1).

Task 1: Work in a Consultation Model

The first task is to work with parents in a consultation model. The therapist works with parents briefly each week, therefore it is crucial that working alliances are

TABLE 9.1. Enhancing Play Therapy with Parent Consultation

Five Key Tasks

1. Work in a consultation model.
2. Define child's problems using a behavioral model.
3. Use solution-focused language.
4. Increase positive reinforcement in the family system.
5. Consult with parents about common reasons children misbehave.

developed quickly. To this end, the therapist strives to provide conditions such that parents feel included, respected, and valued during the therapist's limited time with them. The therapist must also endeavor to facilitate an egalitarian, collaborative relationship with them (Brown et al., 1991; Dougherty, 2005; Noell & Witt, 1996; Zins & Erchul, 1995).

The therapist's role is to work on the behavior problems that concern the parents and assist them in finding workable solutions. The therapist wants to hear the parents' point of view regarding the behavior problems and inquires about what happens before and after the behaviors occur. Brainstorming with the parents about possible solutions, and inviting them to select the solution or the strategy they wish to try during the following week, are also important (Brown et al., 1991; Dougherty, 2005).

Within the consultation system of this model, the parent is the consultee, the child is the client, and the therapist is the consultant (Dougherty, 2005; Mannino & Shore, 1986). In the consultant role, the therapist works with parents with the goal of empowering them to competently address current concerns as well as similar concerns that develop in the future (Dougherty, 2005). Thus, the therapist and parent may discuss responses to specific misbehaviors or strategies for building a stronger parent–child relationship.

It is preferable that play therapists meet with parents prior to initiating contact with the child. Such preliminary sessions provide an opportunity for therapists to inquire about parents' concerns and desires, provide information about play therapy, contract for services, and complete intake procedures. In addition, the play therapists can assist the parents in explaining play therapy to their children. During the initial interactions with parents, it is important to clarify the therapist's diverse roles. The therapist explains that the consultation role is to help parents more effectively respond to the needs of their children. It is appropriate to discuss the differences between the consultation portion with parents and the therapy session with children.

Regardless of the structure or scheduling of the first contact with parents, establishing a working alliance is critical. In order to optimize the benefit of this model, the parents must experience positive regard, caring, and empathic understanding (as outlined in Rogers, 1961). They must have a sense that the therapist is listening to them and that their concerns are being understood. Thus, the therapist needs to reflect feelings about frustration and discouragement as well as pride and relief, to let them know that the therapist is listening intently.

In the consultant role, the therapist does not provide therapy for parents. The purpose of consultation is to help parents to be more effective with their children. The goal is to improve parenting skills and strengthen parent–child relationships. Consultants, "even if they are trained therapists, never provide counseling or psychotherapy to consultees [parents]" (Dougherty, 2000, p. 15).

If a parent needs therapy, he or she should be referred to a separate therapist for work on personal problems.

Having previously met with the parents during the preliminary meeting, the therapist can then focus full attention on the child when he or she first comes to the office. Garry Landreth (2002) suggests that the therapist should approach the child first, kneeling to facilitate eye contact, and initiate an invitational conversation. Then, the therapist can take the child to the playroom when he or she believes the child is psychologically prepared.

At the conclusion of the first session, it is important to explain to the child the format for subsequent sessions. For example, "I will see you again next week. When you come then, I will spend a few minutes with your parents while you stay in the waiting room. Then you and I will go to the playroom for the rest of the time. We'll do that each week when you come."

Some play therapists might think to themselves, "I don't know enough about parenting to be a consultant" or "I don't have any business telling people how to be better parents to their children. They know their problems better than I do." In a consultation model, the therapist works from an assumption that the parents *do know more* about their children than we can possibly know. They do know more about the problems they are having, and often what might work best, than we do. In a consultation model, therapists do not tell the parents what to do. They are cautious about giving advice and finding the solutions for the parents. Rather, therapists find ways to empower parents to find solutions for themselves. In Table 9.1, the five main areas of focus in enhancing play therapy with consultation are summarized.

Task 2: Define Child's Problems Using a Behavioral Model

Parents often bring their child to play therapy because they believe that their child's problems are beyond change. Often, they have developed a negative view of the child and see behavioral issues as immutable character flaws.

One of the most important tasks the therapist can perform is to help the parents frame misbehaviors with language that provides specific and measurable goals (Henning-Stout, 1993). By viewing problems from a behavioral perspective, the therapist focuses on principles such as behavior antecedents and consequences of behavior (Skinner, 1953), as well as concrete measurement issues such as frequency and duration of behaviors (Henning-Stout, 1993).

The therapist can reframe behaviors to help parents understand that behaviors are specific responses to a situation rather than character flaws in the child. Parents can then be helped to understand this by focusing on the behavior problems in a specific and practical manner.

In this regard, the combination of essential tenets of behavioral theory (Pavlov, 1910, 1927; Skinner, 1953) and behavioral consultation models

(Bergan, 1977; Bergan & Kratochwill, 1990; Henning-Stout, 1993; Dougherty, 2005) is applicable:

- The focus in on current, not past, behaviors.
- All behaviors are learned responses.
- New behaviors can be learned to replace old behaviors.
- In order to change behaviors, they must first be reduced to aspects that are observable and measurable. This includes the time of the day a behavior occurs and the frequency and length of the behavior.
- Whether or not a behavior continues depends on (1) what stimulus precedes the behavior and (2) the immediate consequences of the behavior.
- By identifying what is causing and reinforcing behaviors, parents can begin to find alternate solutions that do not reinforce undesirable behaviors.
- By identifying what is causing and reinforcing behaviors, parents can begin to find alternate solutions that positively reinforce behaviors they would like to increase.

Behavioral consultation is guided by a simple step-by-step process of evaluation of each kind of problem behavior (Carlson & Dinkmeyer, 2001; Dougherty, 2005; Lutzker & Martin, 1981). This evaluation includes directives for the therapist to ask parents a series of questions about each behavior of concern, as outlined here (Carlson & Dinkmeyer, 2001; Dougherty, 2005).

1. Describe what it is that your child is doing that is concerning you. (Identifying the behavior of concern.)
2. Provide a specific example of when he (or she) did that in the past week.
3. How did you respond when your child did that? (What was the parent's response to the child?)
4. Did your child stop or continue with the behavior after that? (Did the behavior increase or decrease after the parent's response?)
5. What else might you do differently?

Often, identifying the events that transpire right before a misbehavior can lead to a solution. For example, if a child demands excessive attention at approximately the same time in the late afternoon, one theory might be that the child is hungry and that an afternoon snack is important for this child, or that the child is tired. However, identifying the events that happen right after a misbehavior can also be illuminating. For example, a child who cannot get attention by excelling in schoolwork, but always gets appreciative laughter from fellow students when acting as the class clown, has found a way to get the reinforcement he or she is not getting otherwise. By identifying the events leading up to the misbehavior (the antecedents) and the events happening after the misbehavior (the consequences) (Skinner, 1953), the therapist and the parents (and the teacher, for school behaviors) can identify the kinds of situations that trigger or maintain misbehaviors.

From this point on, the therapist and the parent can brainstorm about (1) other ways to prevent stimuli that set off the child, or (2) different ways to respond if the child does misbehave. If the behavior happens at school, the teacher should be consulted as well, with the parents' permission, so that parents and teachers are responding to the misbehavior in the same fashion. The following week, the therapist can ask the parent if the child's behavior improved or escalated. The therapist can continually assess the frequency and duration of the behavior each week with the parents to ascertain the effects.

If there are improvements in behavior, it is extremely important that the therapist reinforce the changes in the child's behavior, no matter how small the changes. A simple comment such as, "Lupe did her math homework on her own 4 days this week!" is an essential anchoring for the parent of the child's behavior change. Parents who are discouraged by parenting are greatly relieved to get this kind of positive feedback from therapists.

Task 3: Use Solution-Focused Language

In the consultation model *the therapist focuses on the parents' perceptions of their children's behavior, as well as directly addressing the behavior.* In addition, the therapist assists the parents in finding approaches that work with their children. This consultation with parents is augmented with powerful, intentional language patterns from a solution-focused approach (de Shazer, 1985; O'Hanlon & Weiner-Davis, 1989). Precision in language allows the limited time with parents to be maximized. Solution-focused questions are utilized to identify characteristics of times when the behavior does *not* occur. Reframing and normalizing are also relied upon.

The most prominent solution-focused strategy used in this approach with parents is presuppositional language, used throughout work with parents and children to send subtle, yet consistent messages that resolution of the current concerns is a foregone conclusion. A simple, yet powerful example is the substitution of *when* for *if* and *will* for *would*, as illustrated in Table 9.2.

However, the intentional use of presuppositional language is not at the expense of basic helping skills such as empathic responding. Comments such as "You love your son and you are worried about him" and "You have your hands full with three active boys so close to the same age" are useful. The goal is for the parents to express their concerns on their terms, to experience positive regard and respect, and to leave with the sense that they have been heard and understood.

TABLE 9.2. The Use of Presuppositional Language

Problem-focused approach	Presuppositional language (solution-focused approach)
"If she could learn to control her tantrums, she wouldn't get into trouble at school."	"When she starts to control her tantrums, she will do better at school."
"If he would start to assume responsibility, that would fix the problem."	"When he starts assuming responsibility, how will you know?"
"So his problem is ADHD."	"So your challenge is to help him to learn how to manage his behavior so he will be successful at school."
"She is a poor student."	"She is having difficulty with science, but has learned ways that work well for her in social studies."
"He can't do math."	"He has not learned to multiply and divide yet."
"Jill is so defiant, she even refuses to put her toys away."	"Jill hasn't learned to put her toys away yet."

Another important aspect of consulting with parents in a solution-focused manner involves normalizing behavior. Sometimes parents have unrealistic expectations for their children, which may be based on inaccurate comparisons with other children. It can be helpful to mention that many 5-year-old children are challenged by tasks that involve a number of steps, such as cleaning a room. Therapists can also point out that some behavior is developmentally appropriate (e.g., "Sometimes we adults forget how enormous the transition from kindergarten to first grade can be for a 6-year-old.")

In this model, therapists can regularly employ scaling. For example, after the parent describes a problem, the therapist may say, "I'd like you to think of Maria's current challenges during the past week on a 1 to 10 scale. Let's say that a 1 is a terrible week. She refuses to do anything you ask. She fights with her brother. She even gets in trouble at her soccer game. That would be a 1. A week when she follows your directions, sometimes even before you give them, would be a 10. She happily shares her toys with her brother, and she behaves well at her soccer game even though her team loses. Where would you rank Maria's behavior during the past week?" (This sequence of questions can be followed with an exploration of exceptions, or days when Maria's behavior was better than on others). The scale's value can be amplified with related questions such as, "OK. You say 6. Let's say you come next week and rank Maria's behavior, overall, as 7. What will she do between now and our next session so that you will be able to say 7?" Revisiting this scale each week can identify and document improvement for parents.

Modifications of the de Shazer's (1985) miracle question is often used as we endeavor to establish goals. As appropriate, the therapist may say something such as, "I'd like you to imagine that one night in the next month—maybe in 5 weeks, possibly in 3—during the night a miracle happens, and the concerns you have shared with me this afternoon are completely resolved, though you don't know about the miracle. What will happen the next morning that will alert you to the possibility that the miracle has occurred? "

As the parents respond, the therapist becomes tenacious in facilitating clear descriptions in behavioral terms. For example, the therapist might say, "Please forgive me. Sometimes I tend to be concrete. What will Dakota do differently when he wakes up and his 'attitude' is gone? . . . What else will he do? . . . Who else will notice? . . . How will you be different?" And then further along, the therapist might say, "Let's imagine that I am watching through a video monitor—what will I notice that morning as I observe your family?"

The therapist then follows this discussion by saying, "Usually miracles don't happen overnight. They take a bit longer. What are some very small first steps that will let you know that the miracle has begun to happen?" The outcome of this sequence of questions often parallels a behavioral plan. First steps are established, and the goal is clarified. The language accentuates that there will be change, and that it will be gradual. In addition, the parents have a frame of reference for recognizing initial steps that lead to the ultimate goal.

The therapist may choose not to ask parents the miracle question because he or she has a hunch that it may not work well. The therapist may reserve the miracle question for a time when meeting with both children and parents. In that case, the therapist would modify the miracle question to talk to them together. "It's important to me that all of you are happy with coming here. I'd like you to imagine that we have worked together for many weeks. And, sometime after that, you say to a friend, 'I'm so glad we did the play therapy with Lia! Things are so much better for our family now.' What will be happening in your family so that you will be able to say that? . . . . What else?"

Another guiding concept is Michelle Weiner-Davis's notion that excellent therapists invite their clients to teach them how to work with them (O'Hanlon & Weiner-Davis, 1989). In this regard, if the therapy with a family is working, don't fix it! When something does work, continue using that approach. And when one approach is ineffective, try something else.

Task 4: Increase Positive Reinforcement in the Family System

Another focus of this model is increasing the amount of positive reinforcement in the family system. As discussed earlier in regard to Adlerian theory, both children and parents need encouragement (Dreikurs, 1964/1990; Lew & Bettner, 1996/2000; Kottman, 1999). Sometimes a family has a child who has been labeled as a troublemaker or the scapegoat. This child may receive an abundance of negative attention and a dearth of positive attention. In these cases, interventions can be set up that result in positive attention for the child.

A number of options can be used by parents to "catch the child" performing a good behavior so that it can be reinforced (Severe, 1997/2000). Parents can make a chart that identifies two or three desired behaviors, to keep track of over a period of a week. For a preschooler, the behaviors may include getting dressed in the morning, putting dirty clothes in the hamper, and washing hands before dinner. When children perform these behaviors on their own, they get stickers or stars on the chart. At the end of each week, they may receive an additional reinforcement, such as a special event with a parent, like watching a movie together or going for a bike ride together (Severe, 1997/2000). In this way, the parents and children learn that good behavior can result in positive outcomes for all.

Another simple form of intervention involves keeping a log of desired behaviors that rarely occur. In this instance, it may not be helpful to keep track of how many times a child performs the behavior in a week. The therapist can make a "chart" that consists of about five to ten items to color on a page. These items may be different animals. Each time the child performs the desired behavior, he or she gets to color in a new animal. When all of the animals are colored, the child receives reinforcement, such as a special event with the parent. In this way the focus is on reinforcing the behavior whenever it does occur, without putting a time limit on it.

For example, a parent may be concerned that his or her 5-year-old child is rarely using manners. The therapist can suggest that the parent make a chart to specifically note when the child *does remember*. The therapist can suggest keeping track of when the child uses words like "please" and "thank you" by allowing the child to color one of the five to ten items on a chart. The child is thus reinforced any time that he or she chooses to be polite. The behavior will then likely increase because of the added focus and the reinforcement of the chart. The chart should be focused on a single behavior that the parent wants to stress at a time (Severe, 1997/2000).

In addition to increasing the positive reinforcements for the child, it is crucial that the parents receive positive reinforcements for their successes as well. Parents need to be reminded about what is working for them in their parenting and in their relationships with their children. It is a goal of this model that reinforcing parents will eventually filter down to their providing more positive reinforcement for the children. All of this should help parents and children feel a greater connection (Kottman, 1994, 1995, 1999; Lew & Bettner, 1996/2000; VanFleet, 1994).

Task 5: Educate Parents about Common Reasons Children Misbehave

Eight half-page parent handouts that include typical reasons for children misbehaving are included here (see Figures 9.3–9.10). Therapists need to be aware that there may be barriers to reading the material in parent handouts. Handouts may not be appropriate for certain parents if reading in general is a difficulty. For others, it will be necessary and appropriate to have handouts translated and printed in the parents' primary language.

Typically, one handout is given to parents each week. The purpose is to provide a resource that is useful and understandable, yet not overwhelming or impractical because of length. For example, parents can be advised that behaviors can be reinforced or punished and provided with strategies based on simple behavioral theory (e.g., Bandura, 1977; Guerney, 1995; Pavlov, 1910, 1927; Severe, 1997/2000; Skinner, 1953) for increasing desirable behaviors and decreasing misbehaviors.

Therapists also talk to parents in behavioral terms about what they see while working with the child in play therapy. For example, they talk to parents about how limits are typically set in the play therapy room (Axline, 1969; Landreth, 2002) and how the child responds. The therapist can approach this as a collaborative effort by saying something like, "John seems to respond well to these limits in the playroom. If we use the same language, it would probably become even more effective in helping him control his behavior here and at home" (see Figure 9.8).

When talking about patterns of misbehavior in a child, the therapist can briefly explain Adler's theory regarding the goals of misbehavior and how they may relate to a child's unmet needs. According to Adler, children don't discard or abandon behaviors that are working for them (Dreikurs, 1964/1990; Carlson & Dinkmeyer, 2001). Within this paradigm, when children misbehave, it is because they have a mistaken goal. The therapist can explain that children are trying to fulfill an unmet need; however, their efforts are inappropriate (see Figure 9.9). By examining each behavior, parents are helped to identify ways they can respond to the misbehavior without reinforcing it. In addition, the therapist can assist them in developing strategies that respond to children's needs (Dreikurs, 1964/1990; Lew & Bettner, 1996/2000; Kottman, 1999; see Figure 9.10).

Because the therapist works from a model of parent consultation, it is essential for him or her to proceed collaboratively when speaking with parents about misbehavior and the concept of mistaken goals. The therapist should describe the four mistaken goals first, and then ask the parents to consider how specific mistaken goals might be related to the child's current behavioral problem. It is important that the parent identify the mistaken goal rather than the therapist, if possible. Parents may need time to contemplate these questions; thus, it may be appropriate to continue the discussion during the subsequent session.

Sequence of events:

1. The child does a specific behavior at a particular point in time.
2. The parent responds to the child's behavior.
3. The child's behavior either increases or decreases.

Reinforcement: Any response by the parent that results in an increase of a specific behavior by the child

Punishment: Any response by the parent that results in a decrease of a specific behavior by the child

Two guidelines: The closer in time the response is to the behavior, the more effective; and the more connected the response is to the behavior, the more effective.

FIGURE 9.3. Parent handout: reinforcement versus punishment.

Reinforcement: Give child something positive, or take away something negative.

Punishment: Take away something positive, or give child something negative.

	Something Positive	Something Negative
Take Away from Child	Punishment	Reinforcement
Give to Child	Reinforcement	Punishment

FIGURE 9.4. Parent handout: responding to a child's misbehavior.

When your child does something that you want, be sure to give positive reinforcement.

What is positive reinforcement? Praise, hugs, attention from you. In other words, *anything that is seen as positive by your child.*

List things you could do that you think would be reinforcing for *your child.*

1. _____
2. _____
3. _____

FIGURE 9.5 Parent handout: increasing desirable behaviors.

Identify behaviors that your child is currently showing that *you want to continue.* Your child rarely shows the behavior. You wish that he or she would do it more often.

Examples: Using good manners, putting own dishes away.

1. _____
2. _____
3. _____

FIGURE 9.6. Parent handout: identifying good behaviors.

Parents are often concerned that the only way to reduce a behavior is to punish.

Other ways to decrease a behavior:

1 Notice when your child is behaving in ways that you desire, and reinforce!!!
2. Make sure you do not reinforce negative behavior (example: your child seems to be trying to get you upset, or cause you to get angry).
3. Take away a privilege (no TV for a half-hour, no desert tonight, etc.).

Note: When focusing on negative behaviors, pick only one or two priority behaviors to address at one time.

FIGURE 9.7. Parent handout: decreasing negative behaviors—what are the options?

Using the three-part limit that is often used in play therapy:

1. Clearly state the limit, and provide an alternative if possible.
2. If your child repeats the behavior, repeat the limit. Then add the consequence that will follow if he or she does repeat.
3. If your child continues the behavior, state that he or she chose to break the limit, and follow through on the consequence.

Example:

1. "Walls are not for drawing on. You may draw on the paper if you like."
2. "You chose to draw on the wall again. If you choose to do that again, I will put the crayons away for the day."
3. "You chose to make another mark on the wall. The crayons will be put away for the day."

FIGURE 9.8. Parent handout: setting clear limits with your children. After Axline (1969) and Landreth (2002).

When children behave a certain way, they have a purpose. Any pattern of repeated misbehavior should be analyzed by asking, "What is the child trying to accomplish?"

Four reasons that children misbehave:

1. To gain attention.
2. To have power.
3. To get revenge.
4. To avoid having to do something difficult.

Think of a pattern of behaviors your child exhibits, and identify the reason (or reasons) that might fit.

FIGURE 9.9. Parent handout: patterns of repeated misbehavior. After Adler (1957, 1963) and Dreikurs (1964/1990).

Once the parents and the therapist have identified the mistaken goal, the parents will have a clearer idea of what the child is actually trying to accomplish and how these needs can be better met (see Figure 9.10). The aim of this exploration is to discover ways to help reduce misbehavior, continuing the behavioral focus on specific and measurable aspects of the child's actions.

Lew and Bettner (1996/2000) provide a number of excellent charts that can be shown to parents to help them identify the pattern behavior that seems to match their child's misbehavior. In addition, Kottman (1999) beautifully described the ways in which all misbehaving children are striving to connect with one or more of the Crucial Cs.

It is essential to keep in mind that some parents are already frustrated and overwhelmed with parenting responsibilities. It is important to avoid overwhelming them with information. As they become more comfortable and involved in the process, some parents may gain interest in certain subjects. When parents express interest in getting more information, therapists can suggest resources.

For these parents, therapists should keep a library of favorite books for them to borrow. Therapists shouldn't overload parents, but should instead lend one book at a time so that they have time to assimilate the information and identify parts that are useful to them. It is also helpful to focus on a single brief topic or chapter a week, rather than an entire book. During subsequent consultation meetings, parents can be asked what was most useful for them.

1. *If your child is trying to get attention with negative behavior . . .*
   The behavior will decrease if he or she can get positive attention for good behaviors.
   Children attempt to gain attention with negative behavior if they are not getting positive attention in other ways.
2. *If you think your child is trying to get power . . .*
   Find ways to give him or her more choices and possibly more responsibility. Help your child feel capable.
3. *If you think your child is trying to get revenge . . .*
   He or she may not feel connected to the family. For some reason, your child may feel as if he or she doesn't belong or count as much as others. Find ways to demonstrate and communicate that your child is an important and unique part of your family.
4. *If you believe that your child is avoiding activities that are hard for him or her . . .*
   Your child may be discouraged. Find ways to reinforce what he or she is doing well and encourage him or her. Work with your child on difficult tasks until he or she gains more confidence. Express your confidence in his or her ability to complete tasks.

FIGURE 9.10. Parent handout: reducing a repeated misbehavior. After Dreikurs (1964/ 1990), Lew and Bettner (1996/2000), and Kottman (1999).

There are many excellent parenting resources. The following three books are especially helpful with behavioral issues and encouragement. They are also easy to read and provide practical, useful exercises:

- *Parenting: A Skills Training Manual* by Louise F. Guerney (1995).
- *A Parent's Guide to Understanding and Motivating Children* by Amy Lew and Betty Lou Bettner (1996/2000).
- *How to Behave So Your Children Will Too* by Saul Severe (1997/2000).

As parents express continued interest, they can be provided with books that are more complex. In such cases, the following books are helpful:

- *How to Talk So Kids Will Listen and Kids Will Talk* by Adele Faber and Elaine Mazlish (1980/1999).
- *Children: The Challenge* by Rudolph Dreikurs (1964/1990).
- *Raising a Thinking Child* by Myrna B. Shure (1994).

Obviously, many other books addressing special subjects of interest, such as behavioral problems related to parents' separation, divorce, illness, and legal issues are readily available.

LIMITATIONS OF THE ENHANCING PLAY THERAPY WITH PARENT CONSULTATION MODEL

Because this is a brief model of working with parents, parents who remain uncommitted may not benefit a great deal. Consultation involves cooperation, and unless parents are involved during the 5- to 10-minute consultation period, it can function as little more than a brief check-in about the child's behavior for the week. The success of this model lies in motivating and involving parents, and much depends on establishing a positive working relationship with them.

Indeed, it can be frustrating to work with parents who do not seem invested in the therapeutic process or in nurturing their children. In this regard, we appreciate and endeavor to remain cognizant of Axline's (1964) reminder:

> Sometimes it is very difficult to keep firmly in mind the fact that parents, too, have reasons for what they do—have reasons locked in the depths of their personalities for their inability to love, to understand, to give of themselves to their own children. (pp. 80–81)

This approach is not appropriate for every family. Some parents need more assistance than we can provide during this brief consultation. For some parents, consultation may not be feasible if the therapist cannot converse in their primary language and another, more appropriate therapist cannot be found. Other parents are not able to participate at any level for a variety of reasons, about which we may not know.

At the same time, in order to endeavor to enact greater change for the family and for the child, working with the parents is a must during the play therapy process. In this regard, there must always be the hope that positive change in a family system will have a lasting and essential effect. Sometimes the greatest work that therapists do is never completely visible, yet they may have facilitated a shift in a family system that is powerful and immutable.

STRENGTHS OF THE ENHANCING PLAY THERAPY WITH PARENT CONSULTATION MODEL

For parents who are willing to participate, the brief consultation approach can be quite helpful. As parents become more involved, they learn about the play therapy process and they have weekly support in coping with their parenting stress. They get reinforcement as they become familiar with new parenting practices, and they receive assistance in identifying their own solutions to the challenges they encounter with their children.

As parents become more accustomed to consultation, their stress level may be reduced. They may also begin to see their children's behavior in a more manageable and positive light. They may become more empowered as parents and feel a stronger connection with their children. As they recognize the advantages of their involvement, parents may decide to participate in more intensive programs such as filial therapy or parent–child interaction therapy.

And that is the overriding hope during work with parents in a brief consultation model. Even working with parents each week may provide catalysts for positive paradigm shifts that will eventually ripple throughout the family system (see Table 9.3).

TABLE 9.3. Final Summary of Enhancing Play Therapy with Parent Consultation

Overall objectives of working with parents:

1. Motivate parents to have their child stay involved in play therapy.
2. Help the parents to increase positive behaviors in their child.
3. Help the parents to develop a more positive view of their child.
4. Help the parents to reduce the child's misbehavior that motivated them to bring the child to therapy.
5. Encourage the parents. Recognize their efforts throughout the process.
6. Strengthen the parent–child relationship.
7. Help parents effectively meet the needs of their child.

REFERENCES

Adler, A. (1957). *Understanding human nature.* New York: Premier Books.

Adler, A. (1963). *The problem child.* New York: Capricorn Books.

Axline, V. (1964). *Dibs in search of self.* New York: Ballantine Books.

Axline, V. (1969). *Play therapy.* New York: Ballantine Books.

Bandura, A. (1977). *Social leaning theories.* Englewood Cliffs, NJ: Prentice-Hall.

Berg, I. (1990). *Solution-focused approach to family-based services.* Milwaukee: Brief Family Therapy Center.

Bergan, J. R. (1977). *Behavioral consultation.* Columbus, OH: Merrill.

Bergan, J. R., & Kratochwill, I . R. (1990). *Behavioral consultation and therapy.* New York: Plenum Press.

Brown, D., Pryzwansky, D. J., & Schulte, A. C. (1991). *Psychological consultation: Introduction to theory and practice* (2nd ed.). Boston: Allyn & Bacon.

Carlson, J., & Dinkmeyer, D. (Speakers). (2001). *Consultation process and skills: Working with teachers and parents* (Video Recording). New York: Brunner-Routledge.

Carroll, J. (1997). *Introduction to therapeutic play*. Blackwell Science.

Davis, T. E., & Osborn, C. J. (2000). *The solution-focused school counselor: Shaping professional practice*. Philadelphia: Accelerated Development.

de Shazer, S. (1985). *Keys to solution in brief therapy*. New York: Norton.

Dinkmeyer, D., & Carlson, J. (1973). *Consulting: Facilitating human potential and change processes*. Columbus, OH: Merrill.

Dinkmeyer, D., Dinkmeyer, D., & Sperry, L. (1987). *Adlerian counseling and psychotherapy* (2nd ed.). Columbus, OH: Merrill.

Dougherty, A. M. (2000). *Psychological consultation and collaboration* (3rd ed.). Belmont, CA: Brooks/Cole.

Dougherty, A. M. (2005). *Psychological consultation and collaboration* (4th ed.). Belmont, CA: Brooks/Cole.

Dreikurs, R. (1958). *The challenge of parenthood*. New York: Duell, Sloan and Pearce. (Original work published 1948)

Dreikurs, R. (1990). *Children: The challenge*. New York: Penguin Books. (Original work published 1964)

Erickson, M. (1980). Hypnotic psychotherapy. In E. L. Rossi, (Ed.), *The collected works of Milton H. Erickson on hypnosis* (Vol. 4, pp. 149–173). New York: Irvington. (Original work published 1948)

Faber, A., & Mazlish, E. (1999). *How to talk so kids will listen and listen so kids will talk*. New York: HarperCollins. (Original work published 1980)

Guerney, B. (1964). Filial therapy: Description and rationale. *Journal of Consulting Psychology, 28*, 304–310.

Guerney, L. (1991). Parents as partners in treating behavior problems in early childhood settings. *Topics in Early Childhood Education, 11*, 74–90.

Guerney, L. (1995). *Parenting: A skills training manual*. North Bethesda, MD: Institute for the Development of Emotional and Life Skills.

Guerney, L. (1997). Filial therapy. In K. O'Connor & L. Braverman (Eds.), *Play therapy theory and practice: A comparative presentation*. New York: Wiley.

Hembree-Kigin, T. L., & McNeil, C. B. (1995). *Parent and child interaction therapy*. New York: Kluwer Academic/Plenum.

Henning-Stout, M. (1993). Theoretical and empirical bases of consultation. In J. E. Zinz, T. R. Kratochwill, & S. N. Elliott (Eds.), *Handbook of consultation services for children* (pp. 15–45). San Fransisco: Jossey-Bass.

Jernberg, A. (1973). Theraplay technique. In C. Schaefer (Ed.), *The therapeutic use of child's play* (pp. 345–349). New York: Aronson.

Jernberg, A. (1979). *Theraplay*. San Francisco: Jossey-Bass.

Kerr, M. E., & Bowen, M. (1988). *Family evaluation: An approach based on Bowen theory*. New York: Norton.

Kottman, T. (1994). Adlerian play therapy. In K. O'Connor & C. Schaefer (Eds.), *Handbook of Play Therapy* (pp. 2, 3–26). New York: Wiley.

Kottman, T. (1995). *Partners in play: An Adlerian approach to play therapy*. Alexandria, VA: American Counseling Association.

Kottman, T. (1999). Integrating the Crucial C's into Adlerian play therapy. *Journal of Individual Psychology, 55*, 289–297.

Kraft, A., & Landreth, G. (1998). *Parents as therapeutic partners: Listening to your child's play*. Northvale, NJ: Aronson.

Landreth, G. (2002). *Play therapy: The art of the relationship.* New York: Brunner-Routledge.

Lew, A., & Bettner, B. L. (2000). *A parent's guide to understanding and motivating children.* Newton Centre, MA: Connexions. (Original work published 1996)

Littrell, J. M. (1998). *Brief counseling in action.* New York: W. W. Norton.

Lutzker, J. R., & Martin, J. A. (1981). *Behavior change.* Pacific Grove, CA: Brooks/Cole.

Mannino, F. V., & Shore, M. E. (1986). Understanding consultation: Some orienting dimensions. *Counseling Psychologist, 13,* 363–367.

Minuchin, S. (1974). *Families and family therapy.* Cambridge, MA: Harvard University Press.

Noell, G. H., & Witt, J. C. (1996). A critical re-evaluation of the five fundamental assumptions underlying behavioral consultation. *School Psychology Quarterly, 11,* 189–203.

Oaklander, V. (1978). *Windows to our children: A gestalt approach to children and adolescents.* Moah, UT: Real People Press.

O'Hanlon, W. H., & Weiner-Davis, M. (1989). *In search of solutions: A new direction in psychotherapy.* New York: Norton.

Pavlov, I. P. (1910). *Lectures on the work of the digestive glands* (2nd. ed). (W. H. Thompson, Trans.). London: Charles Griffin.

Pavlov, I. P. (1927). *Conditioned reflexes.* (G. V. Anrep, Trans.) London: Oxford University Press.

Presbury, J. H., Echterling, L. G., & McKee, J. E. (2002). *Ideas and tools for brief counseling.* Upper Saddle River, NJ: Merrill Prentice Hall.

Ray, D., Bratton, S., Rhine, T., & Jones, L. (2001). The effectiveness of play therapy: Responding to the critics. *International Journal of Play Therapy, 10,* 85–108.

Rogers, C. R. (1961). *On becoming a person.* Boston: Houghton Mifflin.

Severe, S. (2000). *How to behave so your children will too.* New York: Viking. (Original work published 1997)

Shure, M. B. (1994). *Raising a thinking child.* New York: Pocket Books.

Skinner, B. F. (1953). *Science and human behavior.* New York: Macmillan.

Sklare, G. B. (1997). *Brief counseling that works: A solution-focused approach for school counselors.* Thousand Oaks, CA: Corwin.

VanFleet, R. (1994). *Filial therapy: Strengthening parent–child relationships through play.* Sarasota, FL: Professional Resource Press.

Walter, J. O., & Peller, J. E. (1992). *Becoming solution-focused in brief therapy.* Levittown, PA: Brunner/Mazel.

Watts, R. E., & Pietrzak, D. (2000). Adlerian "encouragement" and the therapeutic process of solution-focused brief therapy. *Journal of Counseling and Development, 78,* 442–447.

Zins, J. E., & Erchul, W. P. (1995). Best practices in school consultation. In A. Thomas & J. Grimes (Eds.), *Best practices in school psychology* (3rd ed., pp. 609–623). Washington, DC: National Association of School Psychologists.

PART III

GROUP PLAY THERAPY

CHAPTER 10

A Creative Play Therapy Approach to the Group Treatment of Young Sexually Abused Children

LORETTA GALLO-LOPEZ

The impact of trauma on young children can be profound and far-reaching. Sexual abuse is among the most potentially damaging sources of trauma and emotional distress in young children. According to the most recent National Incidence Study of Child Abuse and Neglect (Sedlak & Broadhurst, 1996), children as young as 3 years of age are as proportionately vulnerable to sexual victimization as older children and adolescents. Treatment protocols for younger children who have been sexually abused, however, are not as readily available as programs for older children. In most cases, children traumatized by sexual abuse require, at minimum, a brief therapeutic intervention, and in the most severe situations, more extensive treatment may be necessary. The majority of children however, will benefit from a shorter-term intervention that is focused and abuse-specific. Such an intervention is presented here.

This chapter presents a comprehensive, abuse-specific, time-limited group treatment program for young survivors of sexual abuse. This work aims to provide the reader with a framework of healing opportunities to meet the complex needs of the young sexually abused child. Sexual abuse has been found to have both an immediate and long-term impact on most child victims. Most children requiring treatment are likely to have symptoms consistent with either posttraumatic stress disorder (PTSD), acute stress disorder (ASD), or one of several types of adjustment disorders. Symptoms and their severity may vary widely and are believed to be affected by multiple factors, including the severity and duration of the trauma, multiple traumatic experiences, parental response to the traumatic event, developmental stage of the child, and continued exposure to the traumatic stressor (Cohen, Berliner, & March, 2000). In young children, several categories of symptoms may be observed. Anxiety-related symptoms may include nightmares and sleep disturbances, fear of monsters, anxiety related to separation, distractibility, hyperactivity, and highly sexualized behaviors. Regressive behaviors such as clinginess, increased dependency, loss of premastered skills, and developmental lags or delays are common responses to trauma in young children. Symptoms related to self-identity and self-view, such as a distorted sense of body image and integrity, and feelings of guilt and shame, may lead to social isolation or, in the most extreme cases, to self-hurting behaviors. Other trauma-related symptoms often seen in young children include repetitive traumatic play, intrusive thoughts, mood instability, boundary issues, somatic complaints, a loss of trust in the safety of their environment and their caretaker's ability to protect them from harm, and a range of dissociative responses.

Mental health professionals continue to search for effective treatment approaches that can address the significant behavioral and trauma-related symptoms of this population. Group treatment has long been considered the treatment of choice for latency and adolescent victims of sexual abuse (Mandell & Damon, 1989; Powell & Faherty, 1990). Younger children, however, have historically been treated via individual therapy, based on the belief that a group treatment modality was not developmentally appropriate (Salter, 1988).

Steward, Farquhar, Dicharry, Glick, and Martin (1986) describe a group treatment model for young victims of physical and/or sexual abuse that is open-ended, allowing new group members to begin at any time in the treatment process. The model utilizes a nondirective play therapy approach and identifies treatment length as 8 months to 2 years. This approach appears sound, and the treatment goals outlined focus on both healing the wounds of the past and meeting the child's emotional needs in the present and future. However, a directive approach with sexually abused children has been endorsed (Salter, 1988; Rasmussen & Cunningham, 1995, Cohen et al., 2000) as a means of ensuring that trauma issues are specifically addressed in order to bring about a decrease in symptoms and in the child's risk of further abuse. Friedrich (1991) advocates a treatment approach that is "specific, should be sensitive to the child's needs, and should emphasize the interpersonal" (p. 5).

The model proposed in this chapter attempts to integrate the most essential elements of treatment into a single model. The target population includes both boys and girls, ranging in age from 3 to 10, separated into groups according to age and developmental ability. Although it may be effective to mix genders in groups with children through age 5, girls and boys should be treated in separate groups from age 6 onward in order to increase the level of comfort with issues of sexuality, decrease anxiety-related acting-out behaviors, and allow for gender-specific issues to be explored more fully. The treatment model is presented in a time-limited, 16-week format. It relies on group process as a means of targeting the feelings of isolation and stigmatization experienced by many sexually abused children. Nondirective play therapy, directive play therapy, and other abuse-specific strategies are incorporated to meet the complex needs of this population. Such a model is supported by others, such as Ramussen and Cunningham (1995), who advocate the integration of nondirective and focused strategies in the treatment of sexually abused children. This enables the therapist to address trauma-related issues effectively, while providing the child with the emotionally safe environment necessary for the process of healing to begin.

The treatment model is influenced by three distinct but interrelated treatment approaches. The first is based on the long- and short-term impact of trauma on young children. The model of traumagenic dynamics presented by Finkelhor and Browne (1986) is helpful in the formulation of treatment goals related to symptoms of traumatic stress. The four dynamics—traumatic sexualization, stigmatization, betrayal, and powerlessness—are believed by Finkelhor and Browne to lead to emotional trauma by "distorting a child's self-concept, world view, and affective capacities" (pp. 180–181). The treatment model presented here directly addresses each of these areas with the goal of decreasing trauma-related symptoms and behaviors.

The second element of this treatment model is based on developmental theory. This approach is formulated to meet the developmental needs of the young child, providing opportunities for mastery of age-appropriate tasks as well as interventions that allow exploration of regressive themes.

Finally, the model incorporates systems theory, focusing on interpersonal relationships and children's view of themselves within their immediate world.

Although this chapter presents only the treatment protocol for a children's therapy group, concurrent parent treatment serves to support a child's progress and enhances and strengthens the parent–child relationship. Group counseling should be made available for the nonoffending parent/caretaker as well. The ideal situation would allow the parent to attend concurrent group sessions while the child attends a separate group. The parental component should address child development, child sexual development, abuse dynamics, the potential impact of abuse on children, parenting issues, safety issues, family roles and relationships, and should include interventions that serve to enhance and strengthen the parent–child relationship. Families in which sexual abuse has occurred experience stress and anxiety related not only to the trauma but also to its aftermath. They have difficulty trusting people they perceive to be in authority and have a need to move beyond the abuse. Family interventions should help counter these concerns and enhance the family's ability to cope with life stressors.

In families in which the parent–child relationship appears to be particularly problematic, filial therapy may be an appropriate intervention. Costas and

Landreth (1999) found that the use of filial therapy with nonoffending parents of sexually abused children increased the parents' "level of empathy in their interactions with their children, significantly increased their attitude of acceptance toward their children, and significantly reduced their level of stress" (p. 43).

Working directly with the child's primary caretaker is essential to the success of the child's treatment. Cohen et al. (2000) identify parental involvement in treatment as clearly important for the resolution of children's trauma symptoms. When nonoffending parents are involved in their child's therapy, they more successfully align with the treatment process and the treatment providers. Parents may intentionally or unintentionally sabotage their child's treatment if they feel they are in competition with the therapist, or because of their own feelings of guilt and inadequacy. Emphasis should be placed on the important role parents play in a child's healing. Empowering parents in this process decreases their feelings of inadequacy and enhances their ability to parent their children more effectively. In addition, parents tend to respond positively to the time-limited treatment approach. Although parents should be informed that their children may need to continue in treatment beyond the 16-week program, having a sense of the range of treatment length appears to ease parents' stress and anxiety and increase feelings of hopefulness.

ASSESSING APPROPRIATENESS FOR GROUP

Prior to placement, each child should be individually assessed to determine that child's appropriateness for the group. Assessment should include examining the child's developmental history as well as completing a clinical interview. The evaluator should attempt to determine the child's developmental level and needs, giving consideration to the possible regressive impact of the abuse. During this initial interview, the therapist must assess the child's level of trauma and evaluate his or her coping skills. It is essential at this point that the therapist ascertain whether the child has given a clear abuse disclosure. A child who has not disclosed abuse, in at least limited detail, is not an appropriate candidate for group treatment. Very often, children are referred for sexual abuse treatment when there are allegations of sexual abuse or when they display symptoms such as sexual preoccupation, age-inappropriate sexual knowledge and/or behaviors, or excessive masturbation. Children who have such symptoms, but have not disclosed sexual abuse, should be seen in individual therapy so that symptoms can be treated and the possibility of sexual abuse can be assessed. This is also true for children who have provided limited details about their sexual abuse but have not made an adequate disclosure. If such children were seen in a group treatment setting, they would be highly susceptible to contamination by the disclosures of other children in the group. Following individual therapy, children can be reevaluated to determine whether group treatment would be an appropriate intervention. It is important to note that a child who completely denies being sexually abused is not appropriate for group treatment, even if the perpetrator has confessed to the sexual abuse.

It is not necessary to exclude from group treatment children whose condition is diagnosed as attention-deficit/hyperactivity disorder (ADHD) or those who exhibit ADHD-type behaviors. Sexually abused children may experience such extreme levels of anxiety that they display symptoms similar to those of ADHD, which are often diagnosed incorrectly. As issues are addressed and resolved in treatment, the anxiety-related behaviors usually decrease. These children can be successful in group treatment as long as the therapist is able to provide the necessary structure and limit setting within a safe therapy environment. It is essential that therapists monitor the level of stimulation the children experience, appropriately intervene when overstimulation occurs, and provide adequate time for closure exercises.

Children who are highly sexualized and impulsive may not be appropriate candidates for a group because of the risk that they may victimize the other children. It is recommended that these children initially be seen individually, with the goal of enhancing their impulse control skills and formulating strategies to manage the sexualized behaviors. Until this occurs, the focus on sexuality and sexual abuse issues in a group setting may be too highly stimulating for these children. A child who has previously acted out sexually against other children will need to be involved in group or individual treatment that directly addresses the sexual acting-out behaviors as well as victimization issues (Gallo-Lopez, 2005a). It is important to keep in mind that many sexually abused children engage in age-inappropriate sexual behaviors such as excessive masturbation, preoccupation with body parts, and mutual genital touching with other children. For many children these behaviors represent an effort to understand and make sense of what was done to them. For others it is similar to traumatic play. Children who exhibit these behaviors, however, should not automatically be ruled out as group participants. The ultimate consideration must always be the safety of the other children and the integrity of the therapeutic process. This is also true with extremely aggressive children. Children whose aggressive behaviors are so unmanageable that they place others at risk may have to be seen individually in order to learn to manage their aggression and respond more appropriately to anger triggers. They may then be determined to be appropriate for group treatment.

It may be necessary for children who engage in self-injurious or self-hurting behaviors to be seen in individual therapy, in addition to group treatment, so that their safety may be more closely monitored. The same is true for children who have engaged in the abuse of animals, who express suicidal ideation, or who experience significant levels of dissociation. These children should be closely monitored and may require intensive individual therapy and psychiatric support.

Children in foster care, although presenting a distinct set of issues and concerns, should not be excluded from participation in a group. Foster children can reap great benefit from involvement in the familial type of activities involved in group treatment. They may, however, need the ongoing support of an individual therapist to provide them a greater opportunity to bond and connect with a significant adult. As this treatment protocol incorporates parent–child sessions within its framework, if deemed appropriate the foster parent should be invited to attend. An alternative approach is to adapt the protocol presented here for use with groups of children in foster care. The parent–child sessions could be eliminated, and alternative interventions could be utilized to address the general goals of this therapy as well as other goals specifically relevant to children in foster care.

SHORT-TERM PLAY THERAPY APPROACH

Setting Up the Group

One of the first considerations in setting up a group is its size. Children benefit most from small groups. A generally accepted rule is that the number of children should not exceed the age of the youngest child in the group. In other words, a group whose youngest member is 3 years old should have no more than three children, a group whose youngest member is 4 should have no more than four members, and so on to a maximum of six to eight children. Consideration should be given to the makeup of the group and the expertise of the therapist. The presence of an extra group facilitator does not warrant an increase in the number of group members.

Group sessions should be an hour in length, with sessions beginning and ending on time. Predictability is paramount. Group rituals are a means of providing a predictable structure that leads to a naturally developing sense of safety and containment within the therapy environment. Beginning and ending rituals contribute to the establishment of trust and security, as anxiety is reduced when children can anticipate what will happen next. "Beginning and ending rituals help to establish a sense that there is something in common that is being shared" (Gallo-Lopez, 2005a).

Beginning rituals should be the focus of the first 10 minutes or so of each session. Rituals may include grabbing a pillow or mat and taking a place in the group circle. This may be followed by a check-in, a group trust-building game, or a welcome song. One beginning routine involves group members, in turn, explaining why they come to group. This serves to strengthen the connection between group members and to decrease the stigma and shame harbored by many child victims.

Structured group activities (discussed later in this chapter) should follow the beginning rituals and take up approximately 20 minutes of the session. The next 20 minutes should be reserved for nondirective play therapy.

The final 10 minutes of the session are reserved for closure and ending rituals. Ending rituals should help provide a sense of closure by offering a chance to process issues that surfaced during the session. Group members are then better prepared to exit the therapy environment intact. Ending rituals may include a song, a movement activity, or any combination of activities that provide a sense of calm and focus. Most children enjoy attending their therapy sessions and may resist leaving when a session is over. Providing a separate area of the room for ending rituals may ease the transition by allowing children to physically move from one area of the room to another to trigger the change of focus.

Some therapists may choose to provide a snack as part of the group's ending rituals. Food is helpful for two reasons. First, it provides an effective form of tangible nurturance. Even a simple snack of cookies and juice shows children that their group is a place of care and support. Second, snack time parallels a family meal in ways that often facilitate treatment. Because many of the group activities center on domestic issues, members of groups often end up relating to each other in more or less familial ways. Just as shared meals help strengthen bonds within functional families, snack times provide the group members with opportunities to process issues, talk through problems, share feelings, and resolve conflicts together.

For therapists unable to conduct the program within an hour's time, adding 10 extra minutes for closure and ending routines may prevent the pace of the group from seeming too rushed. Closure tends to be the most difficult time for children, and it takes a good deal of skill for the therapist to effectively redirect the children to the closure activities. It is not advisable to lengthen the group time much beyond this, however, because the session may then begin to lose its focus and become more like free play or day care than therapy. Whatever length is chosen, time limits should be set and should not vary from week to week.

The Group Treatment Model

The group treatment model is presented here as a 16-week program. Cohen et al. (2000) assert that children with uncomplicated PTSD have been noted to demonstrate significant positive change "with 12–20 sessions of PTSD-specific psychotherapy." The model presented here can be easily lengthened, however, to meet the needs of those children requiring a more extended treatment intervention. The program is divided into four 4-week modules. The following paragraphs give the primary objectives of each module, as well as a description of several activities that effectively help achieve these objectives. The various activities are listed in the order in which they are typically sequenced for the groups. Meeting modular objectives, however, is more important than following a specific sequence, and clinicians may wish to add and/or delete activities according to their own treatment style.

In each session, the structured activities are followed by a period of nondirective play therapy. Themes established through the structured activities are often further explored in the nondirective play therapy that follows. This naturally flowing progression may lead to more purposeful play during nondirective play therapy. Of course, therapist intervention, feedback, and interpretation are essential to facilitating this process.

Within each module, specific themes are identified. The themes of safety and empowerment, however, are arguably the most essential in the treatment of sexually abused children of this age range. Accordingly, these themes are woven into each of the structured activities and are continually reinforced via therapist interventions in the nondirective play therapy portion of each session.

Enhanced feelings of safety and empowerment must also be fostered by the manner in which the therapist interacts with the children. Suzanne Long (1986) stresses the importance of the therapist's consistently communicating a sense of "respect, acceptance and faith" in the children being treated (p. 222). This is a wonderfully simple way of characterizing the essential elements of the therapeutic relationship. The therapist must communicate "respect" for children, as well as for children's rights to their own feelings, thoughts, and ideas. "Acceptance" enables children to feel confident that they will not be rejected. Finally, "faith" conveys the therapist's belief in a child's power to grow, change, and seek resolution.

Sessions 1–4

The tasks of the first 4 weeks of treatment are to set boundaries and establish the group structure, routines, and rituals. Other tasks include encouraging children to bond, increasing their comfort and trust level with each other and the therapist, and forming a sense of group identity. As treatment begins, it is important to talk about feelings and to give children the words to express what they feel, while continually reinforcing the view that group is a safe and supportive place for self-expression.

From the start of treatment, it is important for children to understand that they share similar reasons for inclusion in group. This serves to decrease children's feelings of isolation, alienation, and negative stigmatization. Shame and the abuse dynamic of secrecy are reduced when this commonality is discussed at the start of each session. Children should be consistently reminded that they have permission to talk about their sexual abuse within the group.

Statements such as "Everyone in this group was touched in private places by someone, or was made to touch someone else's privates" help to set the tone for the group. It is preferable to stay away from the term "bad touch" to avoid increasing feelings of guilt in the children who may have enjoyed the touching or attention. Therapists should take care not to inadvertently reinforce any negative thoughts or feelings children may have about themselves.

Children are not expected, or asked, to disclose the details of their sexual abuse during the first few sessions. Disclosure in group should not take place until the children have developed an adequate level of trust in the group and the therapist. In addition, children need to understand when it is an appropriate time to talk about their abuse. Because many sexually abused children do not have a clear sense of appropriate boundaries related to these issues, they often disclose information about their abuse to anyone they meet, whether they are strangers or other children at school. The therapist can make comments such as, "We'll talk more about this when we know each other a little better," allowing the children to begin to understand the need for boundaries and limits regarding disclosure of their abuse. In this respect, treatment is clearly distinguished from a forensic evaluation or interview in which children are expected to disclose the details of their abuse to complete strangers.

Safety is a primary concern both in and out of the therapy setting. Not only must the therapist work to provide a safe environment for treatment, he or she must work with the parent or caretaker to ensure that the child is safe within the home as well.

Themes and Objectives

- Group joining, establishing group structure, introducing ritual.
- Setting boundaries and limits within the group.
- Setting the stage for the corrective relationship between adults and children.
- Begin differentiating, identifying, and expressing feelings.
- Begin to establish a sense of safety and basic trust within the group.
- Continue to asses each child's developmental and attachment needs, level of trauma through the presentation of trauma-related symptoms, ability to distinguish reality from fantasy, and ability to engage in symbolic and representational play.

Structured Activities

GROUP POSTER

At the start of group treatment, it is helpful to find mechanisms that enhance group cohesiveness while appreciating the individual's uniqueness. One such activity involves the creation of a group poster highlighting commonalities as well as differences among group members. Areas of focus include likes and dislikes, favorite activities, favorite foods, and so on. Children can be asked to draw pictures, cut pictures from magazines, or make lists. The group may want to choose a group name or theme that can also be incorporated into the group poster. The therapist can create a group ritual by setting up the poster at the start of each session and taking it down at the end. Pictures, photographs, and other items can be added to the poster as the sessions progress.

PUPPET INTERVIEW

The purpose of a puppet interview is to increase comfort and trust by giving children an opportunity to get to know each other better. Each child should be instructed to choose from a variety of puppets set out on the table or floor. Irwin and Malloy (1975) suggest offering both realistic and fantasy puppet choices in therapy. They propose including domestic and wild animals (specifically those with orally aggressive characteristics), as well as witch, skeleton, king and queen, police officer, and doctor puppets. The puppets are then interviewed using a "talk show" format. The therapist is the talk show host, and the children are audience members who take turns asking the puppets questions about themselves. The therapist may direct a child to use a chosen puppet to represent him- or herself, or to create a character. The puppet serves as a distancing tool and vehicle for projection. The therapist should decide on the extent of emotional distance the children may need at the time the activity is employed, keeping in mind that the farther from "self" a character is, the greater the amount of distance.

SAFE PLACE DRAWING

Early in treatment it is important to assess each child's feelings related to safety and to determine appropriate interventions to increase his or her ability to feel protected. Gil (2003) supports the use of art activities as a means of communication for sexually abused children. She asserts that "art allows children to create images that communicate their internal projections about self and the world" (p. 155). At the start of this drawing activity, children are asked to draw a picture of a place where they feel safe and then talk about the drawing. Children who were abused in their own homes may not view home as a very secure place. By discussing the characteristics of a safe place, children may be able to identify alternative safe environments. A young girl who had been sexually abused by her biological father indicated that the only place she felt safe was at school. She believed the people there would protect her and prevent her from being kidnapped by her father. Ideally, home should be the one place where each child is able to feel safe and protected. In some cases, however, it may be necessary for the therapist to work to strengthen the relationship between the child and a nonoffending parent or caretaker and to help the family identify strategies to enhance the child's feelings of safety at home. Both of these issues are addressed in greater detail in subsequent sessions.

SELF-PORTRAIT

A self-portrait can be a telling representation of a child's self-view. Although creating a self-portrait is a simple activity, such a picture can offer therapists a wealth of information. Each child should be offered paper and drawing materials and directed to draw a picture of him- or herself. It is important to have children draw their full bodies, not just their faces, as this gives the therapist more information regarding body integrity and self-image. These self-portraits offer valuable information about issues such as strength and vulnerability, groundedness, and self-worth. Size and placement of the figure and body parts, colors, clothing, and facial features and expression deepen our understanding of how children view themselves. This activity can be repeated toward the end of treatment so that the children's self-views can be compared over time.

PARENT–CHILD COMBINED SESSION: PRACTICING LISTENING SKILLS

In a parent–child combined session, the parent and child are brought together to practice listening skills and enhance communication. This activity begins with the entire group of children, parents, and the therapist playing the game of "telephone." This is the old childhood game in which a phrase is passed along as it is whispered by one person to the next. Finally, the last person says the phrase out loud, and usually everyone laughs at how the phrase has changed since it was first uttered. The emphasis should be on listening to the person who is speaking. After this game of telephone is played a few times, each parent-and-child team can work together in a separate area of the room to make a telephone, using two paper cups and a piece of string. The child then tells a story into one cup (telephone) while the parent listens at the other cup. After the story has been told, the parent repeats what he or she remembers of the story. Next, the parent tells a story while the child listens; the child then repeats the story. It may be helpful for the therapist to model this activity first, along with a child or parent. Upon completion of the listening exercise, parents and children should be instructed to engage in structured play together in place of the regular nondirective play therapy time. This parent–child play usually involves the use of puzzles, drawing materials, nontherapeutic board games, and so on. At this point in the treatment process, therapists should avoid encouraging parents and children to engage in projective or pretend play to avoid the possibility that parents may overtly or covertly censor their child's play. Such censorship may alter the content of the child's nondirective play in future sessions. Through structured play activities, the therapist can observe a great deal about family roles, relationships, and styles of interaction between parent and child that may prove helpful for future treatment planning. In addition, parents are given an opportunity to practice playful interaction with their children—an important step in strengthening the parent–child relationship.

MASK MAKING FOR IDENTIFICATION AND EXPRESSION OF FEELINGS

Appropriate expression of feelings, a basic treatment goal, sets the stage for much of the work to come. To accomplish this, children must first acquire the language necessary to communicate what they feel. The structured activity for this session should begin with a group discussion focused on identifying various feelings. A mirror can be used to playfully explore facial expression related to particular emotions. Children should then be directed to create several masks, each representative of a different feeling. Simple materials such as paper plates or precut cardboard can be attached to craft sticks and used to create masks. A child who has difficulty tolerating a mask placed directly on his or her face is usually willing to work with a mask if it can be held with a stick. When the masks are completed, they can be used for role playing during this session if time permits, or they can be saved for use in future sessions.

Sessions 5–8

At this point in treatment, children usually begin to feel comfortable and accustomed to group routines. Trust in the therapist and group members should be adequately established in order to safely and directly address issues related to sexual abuse.

Themes and Objectives

- Continuing to identify and express feelings, accompanied by modulation of affect.
- Understanding privacy versus secrecy.
- Working toward abuse disclosure within the group.
- Repairing cognitive distortions related to guilt and responsibility issues.
- Identifying appropriate and inappropriate touch.
- Exploring issues that support an enhanced sense of body integrity and awareness.
- Exploring issues related to family roles and relationships incorporating the child as part of a system.
- Enhancing communication within the family.

Structured Activities

COLOR MY WORLD

The Color My World intervention is based on Kevin O'Connor's (1983) Color-Your-Life technique, in which children choose colors to represent certain feelings and then color a sheet of paper to represent the different feelings they have experienced. I developed the Color My World intervention specifically for use with traumatized children. For this activity, a preprinted form (Figure 10.1) with a circle and a list of feelings, is provided for each child. Space to add feelings of the child's choosing is provided as well. Next to each feeling is a cartoon drawing symbolizing the given emotion. Children are asked to choose a color to represent each feeling and to make a mark with the chosen color beside each drawing. They are then instructed to fill in the circle with the amount of each color that shows how much of each feeling they have experienced. Children can be asked to show the feelings they have had in the past week, on a given day, before the abuse, since the abuse occurred, or throughout their lives. The use of the circle provides a sense of containment and an artificial boundary for the child's emotions, which for traumatized children are often overwhelming. That is, the circle provides a safe holding space for the child's emotions. The cartoon drawings offer visual cues and more concrete ways for children to identify and express their feelings. Some children may choose to use only one or two colors, other children may use all the colors. Likewise, some may color in a very systematic and structured way, whereas others scribble in

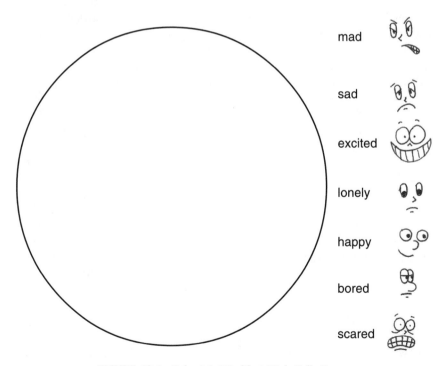

FIGURE 10.1. Color My World. © Nick Gallo Lopez.

and outside the circle. The therapist should not direct the children to color in any particular fashion, as each child's choices can provide a wealth of important information. The therapist should encourage each child to talk about the feelings represented by the colors in his or her circle. This technique can be utilized effectively at different points, and as often as warranted, throughout the treatment program.

PRIVACY BOXES

Many children who have been sexually abused do not understand the concept of privacy. Most have not been afforded much privacy within their own homes. To reinforce the idea that everyone deserves privacy in certain situations, each child is given a cardboard box to decorate (a shoe box works well), which is used to hold the child's group projects. The boxes can be painted or colored with markers and decorated with glitter, feathers, buttons, fabric, magazine pictures, stickers, and so on. The boxes are kept in a safe place in a closet or another secure area in the office or playroom. The box becomes a private place to store projects created in the group. While the children are decorating their boxes, group discussion should revolve around examples of privacy, secrecy, and surprises. Children should be presented with "What If?" scenarios and asked to determine whether a scenario describes an issue of privacy, secrecy, or surprise. Children should be helped to understand that a surprise may be an appropriate kind of secret. An example may be one sibling telling another not to tell Mom what they have gotten her for her birthday. This should be clearly distinguished from a secret about a negative event or incident, such as a child being told not to tell about sexual abuse. The need for and right to privacy can continually be reinforced within the group setting. For example, whenever a group member uses the bathroom, the therapist can remind the child to close the door. Discussion can ensue about the importance of closed doors while dressing, bathing, and using the toilet at home. Parents should be learning about the same issues in their group in order to reinforce these concepts at home.

BODY TRACING

The goal of the body tracing intervention is to guide children toward making a connection between their emotions and what they feel in their bodies. The activity begins with children discussing and listing various emotions. The type and number of emotions should be limited to the simplest and most common—anger, excitement, jealousy, love, happiness, sadness, worry, loneliness, fear, and confidence. Ask the children to talk about what they feel physically when they experience a given emotion. Anger is an easy emotion to begin with. Aim for responses such as, "When I am angry, my hands make a fist," or "When I am worried, my stomach hurts." Once the children understand this concept, each child should be given a set of stickers printed with feeling words and/or the corresponding facial expressions. The stickers can be made by the therapist or purchased through therapeutic activity catalogs. Using a large roll of paper, cut a sheet to accommodate the length of each child's body. Trace the children's bodies by having them stand against a sheet of paper tacked to the wall. This approach engenders less anxiety for children who have been physically violated, than the traditional method of having children lie on their backs on the floor. During the process, it is helpful for the therapist to describe what is being done ("Now I am tracing your arm") in order to decrease anxiety related to physical touch. Children can then fill in facial features and clothes and add anything else they may like. Using the feelings stickers along with the body tracings, the children are guided to identify their physical response to a given emotion. Stickers are then fixed to the body tracing in the area representative of the physical response. Connecting the emotional with the physical increases a child's ability to recognize and identify feelings. The children can then employ newly acquired coping strategies and problem-solving skills to manage and appropriately express their emotions.

PAPER DOLL BODY FIGURES: APPROPRIATE VERSUS INAPPROPRIATE TOUCH

In addition to offering a healing experience, sexual abuse treatment should provide children with strategies for self-protection. It is important that children understand the difference between appropriate and inappropriate touch, as well as their right to refuse unwanted touches. This activity utilizes a felt board, and male and female figures representing adults and children. The figures can be made of felt or cut from poster board with felt or Velcro glued on the back to adhere to the felt board. The figures are used to identify private parts of the body and to help children distinguish appropriate from inappropriate touches. Clothing can be made for the figures in order to help children grasp the concept that private parts are the parts of our bodies that are covered by underwear and bathing suits. Because this activity directly addresses the dynamics of abuse, children may easily become overstimulated and avoidant. The felt board provides an area of focus with distinct boundaries, similar to those of a sandtray, thereby minimizing stimulation and anxiety.

TELLING EACH OTHER WHAT HAPPENED

An effective way to facilitate disclosures of abuse is to highlight the initial statements made by children and to emphasize the bravery it took for them to tell. Children can be asked to draw a picture of the first time they told anyone about their abuse, and then to discuss the drawing. Another approach is to have children use puppets to represent themselves and the person (or people) to whom they disclosed the abuse. The therapist may need to take on a role in the puppet play if a child reported his or her abuse to more than one person. The discussion about initial disclosures should naturally lead to conversation about the abuse itself. It is not necessary for the children to give intricate details about

their abuse if they do not choose to do so. It is essential, however, that the thera
pist correct any cognitive distortions about the abuse, especially those related
to the child's feelings of guilt and responsibility. The therapist should also take
this opportunity to demonstrate acceptance and validation of children's negative and positive feelings regarding an offender.

PARENT–CHILD COMBINED SESSION: SHARING FEELINGS

In a parent–child combined session, the parent/caretaker and child are given
an opportunity to explore feelings and emotions together in order to begin
strengthening their relationship. There are a variety of ways to achieve this goal.
One activity involves drawing, with a focus on feeling words. Each parent–child
pair is given two large sheets of drawing paper, folded to make four equal sections. They are also given markers, colored pencils or crayons, glue, and an
envelope filled with slips of paper showing the following feeling words: "angry,"
"hurt," "proud," "happy," "sad," "worried," "love," and "afraid." The parent
and child each choose four feeling words and glue one feeling word at the top
of each of the four spaces on their papers. They are then asked to draw a picture about a time when they experienced each feeling. When they complete
their drawings, the child and parent share their pictures with each other.

FAMILY ROLE PLAYING

Drama and role play are powerful techniques for helping a child explore family
relationships, as well as his or her role within the family system. In this role-
playing activity, children are asked to enact a role within a family. The therapist structures the play by giving a simple direction such as, "Let's create a story
about a family." In some groups, everyone chooses the role of a child. In other
groups, no one chooses to play a child. In most groups, there is a sampling of
each. It may be necessary, and can be very effective, for the therapist to enact
the roles of missing family members. If a therapist chooses, however, to step
into a role in the drama of a young child, it is important to distinguish between
being in and out of role. Gallo-Lopez (2005a) notes that "for young children,
the lines between reality and fantasy, between 'me' and 'not me,' can be easily
obscured and confused. This ambiguity is often heightened in children who
have been sexually abused, as perpetrators may utilize a distorted version of
pretend play to gain the trust and compliance of their young victims" (p. 142).
Once the roles are established, the therapist asks the group to identify a problem within the family. The children are free to use costumes and props in the
drama and basically determine the direction of their play by the actions of their
characters. The therapist, in character, should take this opportunity to infuse
certain issues into the play that may help to make the play more purposeful.
Such issues include trust and betrayal, separation and loss, abandonment, stigmatization, guilt, secrecy, coercion, and threats. Role play should be followed
by a closure activity, which will enable the children to separate from the roles

they assumed in play. Closure should involve a review of what has occurred and a transition to the "here and now." Themes from this session carry over particularly well to the nondirective play period that follows.

SANDPLAY

Family dynamics can be effectively explored as each child creates a scene in the sand tray depicting his or her family members doing something together. When the scene is complete, the therapist can facilitate discussion by asking simple questions. Like the Kinetic Family Drawing technique (Burns & Kaufman, 1970), this intervention provides insight into the child's personal view of his or her place within the family. It also captures the child's view of family interactions and functions. To facilitate sandplay work in a group setting, it is important to have a separate sand tray for each child. Rectangular plastic storage containers are an acceptable alternative to more expensive wooden trays. The inside bottom of the tray can be painted with blue paint made especially for painting plastic. The paint will adhere more easily if the bottom of the container is sanded before painting. It will also be important to provide enough sand tray figures and objects to enable each child to create a scene. An alternative to this activity is to use the Kinetic Family Drawing technique, followed by questions and discussion.

Sessions 9–12

At this point, the children are midway through the treatment program and are usually feeling safe enough within the group to begin to address and directly confront their fears.

Themes and Objectives

- Identifying and confronting fears and nightmares.
- Enhancing coping and problem-solving skills.
- Reinforcing sense of personal power.
- Safety and protection issues.

Structured Activities

THE NIGHTMARE WALL

Nightmares and sleep disturbances are problems commonly seen in young sexually abused children. It is essential that children be given an opportunity to address and confront their fears and work toward resolution. In this activity, children are asked to discuss and draw their most troublesome nightmares. Some younger children may become frustrated in attempting to draw things in a particular way. The therapist may assist a child in illustrating the nightmare while the child gives specific drawing instructions (location, size, shape, color, etc.). When the drawings are complete, the child is asked to tell the story of the nightmare while the therapist transcribes it on the back of the drawing or on a separate sheet of paper. The pictures are then displayed on the wall under a sign that reads THE NIGHTMARE WALL. Displaying the drawings serves to diminish the power of the nightmares and thus to decrease the child's fear. When groups are facilitated in multi-use rooms, the Nightmare Wall can be made portable by tacking the drawing onto a piece of foam core board or a large sheet of paper that can be rolled up and stored out of sight between sessions. The next part of this activity is focused on helping children to problem-solve by drawing or listing things they can do to feel safe when they have nightmares. Such a list may include sleeping with a special stuffed toy or blanket, using a night-light, getting a hug from a parent/caretaker, and so on. The drawings or lists should also be posted on the Nightmare Wall.

CONQUERING THE MONSTER

For younger children, the "monster" is often representative of things they fear, including the perpetrator or the perpetrator's behavior. There are many effective ways to help children confront the monster metaphor. In this activity, children construct an image of a monster and then destroy it. The activity utilizes a large sheet of paper, water-based washable paints, and spray bottles filled with water. This is a very messy activity that should not be attempted in a space where things must be kept clean and tidy. On a large sheet of heavy paper, approximately 5 feet long and 3 feet wide, children are asked to paint a scary monster. The children can either work together to create one monster, or if space and supervision allow, work separately to create individual monsters. When the monsters are complete, each child is given a water-filled spray bottle. The children then spray the monsters, delighting in watching as water drips from the paper and the monsters are washed away. This activity works especially well outdoors, where the monster paintings can be attached to trees or walls. If that is not an option, large tubs, plastic bags, or old shower curtains can be placed on the floor under the paintings to catch the dripping water and paint.

If it is impossible to attempt such an activity in the therapy space available, dry erase boards offer an excellent alternative. Using a large dry erase board, children can draw monsters and then use the dry eraser to make the monster disappear. This version of the activity actually provides more control to the child who might want to destroy the monster piece by piece until it is totally gone. Children can erase the monster's hands ("so you can't touch me anymore") the monster's eyes ("so you can't see me anymore"), and so on. Many children will engage in this activity over and over again, alternately creating and conquering the monster until they have adequately mastered their fears.

The monster metaphor is often observed in nondirective play and is an important theme for children to explore in treatment. A group of 3- and 4-year-olds engaged in group play that involved capturing, tying, boxing, and hiding a large plastic monster figure. Week after week the monster was conquered and would then "escape" to be conquered again. During one session, the children taped the monster into a box so securely that they had to engage the therapist to assist them in getting the monster out. The following week, the children left the monster in the closet, and it never "escaped" again.

CORRECTING THE NIGHTMARE

A helpful activity focuses on correcting the nightmares. The children are engaged in problem solving in order to create a corrective, positive ending for the nightmares that were the focus of an earlier session. The children are asked to draw pictures of their nightmares with new endings, providing opportunities for children to experience a sense of empowerment and control. These solution drawings are placed over the initial nightmare drawings on the Nightmare Wall. Therapists should also take this opportunity to review the list of coping skills generated in the earlier activity to remind children that they have the power to help themselves to feel safe. The initial nightmare drawing of a 6-year-old girl involved the very common theme of the monster in the closet. Her drawing depicted the monster hiding in the closet while she lay in her bed. In her solution drawing, this child glued the monster inside the closet and exclaimed, "I made the monster scared. I growled at the monster and told him to shut up, and then I glued him in the closet." A 7-year-old child asked to take his solution drawing home. He taped it to the wall next to his bed as a concrete reminder that he had the power to manage his fears and anxieties.

PARENT–CHILD COMBINED SESSION: SAFETY SHIELD

During a combined session, parent and child are given an opportunity to engage in a dialogue about the child's fears and to explore interventions that will enable the child to feel a greater sense of safety and security. Using sheets of poster board or file folders, shields such as those used by medieval knights should be traced and cut. Pipe cleaners can be attached to the sides for handles. A line, drawn about a third of the way down from the top, divides the shield into two sections. The parent and child should be asked to work together to first identify the child's fears and then draw pictures representing those fears on the top portion of the shield. The parent and child again work together to come up with ways to help the child feel safe, and then draw them on the lower portion of the shield. The shield is an obvious symbol of safety and protection, and allowing the parent to join with the child in this endeavor encourages the child to view the parent as a source of support and safety.

PRETEND SLUMBER PARTY

After focusing for several sessions on fears and safety issues, having a pretend slumber party allows children to utilize some of their newly acquired coping skills to confront fears directly in a pretend-play situation. Prior to the session, the therapist should determine whether each of the children is able to tolerate being in the dark for an extended period of time. If so, each child is given a flashlight and the session should take place in the dark. Children should be asked to bring a pillow and something they like to sleep with, such as a stuffed toy or blanket. Blankets are spread on the floor, and the children snack on popcorn and drinks. During this activity, the therapist can lead the play or conversation to focus on fears related to the dark, such as a fear of shadows or sounds. The therapist can guide the children toward finding strategies to confront and resolve those fears. Longo and Longo (2003) describe a similar activity, which entails group members taking turns passing a stuffed animal or pillow and holding the object while sharing something about themselves (i.e., a fear, a wish) with the group. For mixed-gender groups, a pretend camp out may be more appropriate than the slumber party theme. Sheets or fabric can be rigged to make a tent, and snacks can include popcorn and s'mores. An appropriate closure activity for the session might include using flashlights to make shadow puppets on the wall. This activity is both fun and calming and provides one more opportunity to deflate the power of the dark and allow children to feel safe and in control. For many groups, shadow puppets eventually become a weekly ending ritual.

Sessions 13–16

During this period, the group is reviewing and reinforcing themes addressed earlier and preparing for termination. The primary focus is on safety and ensuring that the children adequately understand issues of self-protection (having the right to say no, whom to tell, how to tell, etc.). Activities in this module utilize more cognitive strategies than activities in previous modules. It is also important for the children and their families to begin moving beyond the abuse and to strengthen and brighten their future orientation.

Themes and Objectives

- Abuse dynamics: threats, bribery, coercion, responsibility.
- Continuing to confront cognitive distortions.
- Self-protection skills.
- Establishing a sense of security and protection within the family system.
- Change/loss: working toward termination.
- Future orientation.

Structured Activities

STOP AND TELL SIGN

The goal of this activity is to empower children with words to help protect themselves from inappropriate touching and to identify adults they trust whom they can tell. Using poster board cut into an octagon and colored red like a stop sign, each of the children makes a sign that reads STOP on one side and TELL on the other. Dowels or craft sticks can be attached so that the children can easily hold and turn the signs. After the signs are completed, each child practices holding up his or her sign and yelling, "Stop!" loudly. Lists of trusted adults are generated, and the children rehearse "telling" one of the adults on their lists. The following role-play activity may follow in the same session if time allows.

ROLE-PLAYING "WHAT IF?" SCENARIOS

The focus of the "What If?" role-playing scenes is to continue to confront and correct cognitive distortions, specifically those surrounding issues of responsibility, threats, bribes, coercion, and the imbalance of power that exists between children and their abusers. This is also an effective way to help children to problem-solve and identify strategies and options for given situations. It can be helpful at this point to present a videotape dealing with safety and inappropriate touch. Disney's *Too Smart for Strangers* is one that is appropriate for younger children. The format of the film, presenting a scenario and asking viewers what they think the child in the video should do next, allows children to practice problem-solving skills. Parents can be assigned the task of viewing the film independently and then watching and discussing it with their child.

PARENT–CHILD COMBINED SESSION: SAFE PLACE IN THE SAND

It is important to establish a nonoffending parent or primary caretaker as the child's protector. Both parent and child need to develop skills to enable the child to feel safe and secure and to feel that the parent is capable of protecting him or her. This sandplay activity enables the parent and child to explore creative solutions together. Each parent and child dyad should be provided a sand tray and access to a variety of figures and objects and instructed to work together to create a safe place in the sand. When the sand trays are complete, photographs can be taken, and if appropriate, the group members can share what they have created. One 7-year-old girl worked with her mother to construct a wall between her home and the perpetrator's home. Another child placed herself in her living room on her mother's lap, with a fence and a dog protecting her from the outside world.

POWER MASKS

Learned helplessness and feelings of vulnerability affect children's sense of self-esteem and place them at risk for further abuse. Helping children to identify the source of their personal power reinforces feelings of strength and independence. The session begins with a discussion about power. Power should be defined in terms of inner strength, as well as the courage and ability to enact change and make choices. The therapist presents a variety of magazine pictures of different people—for example, a baby, a boxer, a judge, a school-age child, a teacher, a parent, and so on. Half of the pictures should be of children engaged in various normal daily activities that relate directly or indirectly to the aforementioned definition of power. The children should discuss the power of each person. If they are unable to come up with responses, they should be reminded of the definition.

Examples of correct answers are as follows: "The baby is powerful, because she smiles to get someone's attention or cries to get what she wants," "The child is powerful, because he can keep his room clean or teach his younger sister to play a game." Next, each child should be asked to give an example of how he or she is powerful, and then to create a mask that represents this power. The mask can be made of precut poster board with a craft stick attached at the bottom for holding. The children should be offered a variety of materials for decorating the masks, including markers, glitter, ribbon, beads, feathers, and any other available materials. When the masks are complete, the children are asked to hold up their masks; each is to respond, as his or her mask, by stating "I am powerful because I. . . ."

Termination Activities

To prepare group members for the end of the treatment program, specific termination issues must be addressed. Issues of separation and loss, and fears related to abandonment and change, should be explored. Of equal importance, however, is a focus on growth and healing and movement toward a positive future orientation. Termination activities should, if possible, give the children an opportunity to explore each of these issues. A powerful termination activity asks the children to create their future world in a sand tray. A specific age or amount of time—for example, at age 21 or 20 years from now—can be identified, or the therapist can leave it up to the child to decide how far into the future he or she would like to project. If necessary, the therapist can pose questions such as, "Where would you live?" or, "Who would you want to have in your world with you?"

The final group session should be a celebration of sorts, allowing the children to acknowledge and recognize their accomplishments. Privacy boxes can be reviewed, special goodbye messages or wishes can be added to the group poster, and hugs or special handshakes can be passed around the group circle. A party with festive treats supports the celebratory air of the session. Transitional objects as ending gifts symbolize change and growth. Tabin (2005) notes the value of transitional objects as "extensions of the self, reassuringly proving one's personal continuity, and giving a sense of control." Pocket flashlights or other objects that in some way represent the accomplishments of the group can be appropriate termination gifts.

Play Therapy Toys and Materials

When choosing materials for the playroom, it is important to keep in mind the primary functions of play materials: to enhance thematic and fantasy play, provide vehicles for projection and emotional distancing, promote mastery and self-expression, and support the therapeutic relationship. Although most typical play therapy materials are also appropriate for use with children who have been sexually abused, therapists should carefully choose materials that will make play more purposeful for these children. Because of the nature of the issues with which sexually abused children are dealing and the level of trauma many have experienced related to those issues, materials that support projection and the use of emotional distance are especially useful. Gil (2003) advocates the use of projective play in her belief that "children use projection to both distance and address difficult emotional material. By distancing themselves through symbol they buffer themselves from perceptions, cognitions, or affects that feel uncomfortable, overwhelming, or threatening" (p. 155). A costume box with hats, purses, keys, various other props, and a collection of fabrics in different sizes, colors, and textures facilitates projective play and character development. Providing enough for each child in group allows the children to explore a variety of different roles. Sunglasses are transformational and equip children with a ready disguise and a source of safety (Gallo-Lopez, 2005b). Moreover, sunglasses are wonderful for use in projective play and provide immediate emotional distance for the wearer.

Monster figures are important elements of projective play with younger children. Figures that are not immediately recognizable offer a greater opportunity for use in projective rather then imitative play. Flashlights, though not typical play therapy tools, give children an opportunity to experiment with fears and safety issues in role play and other interventions. Provide enough for all the children in the group. Two dollhouses, along with several sets of family figures, allow children to play out scenes in multiple environments. A variety of art materials should be made available, including materials for mask and puppet making and decorating, large sheets or rolls of craft paper, and spray bottles to be filled with water for the monster-conquering activity. Therapists are advised to provide only materials with which they are comfortable and to practice each activity before using it with children.

Case Illustration

Georgie's wide smile and bright, dark eyes hid deep secrets and intense pain. Just 5 years old, Georgie began attending group therapy only a week after his first day of kindergarten. In school, he learned so quickly that his teacher had to keep finding new ways of challenging him. Within just a few months the school would move him to a first grade class for math and reading. Georgie loved school and was a favorite of his teacher and all the other school personnel. He was friendly and outgoing, and everyone knew him well. At home, however, Georgie's parents were confronted with a very different child. Since his disclosure of sexual abuse by their 15-year-old neighbor Buddy, Georgie had become defiant, destructive, and physically and verbally aggressive. He kicked, hit, and bit both of his parents on numerous occasions, had temper tantrums, during which he threw himself to the ground screaming, and tore his room apart whenever his parents attempted to put him in his room for time-out. One day Georgie's mother walked into his bedroom to find Georgie straddling his 3-year-old brother from behind. Both boys had their pants down around their ankles.

It was just 2 months before beginning treatment that Georgie had disclosed that he had been sexually abused by Buddy, the 15-year-old neighbor, who had been a regular babysitter. The two families were close friends, and Buddy's 6-year-old brother Max had been Georgie's best friend for most of his life. Although at first the goal of both families was to get both boys the help they needed, the situation quickly deteriorated into an ugly battle between the families. Buddy's family eventually moved to another part of town, and the families never saw each other again, except in court.

Their son's disclosure of sexual abuse by Buddy had shocked and infuriated Georgie's parents. Georgie described multiple incidences of anal rape and forced oral sex. He reported having his hands bound behind his back and, on one occasion, being locked in a closet after an attack (in order for Buddy to instill fear and ensure Georgie's silence). Buddy threatened to kill Georgie's little brother and continually warned Georgie that he would be taken away from his parents if he were to tell anyone.

Following this disclosure, Georgie's parents fought all the time. They were distraught over what had happened to their son and worried about what the long-term effects would be for Georgie and their family. They blamed themselves and each other for not being able to protect their child, and they grieved the loss of their best friends. The strain on their relationship was making life at home all the more stressful. As a result, Georgie began to have horrifying nightmares and to fear sleeping in his own bed at night. Aggressive behaviors continued at home. Georgie often kicked, hit, and bit his parents and younger brother. As the case against Buddy progressed, Georgie was referred for treatment by the Department of Children's Services. After his initial assessment, it was determined that Georgie would benefit from group treatment. He was placed in a group with three other 5- and 6-year-old boys. His parents were encouraged to attend the parent support group but were reluctant at first to discuss their problems "with a group of strangers."

Georgie did well in the group right from the start. He enjoyed being with the other boys and was an eager participant in both the structured and nondirective play activities. An extremely creative child, Georgie delighted in leading the group members in the construction of their group poster.

Georgie's self-portrait, created during the second session, began to reveal some of his internal struggle and turmoil. He drew himself as a tiny figure with no hands, floating in the middle of the page. Though he was smiling broadly, his eyes appeared quite sad. On his shirt was a big yellow star. The genital area was circled and the words "bad" and "hate" were scribbled over it. Georgie told a story about his picture, saying that he was happy because he had won a prize at school for reading the most books. When asked about the genital area on his drawing, Georgie indicated that he hated it because of what Buddy had done and it was bad because of what he had done to his brother. The therapist attempted to help Georgie to distinguish between his behaviors and his "self" and to help him to explore sources of his angry feelings other than his own body.

During the third group session the children created their safe place drawings. Georgie drew a picture of himself at school, sitting at his desk surrounded by his classmates and teacher. Georgie said that he felt safest at school because "no one yells at me there, I win prizes, and Buddy can't ever find me there; he doesn't even know where my school is." Georgie described feeling scared at home when "Mommy and Daddy scream at me and at each other" and indicated that he constantly feared that Buddy would try to kill him as he promised. He also reported that he and his brother cry when their parents argue and that he worries that his parents will get divorced and he will then be taken from his parents as Buddy had threatened. This information was shared with Georgie's parents, and they were advised that their stress and conflicts were having a negative impact on their children. The parents agreed to participate in the parents group together and to seek marital counseling to help them repair the damage that been done to their relationship.

Georgie's Color My World drawing, created during the fifth session, included only the colors for mad and sad. Georgie chose red for mad and black for sad and then used markers to write the words in the circle rather then filling the circle with color. "Mad" in large letters filled about one-third of the circle, while "Sad" in even larger letters filled the other two-thirds. Georgie described feeling mad and sad about not being able to see his best friend, Max. He was able to talk about some memories of playing with Max and to verbalize his feelings over the next several sessions. As a result of Georgie's ability to explore and express some of his negative emotions in a safe and appropriate way, his aggressive behaviors at home gradually decreased.

During the tenth session, Georgie painted a large monster with big red eyes, sharp, pointy teeth, and long, sharp claws. This was the monster, he reported, who inhabited his nightmares. Georgie enlisted the aid of other group members in conquering his monster with spray bottles filled with water, the one thing all monsters feared. Georgie watched with wide eyes and a huge grin as his monster dripped from the large sheet of paper and finally disappeared. He then moved on to help other group members conquer their monsters.

Georgie's mother participated with him in the combined parent–child session to create a safe place in the sand tray. Together they created several rooms in the family's home. Georgie put figures representing his parents sitting together on a sofa in the living room with their arms around each other. Figures representing Georgie and his little brother sat in their laps. Georgie said the family would be watching cartoons together, expressing an apparent need to normalize the family's functioning. He was able to verbalize to his mother his fear that his parents would divorce and that then he wouldn't be able to see them again, just as he couldn't see his friend Max or, even worse, that he would be taken away from them as Buddy had threatened. Georgie's mother assured him that she and his dad were working on their problems and that no matter what, he would never be taken away from them. Georgie then had his mother help him create his bedroom in another area of the sand tray. Next to his bed he placed the spray bottle he had used to conquer his monster. When his mother asked about it, Georgie responded, "Just in case that monster comes back, I'll be ready."

During one of the final sessions, the group created their power masks. Georgie's mask was bright, colorful, and decorated with lots of glitter. The mouth was a broad smile. Georgie indicated that he was powerful because he was smart and strong: "I can write lots of words and I can get rid of monsters."

After the treatment group ended, Georgie and his family participated in several family therapy sessions to attempt to heal some of the wounds they had suffered as a family and to strengthen the family relationships. Georgie's parents involved him in several activities, including Cub Scouts, in which he was able to begin to develop new friendships.

CONCLUSION

In this chapter, a time-limited group treatment program is presented for use with sexually abused children ages 3–10. The program combines the essential elements of therapy with sexually abused children into a treatment protocol that has been found to be well suited for this population. It offers a time-limited approach that directly addresses symptoms of trauma, developmental issues, and the impact of sexual abuse on interpersonal relationships. Though much of the program is directive and abuse-specific, it utilizes the healing power of child-centered, nondirective play therapy to enhance the potential for growth and change.

REFERENCES

Burns, R. C., & Kaufman, S. H. (1970). *Kinetic family drawings.* New York: Brunner/ Mazel.

Cohen, J. A., Berliner, L., & March, J. S. (2000). Treatment of children and adolescents. In E. B. Foa, T. M. Keane, & M. J. Friedman (Eds.), *Effective treatments for PTSD: Practice guidelines from the International Society for Traumatic Stress studies* (pp. 106–138). New York: Guilford Press.

Costas, M., & Landreth, G. (1999). Filial therapy with nonoffending parents of children who have been sexually abused. *International Journal of Play Therapy, 8*(1), 43–66.

Finkelhor, D., & Browne, A. (1986). Initial and long-term effects: A conceptual framework. In D. Finkelhor (Ed.), *A sourcebook on child sexual abuse* (pp. 180–198). Newbury Park, CA: Sage.

Friedrich, W. (1991, Spring). Child victims: Promising techniques and programs in the treatment of child sexual abuse. *The APSAC Advisor,* pp. 5–6.

Gallo-Lopez, L. (2005a). Drama therapy in the treatment of children with sexual behavior problems. In A. M. Weber & C. Haen (Eds.), *Clinical applications of drama therapy in child and adolescent treatment* (pp. 137–151). New York: Brunner-Routledge.

Gallo-Lopez, L. (2005b). Drama therapy with adolescents. In L. Gallo-Lopez & C. E. Schaefer (Eds.), *Play therapy with adolescents* (pp. 81–95). New York: Aronson.

Gil, E. (2003). Art and play therapy with sexually abused children. In C. A. Malchiodi (Ed.), *Handbook of art therapy* (pp. 152–166). New York: Guilford Press.

Irwin, G., & Malloy, E. (1975). Family puppet interview. *Family Process, 14*(2), 179–191.

Long, S. (1986). Guidelines for treating young children. In K. MacFarlane, J. Waterman, S. Conerly, L. Damon, M. Durfee, & S. Long (Eds.), *Sexual abuse of young children* (pp. 220–246). New York: Guilford Press.

Longo, R. E., & Longo, D. P. (2003). *New hope for youth: Experiential exercises for children and adolescents.* Holyoke, MA: NEARI Press.

Mandell, J. G., & Damon, L. (1989). *Group treatment for sexually abused children.* New York: Guilford Press.

O'Connor, K. J. (1983). The color-your-life technique. In C. E. Schaefer & K. J. O'Connor (Eds.), *Handbook of play therapy* (pp. 251–258). New York: Wiley.

Powell, L., & Faherty, S. L. (1990). Treating sexually abused latency aged girls. *Arts in Psychotherapy, 17,* 35–47.

Rasmussen, L., & Cuningham, C. (1995). Focused play therapy and non-directive play therapy: Can they be integrated? *Journal of Child Sexual Abuse, 4*(1), 1–20.

Salter, A. (1988). *Treating child sex offenders and victims.* Newbury Park, CA: Sage.

Sedlak, A., & Broadhurst, D. (1996). *Third national incidence study of child abuse and neglect.* Washington, DC: National Clearinghouse on Child Abuse and Neglect Information.

Steward, M. S., Farquhar, L. C., Dicharry, D. C., Glick, D. R., & Martin, P. W. (1986). Group therapy: A treatment of choice for young victims of child abuse. *International Journal of Child Psychotherapy, 36*, 261–275.

Tabin, J. K. (2005). Transitional objects in play therapy with adolescents. In L. Gallo-Lopez & C. E. Schaefer (Eds.), *Play therapy with adolescents* (pp. 68–80). New York: Aronson.

CHAPTER 11

Group Sandtray Play Therapy

LINDA B. HUNTER

The need for relevant mental health interventions for children is clear. Publicized examples of violence in schools have brought new attention to the impact that the emotional and social aspects of students' lives have on their learning and behavior. Studies in the United States show that one in every ten children has mental health problems that impair the child's emotional, social, and intellectual functioning and less than half of that number receive treatment. Interventions that can be delivered in schools and other settings where children are already present and can serve many children in a timely, accessible, cost-effective way are clearly needed (Packman & Bratton, 2003).

A group model that uses the expressive arts play therapy technique called sandtray play has been shown to be highly successful in meeting this need. This approach combines client-centered attitudes and techniques of creating "free and protected space," witnessing the play, and facilitating the group, with a Jungian emphasis on the power of imaginative symbolic meanings and the dynamics and benefits of group therapy. This technique can successfully "travel" to schools, preschools, after-school programs, shelters, camps, and other locations where children spend most of their time.

During much of their day children are expected to conform to structures created by others. An empowering child-centered group environment is so different from this norm that it has tremendous impact. The power of this model comes from the creation of an environment that is both free and protected, allowing each child an opportunity to make many choices, practice skills to resolve both personal and interpersonal problems, experience self-control, and develop confidence, trust, and hope. Because this opportunity is available in children's real-world settings, the learning, growth, and change it fosters easily generalize to the classroom and playground.

A multileveled (physical and emotional) free and protected space provides safety to express true feelings, concerns, and emotional pain. A resiliency model focusing on strengths is used to evaluate and describe children's progress. Cultural sensitivity is accomplished by connecting into the universal spirit of creativity and providing toys relevant to diverse groups. This nonverbal process encourages storytelling, makes possible identity exploration, and works effectively on both intrapsychic and interpersonal levels.

THE WORLD TECHNIQUE

Margaret Lowenfeld (1979, pp. 3–4), a pediatrician in post-World War I England, was intently interested in understanding the causes of war and violence in the human mind. To facilitate real understanding, she worked to devise a method by which "children can demonstrate their own emotional and mental state without the necessary intervention of an adult."

In the safe and playful clinic that Lowenfeld created, the children themselves developed the method she was looking for. By spontaneously combining carefully selected miniature toys with trays of sand and water, children created what they called their "worlds." As she saw the tremendous value of the process, standards were developed. Trays were positioned at a child's waist level for ease in placing and moving objects. The dimensions were defined so that a tray filled a single field of vision. The inside bottom was painted blue to represent water, and real water was available to wet the sand. Drawings were made of the scene the child created to record the work for further study.

Thus, Lowenfeld succeeded in developing a process (the World Technique) that allows the expression of nonverbal, metaphorical, visual, and active states of being and happenings within the psyche. One participant concluded, "It is as if I had previously been trying to describe colors in words and had now, for the first time, been handed brushes and paints" (Lowenfeld, 1979, p. 269).

SANDPLAY

As a student of Carl Jung's who was intensely attracted to working with children, Dora Kalff built Lowenfeld's process into today's system of sandplay therapy. To the communication potential of the World Technique, Kalff added Jung's view of a psyche that contains strong spiritual and symbolic unconscious forces. With sandplay she extended the range of Jungian active imagination techniques into a concrete modality that does not require practice or insight, and thus introduced child therapy into the work of Jungian analysts. She integrated Eastern philosophical ideas of the power of silence and receptive openness into the process. She taught that the therapist's development as a person is equally important as knowledge of symbols in creating the "free and protected space" in which healing occurs.

Kalff (1980) advocated having many and varied figures available as an invitation to free expression of the "inner creative manifoldness which is hidden in every person." She stressed the healing power of a symbol as it evolves through a series of sandplay scenes.

SANDPLAY AS THE LANGUAGE

Sandplay provides a language that is active yet safe, silent yet resonant. It can make the mysterious and unspeakable vividly visible and understandable. Sandplay, like story and the visual arts, provides the language of a country where fantasy and reality meet, where metaphor and image rule over fact and word. Symbols and images create the "language of magic," connecting emotions and intellect.

The language of sandplay bridges the *having* of the experience, and the *recollecting* and *reshaping* of it in imagination. Because sandplay involves the body in the placing of figures and the moving of sand, it is actual experience that creates neural pathways, memories, and resources in the child's brain. Once a child has created a significant image in a sand tray, its power becomes available to enrich everyday life. When the child confronts the image he or she has made, the mirror is being held up by the self. Communication is in the native language (Hunter, 1998). No translation or interpretation is needed for this thinking that can be seen out loud (child's comments).

Thus, sandplay provides a way in which even nonverbal children can "tell" their stories to an observer/listener. For the therapist, Harriet Friedman (1997, p. 19) writes, "a Sandplay picture is to the psyche what an x-ray is to the body," helping us to understand the child and the play process. Sandplay therapy combines the use of sand, water, and miniature figures and a well-defined role for the therapist.

THE MATERIALS

Sand

Sand is both a common and a unique material. It has been used throughout history in rituals of "visioning" and releasing healing powers. Formed by the action of wind, fire, and water on rock, sand represents the elements combined, the *prima materia*. Tibetan Buddhist sand mandala-making ceremonies and Japanese Zen sand gardens create symbolic space. Navajo sand paintings connect to divine healing.

Playing in sand brings memories of sandboxes and the enjoyment of beaches. Sand can be soothing and comforting, like a gentle, nurturing touch, creating a meditative focus and calm energy. Sand, like clay, is good for children who are afraid of making mistakes because it is easily fixed and guarantees success. Burying and finding figures in the sand allows older children to revisit the infant's task of discovering object permanence (Stewart, 1990). Sand focuses the energy of those with hyperactivity and attention difficulties, encourages regression in a playful way, provides a sensory experience for the desensitized, and allows the angry to make positive use of aggressive energy. Sand can be used constructively to make mountains and caves, and destructively to pull figures under, as into quicksand. Sand is symbolically the perfect medium for the work being done in therapy: earth at the border between the unseen, unconscious depths of the sea and the consciously visible shore (Ryce-Menuhin, 1992).

Water

Water represents the unconscious, the feminine, the unknown. Water cleans and cools and drowns. Water is symbolically represented by exposing the blue bottom of the tray or imagining the dry sand as waves or falling rain. When possible, having wet sand or water available for use can allow sculpted sand to hold its shape, thus adding dimension to the landscape.

The Miniature Collection: Symbols of the Real and the Imaginary

Miniature figures, representing many diverse aspects of life, add meaning to the use of sand and water. Nurturing, scary, aggressive, fantasy, familiar—the toys become words for the child's language of play, offering a large vocabulary for the expression of feelings and thoughts, events and wishes. "From time immemorial children have found in their native soil and in the miniature objects in the world around them, the basic tools for structuring their imagination" (Stewart, 1982, p. 204). In antiquity, toys were amulets to protect children against evil influences. Children use toys to externalize their unconscious processes, and to embody and control complex, unacceptable, contradictory parts of themselves. Toys become symbols that connect children to the collective wisdom of humankind and facilitate the development of a sense of meaning and hope for the future. A room with accessibly displayed toys offers the child a familiar and understandable environment and engages even those who intend to be resistant. Figures can be arranged on shelves or in containers. They are categorized according to type:

- Animals—farm, pets, wild, ocean, insects, birds, reptiles, fantasy, prehistoric.
- Vehicles—cars, planes, boats, military, rescue, trains, wagons, skateboards.
- People—family, working, fighting, spiritual, fantasy, hero, babies, cartoon, community, ethnic.
- Landscape—buildings, bridges, trees, flowers, fences, signs, wells, screens, sun, moon, fire, globe.
- Accessories—toilet, telephone, badge, fire extinguisher, first aid kit, keys, tools, mirror, lamp, musical instruments.
- Large shadow figures—monsters, snakes, alligators, sharks, dinosaurs, dragons, bad guys, witches.
- Power/ego protector figures—Batman, Superman, wrestler, Indian chief, king, pilot.
- Magic—fairies, angels, wands, rings, crystals, jewels, wizards, stars, masks.
- Treasure—beads, gold, colored glass, pyrite, costume jewelry, chest/bag, coins, money.
- Natural materials—stones, shells, driftwood, seeds, coral, pine cones, geodes, sticks, feathers, rocks.

Mythological, primitive, and fantasy figures, from a wide range of cultures and historical eras, are often used to express deeply unconscious archetypal meanings.

Many cartoon figures are useful. Although children may initially choose Batman or "the Beast," with the movie in mind, their interior processes soon change the meaning to something personal and significant.

With the large number of toys available, children have a great deal of choice. Broken toys can remain to represent the broken parts of a child's life. Miniature weapons at the scale of the figures can be used to represent violence and protection without play becoming overtly aggressive.

For special populations, figures can be selected to represent specific aspects of life: rural/urban buildings and implements; figures with ethnic features or skin tones; cultural, religious, or national items. Adolescents appreciate figures that are musical, technological, ambiguous, "real," intricate, or to scale. Collections can be tailored to the needs of special settings such as hospitals, shelters, homes, or schools. Portable collections can have some figures from each category, including a few that are large and scary.

Sturdy, inexpensive figures can be purchased in toy stores, dollar stores, and gift shops, as well as at flea markets, yard sales, thrift shops, craft/hobby/ train and hardware stores, pet shops, Christmas and cake decoration stores, party supply and dollhouse stores, and can be found on walks to the beach or through a forest.

The Sandtray

A tray contains the scene and provides boundaries for the work being done, helping children to accept, create, and expand limits. Regulation-size trays are approximately 20" × 30" × 3" deep to encompass the visual field. They are painted blue on the bottom and sides to represent water/sky.

The empty space of the sand tray activates the imagination and becomes a "doorway" to a magic realm. By the child's own actions, abstract ideas and feelings are made visible for which he or she is clearly responsible. A completed tray acts as a mirror that shows the child the real inner self, producing an image that is both internal and external, transitory and permanent, a product of both the unconscious mind that selects the figures and the conscious mind that creates the scene (Bradway, 1986; Bradway & McCoard, 1997).

To create boundaries for a miniature play space when standard trays are not available, it is possible to use makeshift trays of plastic or cardboard boxes, drawers, cafeteria servers, or cookie sheets. When not using trays or sand, a space can be outlined by the builder with yarn or string, a mat or paper, a rug, scarf, or fabric, defined with blocks, fences, train tracks or beads, or drawn outside in the dirt or sand.

THE THERAPIST'S ROLE

Carl Rogers's (1951) and Carl Jung's beliefs in the individual's capacity for growth and self-direction provide the foundation for the therapeutic relationship. An atmosphere of acceptance and permissiveness is established in which the child feels safe to choose to do or not do, say or not say, whatever he or she wants, subject to only minimal limits to prevent injury to persons or significant property.

Because a child's inner experience is constantly changing and reorganizing, only the child knows the work he or she needs to be doing at any given point. The child takes the time he or she needs and moves on when ready. The child interprets for self and therapist. The therapist accepts, reflects, and sometimes comments. In the safety of the therapeutic relationship thus created, the structure of the child's self relaxes, new experiences can be integrated, and change can take place.

Sandplay combines the accepting attitude of client-centered therapy with an analytical awareness of the power of symbols, a holistic emphasis on the mutual interaction of mind, body, and imagination, and a strengths focus on the attributes of a resilient child. Children "talk" through play, structuring their play activity like a conversation. As the child selects symbols and invests them with personal meaning, pictures are created that are attempts to communicate with adults outside the language of words. In this way, the child works on contact and building trust, healing and growth.

Because play is the "royal road to the child's inner world" (Bettelheim, 1987), the therapist learns to walk that road and imaginatively align with the child. The therapist creates a holding environment based on understanding, accepting, and affirming the child. A mutual "co-transference field" is established (Bradway & McCoard, 1997).

The therapist's role is to observe/listen to the child, to receive the child's communications with respect for the inner worth, potential, healing, and growth possibilities valued by both Rogers and Jung. The therapist is both the witness, attending with mindful awareness, silent attention, and nonjudgmental presence at each moment, and the participant–observer, attempting to see from the child's perspective, build the relationship, convey caring and encouragement, and facilitate decision making.

Using Jung's four functions the therapist *observes* (sensate), pays attention to impressions (*feeling*) and hunches (*intuition*), then *thinks* (reasoning) about the child's "world." The therapist accepts expression of the child's feelings and fantasies without minimizing or overreacting, appreciating how the child's imagination and creativity lead to growth and mastery. Respectful attention leads to the child's showing hidden, often positive, aspects of self.

The therapist works to develop and communicate understanding of the intent/purpose of the child's actions and words, the uniqueness, rhythm, and pace of the child's growing and changing, and the child's struggle to deal with challenges, frustrations, and disappointments. The therapist offers reflective listening/observing within the child's metaphor, avoiding verbal interpretation, controlling personal projections, and recognizing that it is the player's experience of the process, not the therapist's understanding, that heals (Bradway & McCoard, 1997).

TECHNIQUES FOR WITNESSING PLAY

I. Structuring play sessions for the group
    A. Expectations: "In here you may play with the toys in *almost* any way you want to—I will let you know if there is something you may not do."
    B. Boundaries: stay in room; give 5-minute warning, then end session on time.
II. Empathic listening responses
    A. Tracking behavior: attention and interest without demands, direction, or labeling. "You are putting those two together." "The little one is in the corner."

B. Reflecting content: restating/paraphrasing verbal statements. "Oh, the big giraffe is the mother and the little one is the child."

C. Acknowledging feelings, wants, ideas: validating the child's internal world.

   1. Feelings cause behavior: All actions and words are motivated by and communicate the underlying feeling, thought, or need. Acknowledging often diffuses the feeling enough so that the child doesn't have to act it out and learns to verbalize.

   2. Good reflections are brief, tentative, neutral; statements, not questions.

   3. Can be in the child's metaphor—"The lion seems angry and the rabbit looks scared"—or direct—"You're disappointed that didn't work out," "You seem upset/ angry/ frustrated."

D. Encouraging/esteem building: Focus on competency, creativity; credit effort. "You worked hard on that and figured it out." "You are able to do that."

E. Facilitating decision making, responsibility: encourages exploration, sense of control. Not answering questions helps the child create internal standards and find his or her own answers.

   1. Child asks: "Do you like what I made?" Response: " You worked hard on your 'world' and want me to see it. In here it's what you like that's important."

   2. Child asks: "What should I build?" Response: "That's up to you to decide."

   3. Child asks: "What is this?" Response: "In here that can be whatever you want it to be."

F. Enlarging the meaning: connecting the play to basic themes:

   1. Belonging: "You're thinking about the differences between people."

   2. Mastery: "You're wondering if it's possible to be strong without being angry."

III. Limit-setting process: three-step model—to *ACT* rather than yell (Landreth, 1991). Teaches child to regulate own behavior, take responsibility for own actions, self-control. Children's ability to test and break limits is an important aspect of their learning and growing.

A. *Acknowledge* the feeling/want/need: make a reflection. "You would like to throw sand."

B. *Communicate* the limit: brief, clear, firm, understandable. Stated as "facts," not personalized. "Sand is not for throwing on the floor" *not* "You can't throw sand on the floor."

C. *Target* an acceptable alternative: way of expressing the feeling that is safe and appropriate. Redirect the feeling into different behavior: "You may throw the sand in the tray."

IV. Choices and consequences: fourth step to limit setting. Wording is important. When we use *choice* words and consistent follow-through, children eventually understand that they are responsible for the consequences of their behavior and choices.

A. "If you choose to *keep the sand in the tray,* you choose to *keep playing with the sand.*"

B. "If you choose to [break limit] *throw sand on the floor,* you will be choosing to [consequence] *not use the sand any more today.*"

C. "Since you chose to *throw sand on the floor,* you have chosen to *stop using the sand.*"

THE POWER OF SANDPLAY

Sandplay harnesses the natural, spontaneous play behavior of children. The materials are familiar and comfortable, inviting the child to play, build rapport with the therapeutic setting, and create a bridge to the adult world. Sandplay is always successful, no talent or technique is needed, and the product is easily changed. Children find the abundant and accessible small toys appealing, interesting, and fun. Exploratory behavior is stimulated by diverse figures and possibilities. As the child leads the play, his or her whole being is involved, including thoughts, emotions, behavior, and the senses of touch, sight, and sound. Abstract concepts are made concrete in the form of tangible symbols that bring inner and outer worlds together through imagination. Figures gathered into clusters communicate many meanings visually and simultaneously.

Combination of Techniques

As a therapeutic modality, sandplay integrates the benefits of many diverse expressive techniques. Like the use of puppets, sandplay combines movement, verbal expression, and an invitation to shift identities. Like storytelling, sandplay identifies and resolves conflicts. Like a doll-house, the use of the realistic people and household figures encourages the child to discuss family issues and to disclose and overcome abuse.

Like the use of art, sandplay concretizes feelings, shifts internal events into the external arena, and produces a tangible product that holds the significance of the child's communication and reduces the need for verbalization (Case & Dalley, 1990). Sandplay often incorporates psychodrama as the child spontaneously speaks for different characters in the scenes. As a miniaturized form of family sculpting, sandplay shows existing and desired relationships and issues of belonging. In sandplay, children easily identify with cartoon and heroic characters, who become powerful imaginary friends and help the children build self-confidence and resolve problems (Mills & Crowley, 1986).

Why It Works

Sandplay is a holistic process that brings together many opposites. Sand worlds express both distress and coping, difficulties and strengths, destruction and reconstruction, concurrently releasing feelings and activating inner resources. Sandplay allows the unconscious to lead, and healing to happen from within (Dundas, 1990). Using both hands simultaneously engages both sides of the brain, increasing visual skills and harnessing imagination, in effect training the "right brain." Noyes (1981) found that this enabled her remedial reading students to become "top-down" readers, connecting the written words to their inner experiences and much improving their reading skills.

Fantasy included in the sand tray becomes reality through conscious acts of choice. There is both freedom (of action) and restriction (limited number of figures to choose from). By being given structure and form, experiences become meaningful. Emotions are not only expressed but become concrete. Nightmare images can be reevaluated in the light of day. The terrific pressure of fantasies decreases as they are creatively expressed. The anxious child calms and focuses.

Sandplay facilitates the process of "synesthesia": inner translation from one modality of receiving and processing information (such as auditory) to another (such as visual). In a very real way, we can see our feelings and touch our thoughts. Using creative, playful means to access traumatic events and difficult feelings combines the positive with the negative in a way that changes the meaning of such events. The power of the feeling dissipates (Lankton, 1980).

The positive power of magical thinking, the sense that what we believe affects our world, that our thoughts make transformation possible, can, in the sand tray, become integrated into tangible reality.

A Quiet Therapy

"I talked lots about everything that happened but here I have been very quiet, I been thinking. Thinking is hard coz no one hears you, but this sand picture is a sort of thinking picture, isn't it, and you can see it out loud."
—CHILD QUOTED IN DEDOMENICO (1988, p. 1)

Ultimately, the power of sandplay is the response it evokes in the child, the "dialogue that takes place between player and play" (Kiepenheuer, 1990, p. 83). A meditative state, relaxed and playful but focused, emerges naturally as the child becomes completely absorbed. Often the body language is trancelike, showing tremendous intensity and duration of concentration. Sandplay taps into the essence of language: the transformation of experience into symbols that can be manipulated and expressed. With play symbols substituted for words, the child can speak without having to give up silence. This silent work/

play can go very deep, tapping into a preverbal mode of image thinking that combines heart, body, and imagination. Spending time with symbols in this quiet meditative way activates their healing potential (Furth, 1988).

HEALING TRAUMA

Healing from trauma begins with telling the story, giving names to the fears, acknowledging the pain and anger as human and universal, honoring what is lost and the humanity of the "enemies" that are seen as causing the loss (Thomas, 2002).

One of the often noted obstacles to telling the story of a traumatic event is the desire and need to avoid reminders that trigger reliving of the horror. Memories of "unspeakable" traumatic events are usually recorded in visual and sensory form. Release of these memories through projective visual and kinesthetic techniques is recognized as both more useful and more humane than allowing traumatic material to emerge in a verbal mode. Techniques that allow the right brain to rework a memory or issue through all sensory systems actually create a new experience at the body–mind level, healing the dissociative splits that occur as a result of traumatic fear and pain, and helping children to find an "emotionally meaningful context into which to place their terrors" (Terr, 1990).

Through play, children express, cope with, master, and move past pain. When adults witness their play, respect and accept it without intrusion, the healing reaches a deeper level. Play allows a potentially damaging secret ritual to heal as it is witnessed by the therapist (Gil, 1991).

In sandplay children can replay the horror and create the hope. They can express the scream (of pain, fear, anger) and find the dream (of beauty, peace, safety). They can re-member, re-experience, and re-work on their own terms.

Imagine children creating miniature worlds that are images of the suffering, fear, and anger that exist in their memories. Imagine the same children creating images of peace, beauty, and unity that exist in their imaginations. Imagine creating these images not only internally or with words, but in actual experience, hands moving figures and sand, solid symbols. Imagine being able to shoot the sand bullets, drop the pebble bombs, destroy the plastic houses, bury the miniature people and animals. Imagine being in charge of the resistance, the rebuilding, the resurrection.

The choices of figures, placement, movement, and story are under the children's control at all times and can be easily changed. Their helplessness can be portrayed, then changed into power. Their fear can be given symbolic form, acknowledged, and transcended by finding support from internal and external resources. Mastery, resolution, control, power, and hope are all hidden in the figures and the sand, waiting to be discovered by any child who can play.

Sandplay makes possible the resolution of both individual trauma and group conflict and allows expression of spiritual, ethnocultural, and political, as well as psychological and interpersonal aspects, in a way that does not retraumatize.

Early pictures often portray devastation, whereas later ones show wishes and hopes for the future. Boys' images often are dynamic and technical, involving planes, cars, or battles. Girls' pictures tend to be more decorative, often focusing on houses, gardens, and relationships. Neither may ever mention the divorce or loss or troubling event that is the reason for their referral, but often they become happier and better behaved.

Shooting the Arrow of Anger

Trauma that is caused by the actions of other people, as in a violent attack or abuse, is most difficult to resolve. Pain is then accompanied and fueled by anger. Sharing the pain is not enough. As Virginia Satir taught (Brothers, 2002), there is a need to "shoot the arrow of anger" to get it out as well, but to shoot it safely, so as not to hurt anyone. Novel means of engaging children are needed to bypass the avoidance factor and allow the expression of intense rage and revenge fantasies in a safe context in which emotional reactions can be validated, mastery increased, and a sense of security regained.

This miniaturized form of play provides a safe outlet for aggressive energy, an opportunity to behaviorally reenact trauma in a nondangerous way. Consequences remain safely in the realm of fantasy, which buffers both the child's and the therapist's connection to what is being expressed. In this small world, the therapist's acceptance and empathy have a much better chance of remaining genuine and thus encouraging full expression.

This active mode of expression is particularly well suited for children who have been deeply wounded. In the sand tray, worst fear scenarios can be played out with different endings, with humor, and with hope. Chaos can be lived with and directed to creative purposes. Ways can be found to accept the unacceptable. Therapeutic relationships can develop with minimal dependence.

The dual nature of play, which both reveals and conceals at the same time, means that issues are revealed symbolically, through image and metaphor, to the trained and watchful eye of the therapist. The same symbols can conceal from the child's conscious awareness that which he or she is not yet ready to acknowledge. For example, a giant male fantasy figure can be murderously fought and repeatedly destroyed. In this way a boy can express his rage at the father who has hurt and abandoned him without having to explicitly own these terrifying feelings (Hunter, 1998).

Thus, the child can maintain defenses and rework conflicts on a deeply symbolic level (Ekstein, 1966), strengthening the ego and dealing with feelings of low self-esteem and helplessness.

SANDTRAY PLAY IN GROUPS

Groups are based on the client-centered theory of respect for the child's innate ability to mature, learn, solve problems, and positively self-direct, given a safe environment, complete acceptance, a respectful, caring attitude, and empathic understanding by therapeutic adults.

In a small-group setting, work is done on both intrapsychic and interpersonal levels, and on inner and outer issues simultaneously. Each group member is both an observer and a participant, a builder and a witness for peers, a giver and a receiver of attention. There is an opportunity for parallel and cooperative play. Children learn to establish individual boundaries, respect those of others, and come together in community (Kestly, 2001). Sand trays and figures are used as the primary mode of communication and vehicle of interaction. Fantasy is given full expression in the sandtray play, and connected to reality by the group. Group sand tray play allows therapy to become a nonlabeling, nonstigmatizing, noncompetitive experience that reduces isolation and normalizes the difficulties with which children struggle.

In the group, children work on social interaction and learn social skills. Group therapy allows for increased participation and vicarious learning, inasmuch as the presence of peers reduces anxiety and makes children more likely to risk expression and try out new behaviors (DeMaria, 1992). Group members experience a relationship, become aware of self and others, learn empathy, appreciate differences, and value uniqueness. They practice life situations, become assertive, develop ego strength, and share their visions. Through feedback from peers, they learn social cues, turn taking, reality testing, and the emotional intelligence to read how others react to their actions. Peers model for less able, more reluctant players.

In group therapy more children can get help in a timely, effective way. Disturbing behaviors can be both more evident and more easily addressed than in the classroom or large program setting. New behaviors can be practiced and more easily generalized. Through participation in groups, children become better able to cope with many stresses in their lives. They experience solving problems through negotiation and compromise. They become more aware of their own and others' feelings and learn to express them appropriately and safely. They develop the skills to communicate and cooperate with peers and adults and the confidence needed to succeed socially and academically.

Group Set-up

Sandtray play groups can be held in diverse settings: schools, preschools, after-school programs, shelters, offices, summer camps, and the like. Eight to twelve sessions, 30–45 minutes in length, with two to six children in each group, is the starting point for planning. Where possible, as in schools, it has been useful to extend the participation of individual children who need and are benefiting from the process, to a second series of group sessions. From preschool through middle school, sand tray play groups have been highly successful.

The composition of the play group is heterogeneous and balanced: boys and girls; active and quiet; with different levels of maturity, social skills, and presenting problems; within a 2-year chronological age span. Both acting-out children (the most referred) and withdrawn children (the least referred) can work on their difficulties in functioning by learning new behaviors as situations arise in the group and by making positive changes (Allan & Bertoia, 1992). Permission forms signed by parents describe the process, goals, and purpose of group treatment.

Providing groups on-site in school or in other facilities brings up the issue of space. The ideal room is one in which very few limits are needed to protect the space or its contents from harm. The room is large enough to handle both active and quiet, individual and interactive, play simultaneously, and is away from major school traffic, offices, and classrooms to ensure privacy and not disturb others with noise. Sand tray play groups have the advantage of being able to work well in smaller spaces than more active play therapy groups. Groups have been held in cafeterias and closets, media centers and offices, in art/music rooms and on stages, in storage rooms and in portable facilities. Setup can be on tables, desks, or floors, or on blue plastic cloths spread on the ground outdoors under a roof that protects the space from sun and rain.

An efficient arrangement is to schedule two to four groups in the same setting during one time period, with perhaps a 15-minute break between groups. In this way, group sessions for 8–16 children can be provided in a morning or afternoon, including driving to and from the site, setup, and cleanup.

Older Children and Adolescents

For children who have experienced trauma, the time period for using pretend play is extended into latency and beyond, making sand tray play therapy an extremely potent way to effect internal change. The groups for older children and adolescents adapt the play process in relevant, constructive ways. According to Landreth (1983, p. 201), "until children reach a level of facility and sophistication with verbal communication that allows them to express themselves fully and effectively to others, use of play media is mandatory" for therapy to happen. Verbalizing feelings and thoughts becomes a goal of the work instead of the entire method, and other means of expression are made available. Members give each other honest verbal, as well as nonverbal, feedback, guiding both the "bully" and the "crybaby" into more useful ways of relating.

For teens, the variety of figures that are available enables many to create scenes without embarrassment or resistance. The less threatening group environment, and the opportunity to interact with peers without adult interference, reduce tension and increase participation and spontaneity. The miniature figures bring the external world down to a manageable size, allowing complete control of the action. The limits of the sand tray help the children set their own limits. There is no technique that has to be learned, no talent that makes a difference in the product. Scenes can be destroyed and remade quickly, so anxiety is reduced and failure is not an issue.

Adult Teams

Teams of therapeutic adults may be utilized in sandtray play therapy. Such teams consist of a counselor or therapist supported by interns, graduate or undergraduate students, or retired volunteers, who, with minimal initial training, can observe as they learn the techniques of nonintrusive witnessing. The advantages of utilizing therapeutic teams are several:

1. Essential elements of both individual and group therapies are combined. Children experience an opportunity for building a trusting, close relationship with positive, safe, accepting adults. Children also learn and practice social skills in a small group of peers, getting direct and clear feedback and many, many second chances to figure out more useful ways of interacting.

2. With a significant adult presence, a loosely structured situation remains safe. An angry, out-of-control child can have one-on-one attention, allowing the maximum opportunity for self-control to develop, while the ability to intervene in any aggressive situation before it becomes dangerous is maintained.

3. The training of new play therapists is facilitated. By working in a group soon after their initial training program, beginning therapists can learn by watching and doing. They observe experienced play therapists in action, try out the techniques they have been taught, and work gradually and comfortably into a more active role. They can process their experiences and ask questions during cleanup time. The most dedicated become the teachers of the next generation of play therapists.

Leaders of sand tray play groups need training and work with individuals before attempting the group setting. Counselors trying to conduct a group alone are advised to start with two children so that they can pay adequate attention to each child's work and maintain a facilitative presence. All are advised to seek training in sand tray play and stay within their own levels of competence (Kestly, 2001).

THE PROCESS OF SANDTRAY PLAY GROUPS

The team arrives 15–20 minutes before the group is scheduled to start and arranges the designated group space to be inviting and child-friendly. The sand trays are smaller, deeper, and less expensive translucent plastic storage boxes that can be stacked and stored from week to week in the various group locations. To make the bottoms blue, we place the trays on bright blue vinyl tablecloth material. Water is sometimes made available in spray bottles so that mountains, caves, and tunnels can hold their shape. The miniature figures are often brought in each week because they are used in several different settings. The most efficient way of handling figures we have found is to use mini rolling storage cabinets with six shallow drawers that can be removed easily from each unit and placed on counter, table, desk, or floor so that the children can make their selections. Toys are organized by drawer in broad categories of animals (wild and domestic), people, landscape, vehicles, and accessories.

Children enter the group room; each sits in front of a tray and uses his or her hands to play in the dry sand while everyone gets settled and says his or her name. When they are introduced to the sand in this way, we find the children more likely to actively use the sand in the constructed "worlds." A small card with a name on it is placed in each tray to make it clear whose world this is and to identify the photos taken at the end of the activity. The children then each take a basket and go to the drawers to select their figures. They play and build, returning to choose more figures as often as they wish, until the counselor gives a 5-minute warning to prepare for pictures and stories. When they are ready, if they choose, a picture is taken, and all listen to the stories they tell about their worlds. At the end of the group meetings each child is given an album with his or her series of pictures to review and take home.

Rules and directions are few. An important rule is to respect the boundaries of the individual trays. Sometimes we explain as follows: "Pretend that I want to use this lion figure that John has in his tray. May I reach in and take it?" Most children will say, "No." "OK, but what if I ask John and he says, 'Yes,' may I then reach in and take it?" Most young children will say, "Yes" to this question, but we explain: "John is the only one who may play in his tray, so he takes the lion out and hands it to me," which he then demonstrates. After all the children work in individual trays for a few weeks and boundaries are established, a larger "together" tray is made available, in which children can build jointly if they want to. Children sometimes choose to put two individual trays next to each other and join their worlds, or create a battle, game, or event using one tray and the surrounding table.

In addition to working on their individual issues and negotiating about the use of the figures, children who are fighting sometimes build in the same tray and then get along better. In one group, two girls with very different personalities, who knew each other well but had a hard time getting along, used a tray together. One would put a figure in, and the other would immediately move or change it. After some time the first girl's assertiveness grew, and the second girl became more aware and in control of her intrusiveness. A new equality and friendship developed.

With groups of young acting-out, energetic boys we include some tension/energy release items: big bears to absorb full body aggression as substitutes: "People are not for hitting or kicking or any other form of hurting, but you can use the bear." Soft fabric balls are available as "soft things for throwing" in place of the hard miniature figures. Styrofoam egg cartons or trays similarly replace toys as things that are "for breaking" when there is a therapeutic need to stomp on or otherwise smash something.

Groups are based on the principles of a client-centered (Rogerian) model. Group sessions are the children's time to talk/play about whatever they choose, practice decision making and self-control, and resolve their own conflicts. The adults pay very close attention to everything said and done by the children, making statements that track behaviors, reflect feelings, encourage growth, and build self-esteem. Limits are therapeutically set to protect the physical safety of persons and property. The freedom to be self-directed, the safe environment, the interaction with other children, the accepting attitude of the counselors and facilitators, and the availability of multiple miniatures and individual trays of sand all combine to produce a powerful therapeutic experience.

Statements that track behavior and reflections of the content of play let the children know that adults are paying attention, are accepting what the children are doing, and are available for more interaction if the children wish. These comments allow the adults to follow the child's lead and stay within the metaphor that the child chooses. This builds the relationship and deepens the individual and group work.

No labels are put on the children's behavior. No effort is made to guide them to work on specific problems. There are no set treatment goals, objectives, or plans. The sessions have no theme or structure. Counselors know little about the children's lives other than what the children show in group. Adults simply arrive; set up the room; get the children from their classrooms; watch, smile, reflect, and protect; set limits when needed; play occasionally when a child requests; observe the children building their worlds; listen to their stories; and return the children to their classrooms at the end of the session.

Unless a child wants to dismantle his or her own tray and put the figures away, which some do as a way of distancing from the meaning of what they have built, we try to leave the scenes intact until the children have left the room. This is to both convey respect for their work and allow them to preserve an internal image of what they have built, which can then evolve over the week until they return to group.

No Verbal Limits

A controversial aspect of the model described here is that counselors prefer to set no limits on verbal behavior. Verbal freedom allows children to release pent-up tension with safety, show anger in a nonphysical way, and make constructive decisions about what vocabulary they choose to use in which setting. Counselors do, however, reflect the feelings of both participants in a verbal conflict, making clear what children intuitively know: that words can be terribly hurtful, and that there are always choices in how words are used and responded to.

One day when a child ran into the group setting and let loose with a string of obscenities, his body visibly relaxed and he said "Whew . . . I've been saving that up all week." It became clear that he was learning self-control. His teacher also gratefully commented that his language in class had become much more appropriate.

Empathy

One of the most important things that is being accomplished in these groups is the development of concern and empathy for others. Empathy has been called the trait that makes people human and makes possible living in community with diverse others. Empathy leads to awareness of how one's actions impact another person. This awareness in turn becomes the reason to modulate the expression of feelings. It is up to the child to take the leap from the externally set limit, "Children are not for hurting," to the internal sequence—"If I yell or hit, my anger is hurting another child. I know it feels bad to be hurt. I care about these children and don't want to do something that feels bad to them."

It is this empathic leap that is the greatest weapon against the wave of violence currently sweeping schools, streets, and children's lives. Sand tray play therapy group teaches moral reasoning through real-life experiences and encourages the caring, sharing part of each child to emerge and blossom into a compassionate awareness of others, based on an internally generated "golden rule."

BUILDING RESILIENCE

The effort to prevent many of the problems confronting children today has led to increased understanding of the reasons that some children manage to thrive despite a negative environment. Asking what is *right* with these children has led to the next question: How can all children be helped to become less vulnerable in the face of life's adversities? Although the nature and intensity of the trauma and the pretrauma level of functioning are significant factors, recent studies have shown that what happens afterward to either counteract or reinforce the devastating images of fear, pain, and/or helplessness, makes the crucial difference. Positive counteracting experiences can come from external support: knowing that people care and are willing to help and having a network of individuals within the family, school, and community to embrace and contain the loss and pain.

Resilience is the "ordinary magic" that allows our normal mechanisms of adaptation and coping to move us out of traumatic stress onto a positive developmental path. Defined as "good outcomes in spite of serious threats to adaptation or development," resilience involves demonstrable risk and observable positive outcomes (external and/or internal).

Specific qualities of resilient children have been identified that can be learned and developed, sometimes by the child acting alone and sometimes with encouragement from others. This encouragement is seen to potentially come from any one or a combination of the systems that primarily shape a child's life: family, school, community, and peers. The factors in the environment that facilitate the development of resiliency include caring and support, positive expectations, and opportunities for children to participate (Benard, 1993). These elements are all present in group sandtray play therapy, creating the possibility for children to develop those qualities that predict resilience and positive growth.

Teach Me to Fish

"Give me a fish and I eat for a day. Teach me to fish and I eat for a lifetime." This African proverb describes a significant aspect of sandplay and resiliency. As children are taught to fish in the unconscious waters inside themselves, to reach into the collective reservoir of symbols and solutions that their imagination contains, they learn a skill by which they can feed themselves emotionally and spiritually throughout life.

Social Competency

Social competency is that combination of prosocial behaviors that allows a child to find and retain people in different systems who are willing to facilitate her or his growth. It constitutes the ability to be liked by others, to get along well with peers, and to be respected by adults. It includes the qualities of empathy, flexibility, and responsiveness, the skills of communication and adaptation, and an openness to diversity combined with a sense of boundaries. In sessions in which adults accept and reflect their feelings, children learn to understand and respect differences and consider others' feelings. The mastery skills needed to safely and appropriately manage and express feelings are repeatedly practiced as children symbolically rehearse and release experiences. Because the adults are not giving advice or proposing solutions, the children help each other and themselves, finding answers within and becoming resources for one another. Thus, they develop communication and social skills, build relationships, and find a sense of belonging and significance.

Problem-Solving Skills

Problem-solving skills involve both the cognitive ability to think abstractly, reflectively, and flexibly and the courage to find and implement alternative solutions. This concerns both internal decisions and issues and social conflicts with others. With freedom of choice, children learn to work and play cooperatively with each other. Because limits on behavior are invoked only when necessary to ensure safety, children learn to resolve their own conflicts with peers through negotiation and compromise.

In making the many choices concerning figures, placement, and story as they play, children learn to use conscious, mindful decision making. Problem-solving skills for developing new and creative solutions are often involved in the process of creating trays as children figure out ways to structure the materials to represent their internal images. Symbolically, problem solving is implied in the use of rescue vehicles, toolboxes, first aid kits, and other resources for handling dangers. The frequent inclusion of representations of the diverse energies of air, earth, and water offer alternative viewpoints and solutions.

Autonomy

Autonomy implies an individual relating to self, acting from an internal locus of control. The concept includes all the "self" qualities, such as self-esteem, self-efficacy, self-discipline, and self-control. A sense of independence is particularly vital when the influence of the immediate environment is negative. This complex quality involves separateness held in balance with relatedness.

Self-Discovery

Sandplay provides children access to their inner wisdom. Through building and "owning" what they have built in a tray, children learn responsibility for their behavior and develop a positive sense of control. They work on self-discovery and identity through mastery experiences from a younger age (pouring, cleaning) and self-statements about what is liked and disliked, chosen or not chosen. Practicing decision making and learning to make constructive choices helps them to say no to impulsive actions.

By exploring and manipulating objects, a child is constantly revising a self-image and creating and holding physical, emotional, and spiritual boundaries. The sand world becomes like a personalized, three-dimensional Thematic

Apperception Test (TAT), which can be easily destroyed and remade as the cycle of discovery and growth evolves. As children observe their own strengths, they begin to integrate them into a more positive self-concept, developing a sense of sovereignty and autonomy, expressing and exploring all aspects of who they are and hope to become. Hidden positive aspects of a child's self often show up in a tray as treasure that has been lost or buried and then found. As children connect to creative and spiritual energies, universal as well as personal, they do not feel so alone in their suffering (Kiepenheuer, 1990). Because they are not being judged or made to perform, children develop confidence in their own abilities and a positive independence, which allows them to separate themselves from negative family situations and peers who engage in risky behavior.

Sense of Purpose and Future

A *sense of purpose and future* includes positive aspirations, anticipation, and the belief that things will probably go as well as can reasonably be expected. Also involved is the motivation to achieve, to set goals, and to believe that they can successfully be reached. Perhaps the most important quality is hopefulness, the ability to imagine a compelling future and a sense that life has meaning (Hunter, 1998).

These are the factors that best predict which children will continue in school to prepare themselves for a meaningful, productive future (Benard, 1993).

A sense of purpose can be seen in the children's sand worlds in the use of construction equipment, with digging and building suggesting goal-directed achievement. A sense of future is portrayed in the placement of eggs and babies, showing the anticipation of something new developing. Once children have imagined positive, resourceful solutions, they are much more likely to achieve them. Once they see themselves as resilient in their imagination, they can in fact become so (Hunter, 1998).

Evaluation

Resiliency checklists measuring social competency, problem-solving skills, and autonomy are completed by older students, teachers, and counselors before and after the group sessions. Report cards and anecdotal comments from teachers and guidance counselors are also reviewed. In most years, 70–90% of the children who attend group consistently show considerable progress.

DIFFERENT POPULATIONS

This type of sand tray play group is suited to a wide range of different settings and problems. School referrals tend to include a variety of social adjustment and behavioral concerns. With a special education group of "emotionally handicapped" fourth and fifth graders with behavior problems, the classroom environment changed from one of the almost constant fighting, disruption, and conflict to one that was much more harmonious and focused, in which positive learning could take place. Another group in the same school included younger mentally challenged students with moderate to severe delays. They too made significant gains in social functioning, and some also advanced in intellectual functioning following the group program. Self-esteem increased as they felt comfortable and confident in building and playing with the miniature figures and made friends with other group members. Children with learning disabilities, struggling with feelings of inferiority, anxiety, and low self-esteem, have been able to increase their social awareness, peer relationships, and academic success.

Perfectionist children like the impermanence of sand tray worlds. The feeling of control allows them to take risks and express concerns they otherwise hide. Children experiencing grief and loss use the metaphoric distance sandplay gives to make abstract ideas concrete and manageable as they are empowered to normalize their family situations and memorialize a lost loved one. Children who have witnessed or experienced violence can express their anger safely while symbolizing and recognizing the real targets.

Children with language skill deficits, those who are selectively mute, or non-English speakers can function well in a setting where verbalizing is not necessary for participation. Their anxiety decreases as they realize that there is no pressure to talk, and their fluency and articulation improve. Crisis work in shelters with abused, neglected, homeless, hurricane surviving, or emotionally disturbed children, shows the value of participation in a sand tray play group to reconstruct the narrative of traumatic events; to express, identify, recognize, and accept feelings; to reduce confusion and increase coping.

Groups that include siblings provide great support in restoring normalcy in a foreign, threatening setting. Siblings can make rapid progress as they know what to expect from each other, make shifts in their communication patterns, develop self-control, and learn to verbalize rather than act out feelings. In a homeless shelter play group, four siblings were self-consciously restrained when alone, but they produced elaborate sand tray scenes about every aspect of their lives when they worked together, showing the true richness of their relationship (Hunter, 1993).

Cultural Responsivity

Group sand tray play provides an important resource for culturally diverse children, increasing self-confidence/esteem/acceptance/control for those who perceive themselves as different from their typical peers. Studies show that these children do best with a therapeutic situation that combines an understandable structure with indirect nonverbal means of communication, includes creativity and concrete natural objects, and is centered on relationships rather than problems (Carmichael, 1991).

Cultural difference is a much less important issue when a child is encouraged to self-generate personally relevant solutions. Using recognizable miniatures from the child's culture crosses barriers of language, culture, and age and promotes a sense of belonging and the ability to identify with the world he or she builds. A cooperative group modality allows for harmonious interaction, especially for children from many Eastern and indigenous cultures who function most naturally and comfortably in group, as opposed to individual, settings.

Nonjudgmental acceptance of silence overcomes resistance. Empathy can develop between children of different backgrounds whose cultures and/or countries are in conflict as they observe and come to understand each other's worlds.

UNDERSTANDING SANDPLAY SCENES

There are many things to watch for as we observe sand tray scenes being built. Attentive appreciation and interest, willingness to "not know," openness to receiving a child's messages, and connecting to the child's inner being are core conditions for all optimum sand tray play experiences. We *do not interpret* and recognize that the adult's understanding of the scene is far less important than the connection that the children make to their own work.

The Children as Creators

Differences in children's processes can be observed in small-group settings. Children immediately show their individuality by responding to the same materials and setting in many different ways, but usually with interest, enthusiasm, and eagerness to explore the possibilities. There is little awkwardness, difficulty in establishing rapport, or confusion about what is expected.

Some work silently and thoughtfully, responding to minimal questions only after they are finished. Others talk continuously, describing all the action, taking on the voices of the different characters, making shooting, driving, and animal noises as they dramatize the scene. Some are uncertain about what they want to do, often asking for help or reassurance, placing and removing figures several times before deciding. Still others work with complete confidence and independence, choosing and arranging figures swiftly and decisively, seeming to have an internal image of what they want to create. Some are spontaneously playful, dynamically moving the figures, leaving them where they happen to fall. Others are artists, carefully crafting a picture to be photographed. Some frequently involve others in their play, creating relationships that become central to their experience. Others relate mainly to figures and sand. Shifts in mood, focus, affect, attention, and verbal comments alert us to changes taking place in the child.

Space

We see trays that are filled to the top with figures, and trays that are totally empty. The most obvious and disturbing are usually those that are overflowing with undifferentiated, confused, disorganized, flooded, chaotic unconscious activity. When children dump many unselected figures into their trays, different dynamics can be in play. Children may be excited in the beginning weeks by the abundance of figures and the freedom to play "almost anyway they want to."

One 6-year-old boy in a school group scooped up a large number of animal figures for his tray in the first session, because they were the first things he saw and closest to him. He played around with them for a few minutes until he noticed the boy across the table, who had been in group the prior year, carefully building a scene with army tents, houses, trees, and so forth. He paused to process what he was seeing, quickly replaced all the animal figures where they had come from, chose some other figures, and began to create an organized story that described the recent hurricanes that had damaged our area, closing the schools for 2 weeks. After several sessions of dynamically showing the effects of wind and water on houses, trees, and cars, he verbally related the play theme to a "hurricane" of anger and violence between adults that was continually blasting his home.

Other children flood a tray after several weeks of exploring the safety and trust aspects of the group setting. They are often graphically describing the chaos of their inner and/or outer life. Nonjudgmentally reflecting the feelings of being overwhelmed and confused that are portrayed, usually helps the child move on. A few children can get stuck in dumping figures, reveling in the knowledge that they are creating a mess that adults will have to clean up. Providing a simple limit, while acknowledging their pleasure in being able to "have" so many things, but stating that the toys are for selecting and playing with, not for dumping, usually contains the behavior. Feedback from other group members who also want to play with those figures often helps to curtail the behavior.

Some children show their depression and discouragement in the early sessions by producing empty, barren, lifeless trays. One such tray was observed; it contained only two snakes, mostly buried in the dry sand, which the builder said were waiting in the desert to attack the people who walk by. Building boundaries in a tray, often with fences, helps to strengthen personal boundaries that are weak and relax those that are rigid. Increasingly organized use of space, and balanced and connected areas with defined but flexible boundaries, show a new level of ego development and life skills.

Use of Sand

The children's use of sand is another aspect to be observed. Some children are reluctant to handle the sand and work entirely on the surface. Others flatten it repeatedly, as if to control their emotions. Some move the sand to get down to the blue bottom, indicating readiness for deeper work and the availability of resources as a clearing is made, treasure is dug up, or something is discovered. The most frequent use of the sand, other than as a foundation for figures, is for burying, which can suggest hiding feelings or parts of self, protecting treasure (potential, promise, incubating something new and important), planting a seed, or holding ugly or scary things down. It is important to pay attention to the part of an item that is protruding and how the buried image emerges in subsequent trays.

When children are encouraged to spend time playing just with the sand before selecting their figures, they seem to make more constructive and creative use of it in building their "worlds."

Aspects to Look For

Choice of figures is the vocabulary children use to elaborate their language of play. Notice the type (soldiers, cars, animals), number, diversity or consistency, and incongruities in their choices. Which figures does the child keep using, and which new ones does he or she add after some weeks? How do the most important symbols evolve over the series of weeks? What allies, models, or power figures is the child attracted to? Is there a "totem" animal that keeps showing up? Are the animals fierce and dangerous or timid and dependent? Do large sharks, dinosaurs, and/or alligators dominate the scene, showing the power of the shadow elements, or is danger more subtly suggested by the scorpion crawling under the fence?

Placement of the figures amplifies their meaning. The most important items often find their way to the center, and opposites into diagonal corners, the farthest distance apart. The left side of the tray often contains unconscious elements, with images representing instincts to the front and spiritual symbols farther away. Figures indicating aspects of conscious, external reality are frequently found on the right side. Movement of figures to or from these areas can indicate the nature of changes taking place (Ryce-Menuhin, 1992).

Figures placed on the side walls of the tray often introduce an observer element. Dramatic action usually centers in and around the tray, with figures falling and diving and being thrown in and out of the tray with great intensity. Fights, accidents, and disasters are contained within the tray. Prone figures suggest woundedness or death.

Shapes, colors, and movement add to the vitality and the emotional energy that each tray holds, as plants grow, machines work, and airplanes take off. Centered mandala shapes can be of jewels and spiritual items denoting the self, or reptilian attacking elements describing wounding.

Is movement freely occurring, as a journey happens along a path, or is it blocked by barriers that isolate or cage individual figures or groups? What direction or pattern predominates? Is it chaotic, as cars and trucks drive anywhere in all directions, or is it contained and orderly as traffic runs smoothly?

Is the feeling that pervades the "world" rigid or chaotic, fragmented or organized, interactive or isolated? How does the story reflect the inner growing that the child is working on? What opposite qualities are being brought together? What themes are repeated with similar activities engaged in by different figures? Themes that can be witnessed in children's play include power/control, anger/aggression, protection/safety, fear/helplessness, loss/death, trust/relationships, rejection/abandonment, nurturing/security, boundaries/identity, intrusion/violation, confusion/conflict, loneliness/sadness, change, empowerment, loyalty, and reunion.

What new elements are being birthed: babies, incubating eggs, construction? Are relationships interactive or separated, dominant or submissive, fragmented or coherent? What elements are connected by a bridge?

Levels of Meaning

The listening/observing of the adult as witness is truly active, developing an openness to receiving messages on several levels.

The first level is the personal meaning of the work to the child, which is expressed in verbal comments and dramatic play. This is the conscious level of associations to the images chosen, which offers important insight. Knowledge of the child's situation, history, and problems is useful here in drawing parallels to the context of the child's life, but because we *do not interpret,* we learn to be very careful with this information.

A very small kindergarten girl played actively with figures of horses, fish, birds, and people week after week in a school group in which we had no information about specific children's issues. Each of her play sessions involved dying, funerals, mourning, burials—memories of the dead in many creative forms. When questioned about this child, the guidance counselor informed us that she was in the group to help her cope emotionally with her mother's terminal illness, and her family had believed that the child didn't know of her mother's condition. The family was then able to handle the situation more openly when it became clear that she, in fact, did know on some very basic level. Having this information about her life however, really did not change how the therapeutic team responded to her play, as we continued to be attentive and interested, to reflect the feelings of the animal families, to encourage and care.

Sometimes this personal level of meaning seems to be in conflict with the second level, the universal, symbolic meaning derived from a knowledge of myths, fairy tales, archetypes, and cultural images—all elements of what Jung called the collective unconscious. This information adds to the depth and richness of understanding and makes room for ambivalence, such as when one child calls the evil queen figure "the protector" or another says he "likes" Freddy Krueger. When figures from distant cultures and eras are used, deep levels of the unconscious are being expressed, whereas more realistic everyday scenes represent elements closer to consciousness (Kalff, 1993).

The third level of meaning is the intuitive sense of the observer, entering into the process as it unfolds and empathically connecting with the playing child. Having empathy for and becoming truly a part of the violent, chaotic interior world of the extremely troubled child, is not easily undertaken. Sandtray play provides a vehicle by which empathy can be both expressed and received. Therapist and child can come together safely in the common ground of the tray and share experiences of all kinds.

Changes over Time

As children build a new tray each week and we take photos that we can refer to, we see changes taking place, some obvious, some subtle. If we spend time with the initial tray (which may be the first one built, or the second or even third if the child is carefully sorting out the process and the group setting), we are often able to see indications of the child's problems, as well as sources of strength and help, possible solutions, and a blueprint of what the child needs to move forward in life.

Over time the child's process may change in that he or she develops a sense of control or of freedom, whichever is needed. Images change, and the play shifts as battles end, crying babies are cared for, scary things are overcome, static scenes start to move, and the roles and/or placements of figures differ. A safe area grows, monsters become smaller, and themes appear or disappear.

Stages

We are often able to see stages in the development of a child's sand trays, portraying chaos, struggle/conflict, and resolution in recurring cycles (Allan, 1988). At a Peace Camp in the Balkans where children from the various ethnic and religious groups come to play in community with each other, sand tray play groups allow them to explore for themselves and with each other the painful, violent events of their countries' wars and how to move past these into a new era of peace.

The "worlds" these children create can be seen to move through the same three stages that have been noted in the work of other troubled children: beginning in chaos and horror, evolving through struggle and conflict, ending in resolution and hope. The images the children choose to express their ex-

perience and feelings combine the universal, cultural, and personal in profound ways.

Chaos–Horror–Violence

In the chaos stage, children may dump large numbers of figures in little or no
order into their trays. Sometimes this is a reflection of a child's chaotic inner
world and sometimes a consciously designed picture of an external world that
is causing him or her great distress.

"Welcome to Hell" screamed the graffiti at the Sarajevo Airport during
the war. An 11-year-old boy set the stage in miniature figures and words:

> "The world is chaos because of one man who opened the gates of hell. Beasts
> have come out after him, killing everyone including children. Monster is
> eating two soldiers. Other men are dying from fear. The big gun kills who-
> ever comes close. Big machines are going wild. Bugs are eating everything.
> The *Titanic* is sinking. A children's bus has crashed. Cars are on top of
> each other. A volcano is erupting in Hawaii."

Some children portrayed the wild beast of evil, the bursts of gunfire, as an angry
red gorilla. "The wild beast is angry, attacking and turning things over. The
children are scared." "Terrible things are happening." "Skeletons and monsters are in our land. Scary bugs are rulers of the world."

Struggle–Conflict–War

The next stage is full of war and scenes of battles between monsters, armies,
aliens, animals, and people of all sorts. At the beginning there is confusion and
destruction, everybody is an enemy, no one wins, all are killed. Gradually, more
equal, organized battles are fought for food, for revenge, for treasure or prize,
for the "good way," to protect the children or save their friends. The purpose
of the Balkan children's battles is primarily defense of land and way of life, often
using American Indians and alien invaders as metaphors for the struggle in their
countries. "The bad guys want to take away the Indians totem and life. The
animals and Indians fight them off." "Modern people and aliens have come to
take the Indian's land and holy objects." Scenes combine reality and fantasy:
"Bomb dropped from a plane started a fire. Soldiers and planes are putting it
out. Monster is trying to tear down the STOP signs." Treasure often represents
the inner self threatened by trauma: "Aliens have come looking for treasure.
Spiders are controlling the attack. People are trying to fight them off."

Eventually, heroes emerge, the good side wins, and the battle becomes a
sports contest in which goals are known and attainable. The needed skills can
be learned, the object is competition, and aggression is contained by rules. Good

and bad indicate greater or lesser skill, the contestants can be friends as well as opponents, and those who lose today can win tomorrow.

Resolution–Hope–Peace

In this phase we see the wars end.

- Normal life is reestablished: "Players make free shot in soccer game. On a farm a cow is eating grass."
- Problems are resolved: "Women each own a farm with a pet, house, and water. Doctor heals a sick cow."
- Relationships are recreated: "The soldiers decided the war was pointless and became friends."
- Hope for the future is regained: "Women get water from the well for a picnic. New house is being built."
- Groups connect: "On the farm and in the jungle, animals are living peacefully with freedom."
- Direction and control are reestablished: "Men are fixing signs. Signs and police keep order."
- Light and safety are found: "Lighthouse keeps the boats safe, goes on at dark so people can see."
- The world is being rebuilt: "Tractor makes a hole to plant a tree. Machines are rebuilding the houses."
- Opposites come together: "Two couples are getting married with the sun shining and music playing."
- Blessings and beauty are found: "An angel came to bless the children. The trees are dancing."

CONCLUSION

Group sandtray play therapy combines some of the most powerful means of facilitating children's healing and growth. Deep inner work can be done in individual trays to explore, express, master, and resolve difficult feelings and events. Cooperative, constructive social learning can result from relating to peers in this intimate yet private way. Locating groups on-site in schools and other settings facilitates generalizing what is learned to new behavior, as well as competence in the classroom and on the playground.

REFERENCES

Allan, J. (1988). *Inscapes of a child's world: Jungian counseling in schools and clinics.* Dallas: Spring Publications.

Allan, J., & Bertoia, J. (1992). *Written paths to healing*. Dallas: Spring Publications.

Benard, B. (1993). Fostering resiliency in kids. *Educational Leadership, 51*, 44–49.

Bettelheim, B. (1987). *The uses of enchantment: The meaning and importance of fairy tales*. New York: Vintage Press.

Bradway, K. (1986). *Sandplay: What makes it work?* Paper preserved at the 10th International Congress for Analytical Psychology.

Bradway, K., & McCoard, B. (1997). *Sandplay: Silent workshop of the psyche*. New York: Routledge.

Brothers, B. (2002). *Satir and trauma*. Presented at the Surviving Trauma with Dignity International Conference, Baku, Azerbaijan.

Carmichael, K. (1991). Play therapy with the culturally different. *APT Newsletter, 10*, 1.

Case, C., & Dalley, T. (1990). *Working with children in art therapy*. New York: Routledge.

DeDominico, G. (1988) *Sand tray world play* (Vols. 1–3). Oakland, CA: GS DeDomenico.

DeMaria, M. (1992) Effects of client-centered group play therapy on self-concept. *International Journal of Play Therapy, 2*(1), 53–67.

Dundas, E. (1990). *Symbols come alive in the sand*. Boston: Coventure.

Ekstein, R. (1966). *Children of time and space, of action and impulse*. New York: Appleton Century Crofts.

Friedman, H. (1997). Sandplay in a play therapy practice. *Sandplay: Coming of age*. LA: (LASA), 17–31.

Furth, G. (1988). *The secret world of drawings: Healing through art*. Boston: Sigo Press.

Gil, E. (1991). *The healing power of play: Working with abused children*. New York: Guilford Press.

Hunter, L. B. (1993). Sibling play therapy with homeless children: An opportunity in the crisis. *Child Welfare, 72*(1), 65–75.

Hunter, L. B. (1998). *Images of resiliency: Troubled children create healing stories in the language of sandplay*. Palm Beach, FL: Behavioral Communications Institute.

Kalff, D. (1980). *Sandplay: A psychotherapeutic approach to the psyche*. Boston: Sigo Press.

Kalff, M. (1993). Twenty points to be considered in the interpretation of a sandplay. *Journal of Sandplay Therapy, 11*(2), 17–35.

Kestly, T. (2001). Group sandplay in elementary schools. In A. Drewes (Ed.), *School-based play therapy* (pp. 329–349). New York: Wiley.

Kiepenheuer, K. (1990). *Crossing the bridge: A Jungian approach to adolescence*. Lasalle, IL: Open Court.

Landreth, G. (1983). Play therapy in elementary school settings. In C. Schaefer & K. O'Conner (Eds.), *Handbook of play therapy* (pp. 200–212). New York: Wiley.

Landreth, G. (1991). *Play therapy: The art of the relationship*. Muncie, IN: Accelerated Development.

Lankton, S. (1980). *Practical magic: A translation of basic NLP into clinical psychotherapy*. Cupertino, CA: Meta.

Lowenfeld, M. (1979). *The world technique*. London: George Allen & Unwin.

Mills, J., & Crowley, R. (1986). *Therapeutic metaphors for children and the child within*. NY: Brunner/Mazel.

Noyes, M. (1981). Sandplay imagery: An aid to teaching reading. *Academic Therapy, 17*(2), 231–237.

Packman, J., & Bratton, S. (2003). A school-based group play/activity therapy intervention with learning disabled pre-adolescents exhibiting behavior problems. *International Journal for Play Therapy, 12*(2), 7–29.

Rogers, C. (1951). *Client-centered therapy.* Boston: Houghton-Mifflin.

Ryce-Menuhin, J. (1992). *Jungian sandplay: The wonderful therapy.* New York: Routledge.

Stewart, C. (1990). Developmental psychology of sandplay. *Sandplay studies.* Boston: Sigo Press.

Stewart L. (1982). Sandplay and Jungian analysis. In M. Stein (Ed.), *Jungian analysis* (pp. 39–92). Boulder, CO: Shambhala.

Terr, L. (1990) *Too scared to cry.* New York: Basic Books.

Thomas, M. (2002). *Understanding Trauma.* Presented at the Surviving Trauma with Dignity International Conference, Baku, Azerbaijan.

CHAPTER 12

Short-Term Group Play Therapy for Children Whose Parents Are Divorcing

WENDY LUDLOW
MARY K. WILLIAMS

This chapter offers an eight-session short-term play therapy group format for use with latency-age children experiencing parental divorce. The format, inspired by several well-researched "children of divorce" groups, is suitable for a school, agency, or clinic setting and can easily be expanded from eight into twelve or more sessions if time permits. Therapists can conduct this group without having extensive play therapy experience. The goal is to provide children going through any stage of divorce a safe and lighthearted atmosphere in which they can simultaneously experience the benefits of group camaraderie and therapeutic play.

Group treatment has been documented as one of the most effective interventions for children of divorce, whether or not there is any identified pathology in a child (Guldner & O'Connor, 1991; Kalter, 1998; Kalter & Schreier, 1993; Pedro-Carroll, 2005). Such a group can serve simultaneously as a preventive and therapeutic intervention. Puppet making, role plays, and structured play activities are utilized in each session, with a unifying theme of the creation of an "Advice Brochure" that is presented in the final group session. Parental involvement is also a key component. The emphasis on playfulness allows children to connect and communicate with one another in a situation that is often painful and isolating.

DIVORCE: A MODERN REALITY

Divorce is a common occurrence in children's lives. Most school-age children are able to name several peers who have divorced parents. Current research (Eitzen & Baca Zinn, 1997) continues to indicate that 60% of all marriages in the United States end in divorce, and 60% of those divorcing couples have children. More than one million children in the United States experience divorce annually (Clarke, 1995), and researchers have estimated that 40% of children in the United States will witness the divorce of parents by age 18 (Barker, Brinkman, & Deardorff, 1995).

Divorce is not a single event in a child's life, and is often the cause of ongoing stressors for a family. Several studies have mentioned, for example, that family income declines dramatically after divorce, that parents often are compromised by mental health disorders such as depression, and that remarriage and multiple divorces often occur within just a few years of the initial divorce (Amato & Keith, 1991a). Divorce is also a difficult concept for children to grasp and a difficult reality to accept, and there is no official ceremony that commemorates divorce, such as a wedding or a funeral.

Despite the high prevalence of divorce, social stigma still negatively impacts the divorcing family. Neuman and Romanowski (1998) note that a widowed parent is more likely to receive praise and validation for his or her commitment and struggle through the transition of becoming a single parent, whereas divorced parents get little recognition for tackling a similar family crisis.

Divorce and parental marital conflict are associated with a variety of long-term problems for children throughout the lifespan, including delinquent behavior, substance abuse, and poorer academic, social, and psychological functioning (Amato, 2001; Amato & Booth, 1991; Amato & Keith, 1991b; Booth & Edwards, 1990). The distress experienced by children involved in a divorce commonly involves feelings of isolation, anxiety, responsibility, helplessness, anger, guilt, confusion, and ambivalence. Estimates are that one-quarter of children develop mental health disorders following parental divorce (Hetherington, Bridges, & InSabella, 1998).

Children in the divorce play therapy group described in this chapter are provided with an environment where feelings can be accepted, expressed, and processed, with the aim of reducing the severity of the impact of the divorce on each child. Neuman and Romanowski (1998) state:

> When these feelings are not expressed and dealt with in a healthy, productive way, they endure and taint children's views of themselves and of others. This is why, decades after the fact, most adult children of divorce view it as the most devastating event of their childhoods, if not their lives. How well a child copes with her family's transition and its far-ranging implications will be a—if not

the—major influence on several important aspects of her life, including the ability to forge and sustain loving relationships and be a good parent herself. (p. 9)

This group offers a child in a divorce situation an opportunity to build resilience and continue developmental progress within the context of this major life transition.

PLAYFULNESS AS THE PRIMARY HEALING ELEMENT

A primary objective of the therapy group is to nurture a child's need for fun and playfulness. Divorce is not fun, and children are often deprived of typical sources of fun and playfulness during the process of the martial breakup. They often become witnesses to arguments, and are frequently forced to move and to leave schools and friends. Children often lack the ability to identify and communicate their thoughts and feelings effectively. Play is a child's natural mode of communication and a means of providing emotional balance. Play therapy is not always immediately recognized by the general public as a preferred intervention for children. Those involved with facilitating and implementing a divorce group, including parents, may need to be informed of the therapeutic value of play. Therapeutic elements worth mentioning include the following:

- Play is lighthearted and fun.
- Play allows children to be free and to lower their guard.
- Children can be the masters of their universe in play.
- Play is a natural way to release anxiety.
- Negative emotions are more easily expressed through play.
- Negative emotions are more readily accepted through play.
- Elation is easily attainable through play.
- Play allows children the means to explore and experiment without criticism.

Play provides children the means to address emotionally charged issues in a way that is gentle to the ego, allowing them to acknowledge and interpret conflicts and emotions as they are prepared and able.

DIVORCE GROUP OBJECTIVES

Each child has a unique situation and set of strengths that he or she brings to the group, as well as his or her own emotional and developmental needs. This group is designed to allow all members opportunities for growth, regardless of the variety of needs and situations. The program has five objectives, described in the following paragraphs, shared by well-researched divorce group formats such as the Children of Divorce Intervention Program (Pedro-Carroll & Cowen, 1985), the Children's Support Group (Stolberg & Garrison, 1985; Stolberg & Mahler, 1994), and the Kalter, Pickar, and Lesowitz (1984) Developmental Facilitation Groups.

Group Membership and Normalization

The divorce group allows children to experience a supportive group environment in which they can feel that they are not alone and can freely communicate about divorce-related issues and feelings with one another. Children often do not realize that they share many problems, feelings, and worries with other children.

Clarification

Divorce groups aid children in establishing the facts of their situations and of the divorce itself, which includes correcting any misconceptions. For example, a common misconception is a child's belief that he or she will be forced to testify in court and choose one parent over the other. Children may also need to be provided with definitions of words such as "divorce," "visitation," "custody," and the like.

Expressing and Reexperiencing

A child is encouraged, usually through indirect means, to identify and express thoughts and feelings associated with the divorce. The play activities in this and other successful divorce groups are chosen to facilitate the reworking of difficult or painful events and allow members to gain a new sense of mastery over previously debilitating situations. Group membership also establishes an atmosphere conducive to this process. The group serves as a facsimile of the family, providing members an opportunity to play out familiar family roles and to experiment with new roles. For example, a child involved with divorce may take on a parental role in the family, which can result in feelings of overwhelming responsibility, worry, and guilt. The group offers the child an opportunity to reverse and experiment with roles in play and in interaction with peers, to express him- or herself both verbally and nonverbally, and to view family conflict from different perspectives. The transitions involved with group participation also have great therapeutic potential. Pedro-Carroll and Cowen (1985) emphasize the importance of a healthy termination for a group, as the ending of a group is an emotional representation of the divorce itself.

Skill Building

The group is designed to assist children in the development of problem-solving skills and coping behaviors that can help in surviving a divorce as successfully as possible. Pedro-Carroll (2005) has identified several important skills, such as the ability to discern between problems that are solvable and those that are not, to elicit help and support, to communicate needs and feelings, and to express anger appropriately. All activities for this group format support the development of such skills through play.

Parent–Child Communication

Group work fosters improved communication between parent and child about the divorce, helps children sustain loving attachments to parents, and facilitates opportunities for children to find appropriate ways to have their emotional needs met. Filial (parent–child) therapy is another play therapy modality that should be recommended to families in need of relationship enhancement when group therapy alone is not sufficient. Most divorce groups for children that have been found to be beneficial have parent education or parent involvement components.

PRACTICE PRINCIPLES

There are several other clinical issues to keep in mind when planning and conducting a divorce group.

Parent Involvement

Parent involvement is a key component of a successful divorce group. It can be quite threatening for a parent to volunteer his or her child for a confidential group in which issues of divorce are addressed. Parents require information and support from group leaders. Group leaders are urged to call each parent before the beginning of the group, during the middle phase of the group, and at the end of the group to check on the child's functioning and progress. These phone calls also provide opportunities to learn about the family's current status and the significant events taking place in the family and to answer any questions parents might have about the group. The leader can share pertinent information with the parent about the child's progress, as well as give the parent support and validation with the hope that he or she will, in turn, do the same for the child. Such contact also provides an opportunity to make outside referrals if necessary.

When done respectfully, parents may appreciate some coaching from the group leader on how to be supportive of the child. Parents also need reminders that the child's confidentiality is of value and that they should not quiz the child about what is going on in the divorce group. When talking to parents, as well as when coaching parents on interacting with their children, leaders should keep in mind that the emphasis should be on open communication, reflection, validation, and playfulness.

Letter to Parents

A letter should be sent to each parent prior to the start of the group explaining the Advice Brochure that the children will be making. Explain to parents that an "Advice Brochure Workbook" will be sent home in a folder with the child after the first group, with a list of topics for them to think about and discuss with the child. Make it clear that they can talk about divorce in general and do not have to talk specifically about their own situations. Each parent will also receive a duplicate workbook in the mail to keep at home. Explain in the letter that this Advice Brochure Workbook offers a way for a parent to communicate with the child about the divorce, stressing the importance of allowing the child to say whatever he or she wants to say and replying with supportive statements. Mention in the letter that the parent praise the child for anything he or she contributes. Parents are also encouraged to present problems or issues on which families going through a divorce might need advice from the group. The first phone call to the parents should explain the Advice Brochure Workbook in detail so that it is not a surprise when their children come home with it. Parents should be encouraged to ask their children about the brochure by saying something like, "I hear you are making an Advice Brochure! Wow, I sure would like to be a part of that. Let's look at our new workbook together!" (See Figure 12.1 for a sample take-home Advice Brochure Workbook.)

Group Development

Awareness of and trust in the natural development of the group is an important tool for the leader. It is well established that therapy groups have a developmental process with associated tasks and challenges of their own (Northen & Kurland, 2001). Ideally, therapists are aware of this process so that interventions can be appropriately tailored to foster the natural development and intrinsic healing power of the group itself.

Latency-Phase Developmental Issues

Latency-age children (roughly ages 6–11) are challenged with a variety of developmental tasks that are potentially compromised by the stressors associated with divorce. A group format is especially appropriate for the latency-age child, as in this phase of development a great amount of learning about the world occurs through experiences and relationships. Children at this age are building

Note: Each page should be left blank after the question, providing space for parents and children to write suggestions together. This will create a multipage workbook. Pages can be stapled together to make a book format. Be sure to leave blank pages at the end for additional ideas/advice.

Page 1

Your child is currently in the process of helping to make an Advice Brochure for families going through a divorce, as well as for anyone working with a child or family going through a divorce. The following are some suggested topics for you to consider when working on this together. Please feel free to list any thoughts you have about this subject.

1. Children often worry that the divorce is their fault. What can parents do to reassure them that divorce is definitely not their fault?

Page 2

2. Children often do not know how to tell their parents of their feelings about the divorce. What can parents do to help them with this?

Page 3

3. Sometimes children overhear their parents having fights. This can be painful for them, and sometimes they don't know what to do at these times. What are some suggestions for children and parents when this happens?

Page 4

4. It is really hard for children to have to go from one home to another home. It gets confusing, and it is hard to know how to set up things in each home. What can parents do to make this transition easier for children?

Page 5

5. Sometimes parents going through a divorce aren't around a lot for their children. This is hard for children, and sometimes they feel as if a parent went away because he or she doesn't love them anymore. What can parents do to help their children know they are loved?

Page 6

6. Think of some families you know that have been through a divorce. What are some things that you think helped them? What are some things that made it hard for them?

Page 7

7. Sometimes there are new boyfriends or girlfriends that moms and dads have when they are going through a divorce. This is very hard for children. What can parents do to make this transition easier for their child?

FIGURE 12.1. Advice Brochure Workbook.

Page 8

    8. Who are some safe people for children to talk to about what they are going through?

Page 9

    9. What can teachers do to help families that are going through a divorce? What should they *not* do?

Page 10

    10. What can friends do to help children and/or parents going through a divorce? What should they *not* do?

The following blank pages are for you to add whatever you want to this workbook.

Figure 12.1. *continued*

a concept of the self that is increasingly independent of the family unit, learning sex roles, and constantly trying out their ever developing identities in new and different ways. Normal play themes involve conquests, battles, and rescues, thus it is expected that these themes will be reflected in group members' choices of puppets and responses to role plays. Teasing, peer rivalry, and the testing of any type of boundary are common behaviors for children in this age group and should not necessarily be interpreted by leaders as indications of deeper emotional problems or resistance to participation in the group. The brains of children in this age group are developing rapidly, and they are faced with higher expectations regarding their performance at home, in their peer groups, and in school. This, in turn, increases the need for skills to manage feelings and impulses. Consequently, their activities often focus on organization, control, achievement, and mastery. Secrecy, which involves controlling information, is a dominant social theme for children of this age group, whether or not divorce is part of their lives. This is one reason that a child experiencing divorce may avoid directly discussing subjects such as a family breakup, but will enthusiastically engage with peers in role plays.

Younger Children

The group will require adaptation for children in the 5–7 age range. A rule of thumb is that the younger the child, the greater the need for introduction, identification, explanation, clarification, and structure. Younger children tend to have more confusion about the concept of divorce itself, greater fear of the loss of the love of parents, and more intense reunification fantasies. When possible, groups for younger children should use a 10- to 12-week format, and more time should be spent on each phase. For younger children, the parent

Advice Brochure Workbook needs modification, with exercises involving photo collage and drawing added. Some discussion and planning will have to be done by leaders working with this age group to ensure that appropriate modifications are implemented.

Techniques of Displacement and Generalized Statements

Displacement techniques and generalized statements require using a particular style of language and play, which can be easily developed but should be reviewed and practiced. Kalter and Shreier (1993) make special mention of the importance of using displacement activities, such as puppet play, and generalized statements such as "Some kids are worried that. . . ." Displacement is a coping defense whereby taboo or threatening thoughts and feelings are redirected from the intended person to someone considered to be more acceptable. The act of displacement allows children to symbolically place unwanted or inappropriate thoughts or feelings about someone or something outside themselves until they are emotionally and cognitively able to reabsorb them and react appropriately. Leaders utilize displacement by taking the subject of divorce out of the realm of the child's own personal experience and placing it in the realm of the "other." In other words, displacement allows the child to bring conscious and unconscious material into the group through puppet play and by talking about "other kids." Care should be taken to avoid direct interpretation of a child's statements or play (such as "Jordan, you seem to be talking about how you feel about your own mother"), as it will likely disrupt this process and violate the sense of safety in the group.

Coleaders

Whenever possible, groups should be conducted by two leaders. The reasons for this are significant. Having two adults working with the group allows for one leader to address behavior management and, more importantly, to provide ongoing positive reinforcement while the other presents the activity. Coleaders also serve as a representation of parental figures, so it is desirable to have a male and a female leader if at all possible. One leader must be a trained professional, but a nonprofessional with some basic training and close supervision can serve as coleader. Leaders should meet between sessions to review individual and group progress and process. Several hours will be needed initially to prepare the materials and organize for the group sessions.

Intervention Style

Because it is time limited and has several objectives, this play therapy group is quite structured and directive. The leader must be observant of individual and group progress and help the group move forward when necessary. Although creativity and play are emphasized, the leader must intervene and shape play and conversation, particularly when the group is becoming stagnant in one phase or coping behavior. Young (1989) suggests five situations that merit intervention in children's divorce groups: (1) when children are emphasizing external sources of problems and solutions—blaming excessively; (2) when a child defends the status quo, such as "That's just the way I am"; (3) when a member is manipulating the communication of the group, such as by asking loaded questions; (4) when the therapist identifies a discrepancy between a child's (or a depicted puppet character's) stated goals and his or her behavior that calls for the child to reevaluate his or her (or the puppet's) motivation; and (5) when there is a need to balance the amount of time and attention given to group members.

Group Notebook

Leaders should consider and record the aforementioned behaviors in a dedicated group notebook. This notebook should also document and include information on the content of role plays, the advice given for the brochure, and other pertinent information so that it can easily be reviewed and discussed between sessions.

Behavior Management

There will likely be times when some type of behavior management is necessary in the group. However, children with significant behavior problems should be screened out (before the group begins) and referred for individual therapy until they are ready for group. Leaders must plan ahead of time how they will handle inappropriate behavior. Transition times, such as when children are entering or departing the group room, or moving from one activity to another, are often the times when behavior problems emerge. The most effective behavior management strategy is to utilize positive verbal reinforcement of desired behaviors often with each child individually, and with the group as a whole throughout every session. Leaders can use statements such as the following:

- "Matt, what a great job you are doing sitting in your chair!"
- "Does everyone see how Will is sharing the markers so nicely?"
- "Wow, this group sure knows how to work together!"
- "I'm amazed! A lot of kids couldn't say that!"
- "Great way to express angry feelings, Olivia!"
- "Why, I just don't know how we would have made this brochure without all the good advice from this group!"
- "Rowan, congratulations on sharing some very valuable information."

SETTING UP THE GROUP

Thoughtful preparation for the group can provide the leader with the highest possibility of having motivated participants, involved parents, and satisfied institutional supporters.

Screening

When possible, a brief pregroup interview should be conducted with at least one parent and the child (separately) for the purposes of informing the family of the group format and content and ensuring that the child is an appropriate candidate for the group. Both parents should be informed about the group and, ideally, included in this process. It is important that the parents have an opportunity to meet with the leader individually to give information about the divorce privately. In addition, information from teachers or other clinicians can be utilized in determining the readiness of children for the group. If one-on-one meetings are not possible, parent consent forms must be mailed, and phone contact is imperative. Parental involvement is vital and should be encouraged every step of the way.

Parent Permission

If at all possible, inform both custodial and noncustodial parents about the group and request their written consent. A written release signed by both parents is necessary unless one parent has sole legal custody, in which case it is recommended that you have a copy of that order on file. Group leaders are cautioned against doing any type of counseling without proper consent, and local laws should be reviewed.

Details regarding when, where, and for how long the group meets, and other important information, should be clearly stated in a permission form. If you are going to be doing any type of audio or video recording of sessions, this should also be included in a release. Leaders affiliated with agencies, schools, or clinics should have such a release approved by their administrators before sending it to any parent, to ensure legal viability.

Group Member Selection

It is widely accepted that four to eight children is an optimal number of members for elementary, school-age children. Younger children (4–6 years old) require a smaller group of four to six members, while older children can participate in larger groups of up to 12 children. Ideally, there should be an equal number of boys and girls who are developmentally similar. An easy way to ensure this population is to form groups from the same grade or age groups.

Children who are in differing phases of divorce can be intermingled in the group, but leaders should ensure that no child is experiencing a divorce situation that is so dramatically different from that of peers that the child will feel isolated. Siblings and close relatives should not be in the same group.

Other Supports and Services

A divorce group does not replace individual or family therapy. Leaders may identify a child during the screening interview or group process who is in need of additional services, such as play therapy, filial therapy, family therapy, individual therapy for the parents, psychiatric care, or case management services.

Attendance

Groups should meet in the same place at the same time, once or twice a week, the same day(s) each week. Regular attendance is crucial, and its importance should be emphasized to all involved. Usually, a school setting allows for weekly sessions only. In general, weekly sessions constitute the recommended format.

Room Requirements

Group members should be able to sit in chairs. When a table is not available, individual desks can be pushed together to form a closed rectangle, with art supplies located in the center. There should also be a large open area available for play activities. Desks or tables can be pushed to the sides of a room for this if necessary.

Time Requirements

In most settings, it is likely that group sessions will have to take place within a 60-minute time span. The format described here adheres to that time limit. However, if more time is available, particularly in the first session, it is advisable to take more time. Ninety minutes should be devoted to session 1 when possible. It is vital that time be saved for the play activity at the end of each session, as this is when a great deal of emotional release and skill building occurs.

GROUP SESSIONS

For the convenience of the leader, this group format is designed around a "phase" system based on the divorce groups of Pedro-Carroll and Cowen (1985), as well as general concepts of group development theory. Identifying group phases can allow the leader to be flexible in choices of activities and to harness the healing power of the group itself. The first phase of the divorce group emphasizes creating an environment of safety and normalization and establishing familiarity with expressing feeling states. The second phase focuses on skill development and enhancement of the child's resilience. The third phase facilitates the implementation of skills and is a prelude to termination. The final (fourth) phase is the termination itself. Each phase has two to four sessions that include an introduction, a puppet show role play, and a play activity. Out of the role-play process, the children will develop an advice brochure on divorce that will ultimately be made to look professional by the coleaders and sent home with each child at the end of the group.

The role-play activities are loosely based on the activities of the divorce groups developed by Kalter and Schreier (1993) that have been formally evaluated for effectiveness for short- and long-term benefits. Although several play activities are suggested, group leaders must be aware of their own unique group process in order to determine the most appropriate interventions. Group leaders are also encouraged to use resources available in other texts and/or to create their own play activities and interventions. Several useful texts for play techniques are referred to in this chapter. By joining the Association for Play Therapy, leaders or agencies will receive announcements of local and national play therapy training programs valuable to this process.

Overview of Session Structure

After the initial session, which includes a general introduction, the first 10–15 minutes of a session is an art time during which members can make a new character for their cast of puppets. During this time leaders also ask members if they have anything from their take-home Advice Brochure Workbook that they would like to share. This is followed by 10–15 minutes of a role-play puppet activity. The leaders use their cast of puppets to begin a brief puppet show about a family going through a divorce (divorce topics typically change with each group). Leaders then facilitate group members in completing the puppet show role play. Role plays should not be dragged on too long or forced; they should be playful and fun. At the end of the role play, each group member is invited to use one of his or her puppets to give advice or to make a comment to someone in the puppet show, or about the puppet family/situation in general. The discussion and advice phase should take about 5 minutes. The final 15–30 minutes is used for a lighthearted play activity. Three to five minutes should be reserved at the very end for members' to organize their materials and to prepare to continue their day outside the group. The time line looks something like this for a 60-minute group:

- Introduction/puppet making: 10–15 minutes.
- Role playing and advice giving: 10–20 minutes.
- Play activity: 15–30 minutes.
- End of group/organization time: 5 minutes.

Regular Interventions

Group leaders need to remember to do the following in each session or between sessions:

- Ask the children about their Advice Brochure Workbooks during the puppet-making time (call parents to support and simplify their participation in this project if necessary).
- Remind group members that the purpose of the role play is to generate ideas for the Advice Brochure.
- Remind the children to bring their Advice Brochure Workbooks to the group and to take them home. Make sure that their workbooks are put in their backpacks.
- Tell group members how many sessions have elapsed and how many more remain.

Clinical Supervision Activities

It is helpful to include these activities when reviewing progress and interventions:

- Review group process and current goal.
- Have the role-play notebook on hand and review current role-play themes.
- Review displacement statements that will be used for the current session, such as "How do you think the son puppet feels about _____?"
- Review intervention strategies to ensure that the group is moving forward in its development.
- Keep a record of parent contact.
- Write individual letters to each child to place in the puppet bag to take home in the last session, making personal statements about his or her own unique contributions to the group.

Puppets

There are many types of puppets to use and/or to make. A simple stick puppet is used in this group format. However, if group leaders have access to a large supply of puppets, it is appropriate to adapt the model to use purchased hand puppets. If using purchased puppets, it is important that there be a large assortment of many different types of puppets so that a variety of emotions, roles, and situations can be represented. Keep in mind that the puppet assembly and decoration time presented here serves as an opportunity for reflection and centering, as well as a time for leaders to validate and connect with individual members. This may naturally evolve into a "sharing time" which should be nurtured but not formalized by the leader. If purchased puppets are used, leaders must take into consideration how they will accomplish this task in other ways.

Phase 1: Sessions 1 and 2

Phase 1 sets the stage for the group experience. The focus is on orienting children to the group, creating an atmosphere of inclusion and safety, finding commonalities among members, and normalizing the experience of divorce. Group leaders must establish their roles by making it clear that they are not teachers, but rather adult leaders who specialize in playing and having fun with children going through a family transition. The emphasis here is that it is safe for kids to pretend, to emote, to express positive and negative thoughts and feelings, and ultimately to be playful. Some children may be reluctant to participate and distrustful of others as they begin with group work, and this may be reflected in the superficial content of their contributions. Members are typically much more dependent on group leaders during this phase than they may be later. Any participation should be encouraged and applauded, but no individual prompting to participate is needed (children are allowed to decline participation). Instead, leaders can prompt the group as a whole by saying something like, "Does anyone in the group have any thoughts about what kids might be thinking or feeling in this situation?" It is important that children leave hopeful about the benefits of the group and are motivated to return. If Phase 1 objectives are met, the group itself will have matured into an entity that allows members to face divorce-related problems in greater depth and address personal issues more boldly.

Session 1

Supplies needed: easel board or giant Post-its and markers; assembled stick puppets (see the next section); art materials for stick puppet faces, such as markers, magazine face and feature (eyes, mouth, nose, hair, etc.) cutouts, glue sticks, glue, google eyes, and yarn; large plastic baggie or box for each child; eight ready-made generic puppets in Ziploc bag for each child; Advice Brochure mock-up for demonstration with a title such as "How to Deal with Your Family's Divorce" or "When Divorce Happens to You" on the front.

READY-MADE PUPPETS

Group leaders must make their own, as well as the children's, puppets prior to the first session. The puppets are a vital component of the group format and should be simply made with some thought and care. Each puppet should have a sturdy head/body attached to a large craft stick (get the biggest sticks you can find). Make the heads out of something like tagboard and make them big enough so that hair, google eyes, and other items can be added by the group members. Vary the types and shapes of the heads/bodies. Group leaders should make the original puppet cast, including (but not limited to) the following members: mother, father, boy, girl, baby, aunt, uncle, neighbor, dog, cat, grandparent, bully, and other adult and child characters to be defined in the initial role play by the group. Puppets should not be elaborate, as the children will use them as examples when given an opportunity to make their own puppets in session 1. Remember that you will make puppets as you go along, so make extra generic puppets to utilize when needed, using your ingenuity.

ROLE-PLAY BOOK

Leaders should keep a separate notebook to record the role plays and advice given by the children during and after each session. This is referred to for future role plays and in the final making of the Advice Brochure.

TAKE-HOME ADVICE BROCHURE WORKBOOK TO USE WITH PARENTS

Children are given their take-home Advice Brochure Workbooks to share with their parents in session 1. The workbook should be nicely placed in a folder with pockets so that it won't fall out and given to each child to take home at the end of the group. See the sample Advice Brochure Workbook in Figure 12.1.

INTRODUCTION OF MEMBERS (10 MINUTES)

Each group leader starts by saying something like:

> "My name is Bob and I am going to be your group leader. This group is about family changes that happen with divorce. It is a friendship group. All of you have parents who are separated, divorced, or who are getting divorced. We are going to have fun together while we talk and learn about how divorce changes families and kids and what we can do about all of this. Everyone needs to know that this group is a private friendship group. That means that we don't talk about what other people say in the group without their permission. Let's start by introducing ourselves. My name is Bob."

The group leader then gives all of the children an opportunity to introduce themselves.

DEFINING GROUP RULES

The leader continues quickly to a discussion of group rules: "OK, now let's make up our group rules." Write down all suggestions. After all the suggestions have been made, simplify them into four to five rules such as:

1. Listen to others respectfully.
2. Hands to yourself.
3. Talk one at a time.
4. Everyone may choose whether or not he or she wants to participate.
5. Group members talk and play outside the group if they want to, but what happens in this group is private.

NAMING THE GROUP

The leader then says, "OK! Great! Now we are going to do some fun things, and at the end we will give this group a name, so I want everyone to think about what this group could be called. We need your ideas!"

During this introduction, it is important that the leader establish that everyone's ideas are valued and that everyone will be heard. The following is a list of statements that can be used to ensure that this happens:

- "Very important idea!"
- "Cool! Did everyone hear that idea?"
- "No one has come up with that one yet!"
- "Yes! Say that again!"
- "We could not have this group without that idea!"

Note: Group leaders need to have character and silliness or distinction in their tones of voice and in their choices of words. This sets the stage for safety and acceptance. In other words, be playful!

FIRST ROLE PLAY: DIVORCING FAMILY (10–15 MINUTES)

Every child is given a baggie or box containing eight puppets with blank faces. Start by telling the group members that they will get a chance to create one of their own puppets later in the session. Then state, "We are going to create a puppet show about a family just starting to go through a divorce." Next, introduce the ready-made puppets as a family and playfully engage the children in naming the cast. Start the story and then give each group member a chance to add to the story. For example: "Once upon a time, there was a family that was going through a divorce. The divorce started because the parents could not get along. Everyone in the family had lots of different feelings about this divorce. It all started when. . . ." Now ask for volunteers to take turns adding to the story, ultimately coming up with an ending to the role play.

Group leaders should elicit divorce-related thoughts, feelings, and issues through the development of the puppet show script and the displacement process. The more the group leaders know about the individual members' situations, the more they can tailor their responses to facilitate displacement in those areas. Members' content during this first role play may be superficial, or they may mention feelings of shock and disbelief, sadness, anger, blame, confusion, and guilt. Violent themes and inappropriate behavior may be presented, which is acceptable but may require the eliciting of group problem solving in later group sessions. Leaders should keep the role play silly, adding to the story to keep the flow moving. They should record all of the content in the role-play notebook. Leaders must also be sure to validate (being careful not to interpret) any thoughts, feelings, ideas, or fantasies that may arise, including ideas of reconciliation.

ADVICE AND PUPPET MAKING

Now tell the group members that they will make their first puppets, which are to be the "advice givers" for the story. Tell them that their puppets can be anything they like and that all types of characters and advice are needed for this story, including bullies, animals, happy puppets, mad puppets, mean puppets, quiet puppets, and so on. Make it clear that this is not an art class. Give them 10–15 minutes to make their puppets, and then offer each member an opportunity to give advice to an individual puppet in the family, or to the family as a whole. Explain what advice is by giving simple examples such as, "Advice is a statement starting with 'You could,' or 'Have you thought about . . . ?'" Tell the group members that all of their advice will be written down and put in an important brochure that will be made about helping families through a divorce. Show the sample advice brochure to the children, stating what a valuable help it will be to other children and families. Make sure they understand that no names will be put on this brochure, so the advice they give will be kept private. Tell them that at the end of the group they will get to take home a final brochure containing all of the advice given during these puppet advice times. Validate whatever contributions a child brings to the story, and write down all of the advice given.

HOMEWORK

This is also the time to tell the children about their folders with their Advice Brochure Workbooks to take home and share with their parents. Tell them that their only homework is to show their parents this brochure and to see if they can come up with any other advice and/or problems to be considered for the final Advice Brochure:

> "Your parents may have thoughts about what might be helpful for this brochure, and we want their input as well. There may also be things that come

up during the week that you think are important for this brochure. For example, if you notice that it is hard to do your homework because you are worried about your parents' divorce, you can write, 'Teachers should not give kids as much homework when they are going through a divorce.' There is no right or wrong advice. We have told your parents about the brochure we are making, and all of your parents have agreed to help you write down anything that you think is important to put in it. Your parents may ask about this Advice Brochure Workbook when you get home, because they know what an important document it is that you are making, and they will probably want to be helpful in this process just like you."

PLAY ACTIVITY (10–15 MINUTES)

Move on to the play activity (see play activity suggestions for phase 1 groups) before ending the session. You may not have as much time as usual for the play activity in this first session, so choose the activity carefully. Make sure to save enough time for this play.

END THE SESSION (5–10 MINUTES)

The conclusion of the session has symbolic power as a representation of the breakup of the family unit and a prelude to the eventual ending of the divorce group. The final minutes of group time should be announced (i.e., "We will get in a line and return all group members to their classrooms in 5 minutes"). To end the session, ask the children to come up with a name for this friendship group and facilitate their ability to make a decision and include everyone's ideas. Naming the group can be postponed until the next session if necessary. In either the first or second session, encourage the children to create a special parting hand gesture, handshake, or cheer.

Session 2

Supplies needed: each child's bag of puppets; puppet art supplies.

INTRODUCTION (10–15 MINUTES)

From now on, every child should be given his or her bag of puppets to work on for the first 10–15 minutes of the session. Art supplies can be set out in the middle of the table, and leaders should facilitate the sharing and passing of these supplies. Group leaders can encourage members to continue to make more characters for their collections of puppets, including puppets that exhibit a variety of traits, as stated in session 1, so that they can contribute in different ways to the role plays. For children who are reluctant to make additional puppets, embellishments to the existing puppets can be made. During this phase, group leaders should also ask members about their take-home Advice Brochure Workbooks, and provide an opportunity for members to discuss matters that are important to them with the group. However, because there will be varied levels of parental involvement in this project, no one should be singled out to discuss his or her workbook.

ROLE PLAYS: PARENTAL ARGUMENT AND
CHILDREN OVERHEARING ARGUMENT

There are two role-play scripts to create for session 2 (based on Kalter & Schreier, 1993). The first is a predivorce argument between parents, with the goal of allowing thoughts and feelings of hostility to emerge. Group leaders start the role play and then encourage group members to raise their hands when they want to contribute to the role play. A second role play is of children overhearing a fight between parents. After the two role plays are produced, group members are once again instructed to use one of their puppets to give advice or make a comment to one of the characters or to the family as a whole. One of the leaders should model freedom of expression by having one of his or her puppets make a comment, in a playful voice, to the parents such as, "You two parents are being a pain in the neck! Don't you know how to talk nicely to each other?" The other leader then says something like, "What do you think about the way these parents are talking to each other? How do you think a kid might feel hearing this?" and "What do you think the kids can do to get through having to hear this?" Leaders can then empathize with the children's responses and facilitate a discussion of maladaptive and adaptive responses, such as getting away from the fighting by playing music, crying, yelling, using positive self-talk, drawing, or a child's going into his or her room and closing the door. All types of responses should be welcomed for discussion so that each can be evaluated and considered. This is an example of when it is important for leaders to know as much as possible about the children's individual situations so that unsafe scenarios can be discussed and prevented. Leaders write down all of the advice given to incorporate in the final brochure.

PLAY ACTIVITY

Choose an activity from phase 1 activities described in a following section.

END GROUP

In each session, mention the number of sessions that have elapsed. If there was not enough time in session 1 to create a hand gesture, handshake, or cheer, do it now. Repeat any ending rituals the members have created on their own.

Play Activity Suggestions for Phase 1 Groups (Sessions 1 and 2)

Phase 1 play activities emphasize group formation and the building of cohesiveness, identification of feelings, and increasing the comfort level of members by reassuring them that the group provides a nurturing and playful environment.

HAPPENIN' HOPSCOTCH

Supplies needed: tape; paper; feeling face cards, either handmade or from the game Emotional Bingo (can be purchased from the Self-Esteem Shop at www.selfesteemshop.com); large coin or similar object; chips or stickers; CD/MP3 player with recording of upbeat instrumental music (optional).

This game can be used for younger or older children. Use tape to make a hopscotch formation on the floor. In each square have a number corresponding to a handmade card with either a silly command or a feelings face or word. Include all six basic feelings: mad, sad, happy, scared, excited, and surprised. For older children, more complex feelings can be used, such as worried, bored, sneaky, frustrated, contented, and hyper. If a feelings card is chosen, members get a chip/sticker/M&M for stating a time they have that feeling. If a silly activity card is chosen, members get a chip/sticker/M&M for doing the activity. Suggested silly activities are:

- Say, "My name is _____" in a low voice.
- Jump three times.
- Pat your head and rub your stomach.
- Turn around three times.
- Finish the sentence: "My favorite food is_____."
- Take another turn.
- Finish the sentence: "The grossest thing ever is_____."

Each player uses a large coin or a similar object to toss into the hopscotch formation and then hops into the square on which it landed. The group leaders should go first and model the activity for the group. Some light and playful-sounding instrumental background music may be added to foster a lighthearted and fun atmosphere. The following directions can be given:

"Now we are going to play the game Happenin' Hopscotch. The idea of this game is to get to know each other, and to have some fun. I am going to show you how to play. [Leader takes a turn.] During this activity when you are watching someone take a turn, it is your job to cheer that person on. After someone finishes a turn, everybody claps. OK? OK. Now I'm going to go again, and when I'm done, everybody clap. [Leader takes a turn again and cues everyone to clap.] Now who wants to go next?"

Play this game until everyone has had several turns. Make sure to tell the group members that they have a choice of whether or not they want to do what is indicated by the card.

Supplies needed: white paper; markers; tape; feelings face poster (can be purchased from www.selfesteemshop.com); ready-made cutout facial features (eyes, nose, mouths) showing mad/sad/happy/scared/surprised/excited.

This activity is a great alternate activity for children ages 6–8, a group of children who have never met, or a group that has many reluctant members. Tell the group members that you need their help to make some face posters. It is particularly fun to use giant Post-its and to make huge faces along a wall if space permits; otherwise, use any white paper available. The paper can be taped on a wall, a table, an easel, or whatever is available, but hang up the paper if at all possible. Tell the group that these faces are supposed to look silly. Have one of the six basic feelings (mad, sad, happy, scared, surprised, excited) written on the bottom of each piece of paper and a circle for the face already drawn. Now show the group the feelings face poster that is available for help with this activity. One of the group leaders can demonstrate putting the eyes on the happy face and then ask for a volunteer to either draw or tape on the nose. Continue with this process, having group members add the mouths, hair, ears, freckles, silly spots, mad dabs, and whatever else comes to mind to make six silly feelings faces. After the feelings faces are complete, have the children name each face and suggest three reasons each face is having the particular feeling. You can also ask for volunteers to show how people with the different faces walk, talk, or move their bodies. Leaders can again demonstrate. For example, if the mad face is called "Mad Max," one of the leaders can stand up and stomp, saying, "I'm Mad Max and I stomp my feet like this!" The faces can be used in numerous ways in this and following sessions.

1. Emotional Bingo game (can be purchased from www.selfesteemshop.com).
2. Dynamic Dinosaurs, as created by VanFleet in (2001a, p. 359).
3. The Gallery of Goofy Art, as created by VanFleet (2001b, p. 359).
4. Any name game.

Phase 2: Session 3

Phase 2 begins as the "getting to know you" phase comes to a close. Phase 2 objectives include achieving a deeper exploration of relationships and authority by group members, further clarification about divorce, and correction of misconceptions. Group work shifts its focus to issues of resilience and the development of the child's coping skills. As the group makes its own developmental progress, it is common for members to challenge leaders, for differences and conflicts to be highlighted, and for members to form alliances with one another. As the session continues, members typically demonstrate increased awareness of their power to apply problem-solving skills to divorce situations. This is a good time for group leaders to review the rules among themselves and to review how problem behaviors will be addressed. *Note*: Group leaders need to stay playful!

Session 3

Start as usual with puppet making and review of the Advice Brochure Workbook. Encourage group members to make a "wild" (hostile/sad/angry) character or object if they have not yet done so. Explain that it is important that all types of feelings are represented and that there are no wrong feelings. Also remind everyone that puppets can be anything from animals to talking objects. Leaders may want to add new characters themselves to demonstrate diversity. Examples include a fly on the wall, a staircase, a lamp, a lipstick tube, or a bowl of cereal.

ROLE PLAY: PARENTS ANNOUNCING DIVORCE

The goal of the session 3 puppet role play is to support a process of expressing thoughts and feelings of vulnerability experienced by the children. Group leaders start the role play with the puppet parents telling the children their plans for divorce. Leaders must remember to respond to members' additions with acceptance and validation. It is also important to point out how difficult this type of role play is, because no one wants to hear that his or her parents are getting divorced and no parent wants to tell this to his or her child. The bigger message, however, is that communicating thoughts and feeling is OK even though it may be uncomfortable. Leaders should model supportive comments. Leaders can also ask the group to suggest various scenarios; they can also support a problem-solving discussion on how children can express their worries to their parents effectively. As usual, this part of the session is ended with advice giving, and leaders record the advice to be used in the final brochure.

PLAY ACTIVITY

Finally, close with a play activity (See phase 2 and 3 play activities, as described later). *Note*: Do not lose sight of the fact that these role plays should be kept lighthearted and playful so that it is safe for children to feel comfortable in the puppet play. This is not to minimize the seriousness of the associated feelings and thoughts, but to keep in mind that children will feel safer in their expression when it is kept in the play.

Phase 3: Sessions 4, 5, and 6

Somewhere between sessions 4 and 6 (and perhaps even starting in session 3), phase 3 emerges. In phase 3, increased cohesion and acceptance among group members is typically observed. The group is likely to be less dependent on the leaders. When a group has successfully achieved phase 3, intimacy has been developed, there is increased disclosure by group members, and it becomes more natural for them to examine conflicts. This phase is valuable because it is at this point that it becomes safer for members to participate and more emotionally intense material can be processed. Leaders must make sure to discuss the group process before and after each session.

Sessions 4–6

ROLE PLAYS: CONTINUING THE DIVORCE STORY

As suggested by Kalter and Shreier (1993), the role plays for sessions 4 through 6 maintain a similar structure, attempting to approximate the general unfolding of the divorce process. The more knowledgeable the leaders are about individual children's situations, the better the puppet script themes can be initiated by the leaders. The following script themes may be considered:

- Loyalty conflict
- Fear of having to choose one parent over the other
- Fear of having to testify in court
- Fear of loss of one parent
- Visitation issues
- The addition of new adults (Mom's new boyfriend, etc.)
- Absence of one parent
- Feelings of loss
- Feelings of being unloved
- Self-blame
- Blaming one parent over the other
- Feeling invalidated and unimportant
- Revisiting fantasies of reconciliation

The goal here for group leaders is to allow the issues to be presented in the role play, and to then ensure that the various feelings experienced by the children are validated, normalized, and demystified via the role play and response activity. The advice giving at the end provides a way for children to feel a sense of control and mastery. The following statements are suggested for starting any role play (using the names of your puppets):

- _____ is a kid who lately has been feeling that . . .
- Lately, this mom and dad have been saying things like . . .
- It's been really hard for_____ when . . .
- Sometimes it seems to this kid that_____ . . .
- _____ just wishes that . . .
- The kids in this story worry that . . .
- The parents in this story worry that . . .

Leaders should not discourage depictions of conflicts or "unsolvable" problems, as long as the group is continuing to develop a supportive environment and individual members are not being singled out as scapegoats.

Play Activity Suggestions for Phase 2 and 3 Groups

The goal of phase 2 and 3 play activities is for children to continue to work to find words and actions that help to identify and express thoughts and feelings, release negative emotion, engage in the process of problem solving, practice new behaviors, and build confidence and resilience.

CHARADES (WITH AN EXPRESSIVE FEELING COMPONENT)

Supplies needed: Kids on Stage game and/or blank cards/cut-up pieces of paper for the making of charade cards; pencils and/or pens; easel.

The board game Kids on Stage can be used for younger children, or the traditional game of charades for older children (can be adapted for younger children). If Kids on Stage is used, leaders should add cards with feeling words. The leaders can either have the group divide into two teams, divide into partners, or keep the group as a whole and have one member act out a card while the rest of the group members guess. Either use premade cards or, if appropriate, have the two teams make their own cards. Keep the game simple, telling the teams that the categories should be either animals, actions (such as jumping or riding a bike), objects (such as scissors or a camera), or feelings. Facilitate this problem-solving process and then initiate the actual game. Have group members practice giving supportive comments to those "acting," such as:

- "Great work!"
- "Way to go!"
- "You really did that well!"
- "Wow!"
- "That wasn't easy!"

Modification: In addition to acting out the cards, members can draw the word(s) on cards mounted on an easel.

ALTERNATE ACTIVITY

Play Trouble, Sorry!, or another simple board game, using teams and a time limit. Facilitate partners' decision making about how they will play as teammates and what the criteria for winning the game will be.

Discussion: During and after the activity, lead a discussion about what it was like being part of a team, verbalizing that teamwork is never easy or problem-free. Reframe negative comments into healthier ones and emphasize the problem-solving skills that were used.

ALTERNATE ACTIVITY: IT'S NOT YOUR FAULT!

Supplies needed: Pictionary Jr. or drawable word cards for older kids; paper; markers; cutout tail; tape.

For this activity, either play pin the tail on the donkey (for younger children), or blindfolded Pictionary Jr., using an easel (for older children). If the game Pictionary Jr. isn't available, leaders can easily make up their own cards with things for kids to draw, such as table, cat, house, boat, roller skates, and the like. Explain to the group members that even though they are blindfolded they should try their best, but emphasize that it is impossible for the drawings not to look silly and that having fun is the point of the game. Have one group leader demonstrate (make sure to falter and make silly, playful noises of frustration). After the demonstration, this leader takes off the blindfold and says, "I did my best, but I still had a really hard time! Sometimes we try our best, but we still can't make things the way we want them to be!" The other leader then states, "Group, let's show Sue [group leader's name] that it's not her fault by saying, 'It's not your fault, Sue!' OK, on the count of three, everybody yell, 'It's not your fault, Sue!'" Encourage the children to yell and chant as if they are cheerleaders. Then have each group member try the same activity and, in turn, have the drawer/pinner state: "I did my best, but I still had a hard time!" and then have the group yell, "It's not your fault, David!" Be sure to use each person's name so that everyone can experience hearing the encouraging statements.

BREAKTHROUGH

Supplies needed: butcher paper or a large roll of any kind of paper.

This activity is to be used at the end of phase 3 with children ages 7–12. The goal of this activity is to support a child's positive self-image and the development of a transformed identity in the context of the transitioning family. It is also a goal to give the children a sense of mastery over their situations by pointing out that they are now experts on family transitions, that they possess knowledge and experience that others do not (despite the fact that it hasn't all been fun and games), and that it may continue to be difficult at times.

Bring up the topic of mountain climbing. Talk about how hikers prepare to climb a mountain by exercising, building muscle, practicing to hike up large hills, and working a little every day at getting in shape for the big day. In fact, hikers literally reshape their bodies and lungs to be able to climb mountains, and sometimes they even have to pitch base camps to adjust to the altitude. This preparation can take months or even years. It is this hard work that transforms a hiker into a mountain climber and enables him or her to reach the summit. Then talk about how getting through family transitions has some things in common with climbing mountains. Talk about how mountain climbers have to change their shapes to be able to reach the top, and how members of families have to work at taking on new shapes as well, when going through a divorce. Continue with the following:

> "This can be hard, like exercise, and can take a lot of practice. It feels funny for a while, something like a new pair of hiking boots. Having two homes and adjusting to being in a different environment with a family is like a base camp, and it takes some getting used to before the members of the family feel as though they have reached their summit and can break through to the other side of their experience. With practice, however, a new shape will be formed, and out of that will come a feeling of accomplishment, excitement, joy, sadness, and pride. Today we are going to practice breaking through to the other side. Each one of you, with support from the group, is going to break through a large piece of paper."

Cut a very large piece of paper for each child, and have two volunteers hold the paper on either side. Cut small tears into the middle edges of the paper so that the child won't have difficulty in breaking through. Tell the group members that while someone is breaking through to the other side, it is their job to cheer that person on by saying things such as, "You can do it!," "Way to go!," "Go all the way!," "You're doing it!," "You are going to go all the way!," "Rock on!," "You go, girl!," Before each child's turn, say, "[Child's name,] you are now going to break on through to the other side. Prepare for transformation!" Then ring some type of bell or make a special sound and say, "Go when you are ready!" Have the group wait quietly while the child gets ready to break through. Once the child is on the other side, lead everyone in applause, then have the child shake hands with everyone, and cue the group to say, "Congratulations! You did it!"

OTHER ALTERNATE ACTIVITIES

1. The Anger Box, as created by Kaduson (2001a, p. 375).
2. Playback Theatre, as created by Ford and Ward-Wimmer (2001, p. 390).

Phase 4: Sessions 7 and 8

Phase 4 not only brings the group experience to a conclusion, it promotes integration and strengthening of the therapeutic benefits of participating in the divorce group and encourages the use of new ideas and skills in the world outside the group. There is a deliberate "backing off" from the emotionally intense material presented in previous sessions. In this phase, children are faced with the impending loss of the group and have an opportunity to experience loss in a more contained and expectable fashion (in comparison to divorce-related losses that have occurred). An important ingredient in this phase is the identification and reinforcement of outside supports, as well as reinforcement of all the skills and insight group members have gained. This is also a phase in which use of skills can be concretely reviewed and members can reflect on individual and group progress both directly and through play.

It was previously stated that termination has great symbolic power for a divorce group. Termination provides an opportunity to rework previous painful or incomplete terminations in the child's life. Group termination may also activate abandonment anxiety, grief, anger, and other feelings. Leaders should view acting-out behaviors in this light and intervene in ways that allow the children to face the reality of the loss of the group, express feelings and thoughts, and use new coping behaviors.

Session 7

ROLE PLAY: EXPERT PANEL

Supplies needed: cell phone headset or some type of microphone; chairs and table; paper; video recording equipment if available.

This session shifts from puppet role play to an Expert Panel role-play activity based on Kaduson's (2001b) technique Broadcast News. Start by telling the group members that in these last two sessions they are going to complete their advice brochure. Explain that they will be doing a different kind of activity called Expert Panel. Group leaders introduce the Expert Panel exercise by explaining that the group is going to produce a special edition show on the topic of divorce. State that they will sit as a panel of experts for this production. Explain that there will be callers who are going to ask questions about handling problems related to divorce. The group leaders will act as callers, who are children and parents currently going through a divorce. These callers will direct questions to the panel for expert advice. The group leaders should arrange the panel and have its members sit in a row, and then introduce them to the "audience." The coleaders should explain to the imaginary audience that callers should specify who they are directing their questions to, but make it clear to the panel that anyone is free to add to the expert advice after the questioned expert is finished speaking. When possible, give every group member some type of microphone or headset. If necessary, one microphone can be used and passed between members.

Group leaders should take turns acting as the show host and callers. The callers should be diverse and should not represent any group member specifically. Because every group is unique, leaders need to tailor their questions for the group at hand and the issues that arose during the group processes. Leaders need to ensure that every group member has an opportunity to be an expert. Leaders must also write down or record the comments made by the panel so that they can be incorporated into the final Advice Brochure. Be sure to ask questions about people children can talk to about their concerns so that this can be incorporated into the final brochure. When possible, it is recommended to record this exercise for viewing during the last session.

PLAY ACTIVITY

Be sure to budget the last 15 minutes of the session for a play activity.

END OF SESSION 7

End the session by telling members that the information needed for the Advice Brochure is complete and that each member will be given his or her own copy to take home during the final pizza party session. Because there was no opportunity at the beginning of the session for members to share anything from their take-home Advice Brochure Workbooks, be sure to allow some time for that during this ending phase so that any new material can be added for the final Advice Brochure.

Session 8

- *Option* 1: If a video recording of the expert panel is available, start by showing the video to the group.
- *Option* 2: Instruct the children to make their last puppets, saying that there is one last role play in need of advice.

Compliment the panel on what a fabulous job they did last week and state:

> "Because of all your advice over these past few weeks, we have been able to complete our Advice Brochure and we have a few copies for each of you to take home. However, we have one last puppet role play we need your help with. [If Option 1 was used at the beginning of the session, simply have the group members use their current cast of puppets.] We are going to start the role play, and then we need each of you to give advice one last time. OK, here goes!"

Group leaders then act out a scene in which two of the children in a family have a discussion about the ending of their own friendship group and their feelings of loss. After getting the group member to complete a short role play, have them each give their final advice. Reiterate this advice as a summary for the puppets so that group members hear it a few times, and point out what great suggestions these are and what a wealth of information the group has created.

Now it is time to congratulate the members of the group on their hard work that resulted in the magnificent Advice Brochure, stating that with their permission it will be shared with other teachers, kids, families, or counselors so that they can help families going through a divorce (remind everyone that no names appear on the brochure). After the children have had time to read the brochure, bring out a pizza and drinks and facilitate a discussion about all the group accomplishments. Mention to the children that they are welcome to exchange puppets with one another if they would like to. Gather each child's puppets and make sure the children have them to take home; write a personal note to each child and place it in his or her puppet bag with an individualized message thanking the child for all of his or her contributions and stating the unique qualities that child has added to the group process.

Play Activity Suggestions for Phase 4 Groups

1. Play Self-Esteem Musical Chairs, as created by Shapiro (1994, p. 151). *Note*: The basic technique is that whoever is left without a seat is given a compliment by each member of the group. For the purposes of this group, members could also say something they learned from or something they appreciated about this member. Another idea is to have them say something they wish for this member.

2. Make power charms. **Supplies needed**: beads, charms, leather string in different colors or plain string if this is not available, shells with holes, and anything that can be made into a charm bracelet or necklace. Tell the group that they are going to make "[name of group]" power charms that they can hang in their rooms or wear as bracelets or necklaces to remind them of their inner power and all the good advice they came up with for the advice brochure. Remind them of their achievements and lead a discussion about the power and friendship they gained from this group. Members can assign a word to a particular bead or item, such as "awesome," "survivor," "problem solver," "star," "phoenix," and then give the bead or item to another member. Leaders can add one bead or item to each member's power charm bracelet or necklace.

3. Decorate plain T-shirts with fabric markers and have everybody draw, or write a "power word," on each person's shirt.

4. Allow group members to select a play activity they enjoyed from a previous session.

CONCLUSION

Group leaders need to remember that this is a short-term therapy group and that the overall goal is to provide a safe environment for children of divorce to have their divorce experience normalized, to experience camaraderie, and to release negative emotion through play. Strict adherence to any group format is pointless without an awareness of the individual and group process that is unfolding within the play.

REFERENCES

Amato, P. R. (2001). Children of divorce in the 1990s: An update of the Amato and Keith (1991) meta-analysis. *Journal of Family Psychology, 15*, 355–370.

Amato, P. R., & Booth, A. (1991). Consequences of parental divorce and marital unhappiness for adult well-being. *Social Forces, 69*, 895–914.

Amato, P. R., & Keith, B. (1991a). Parental divorce and adult well-being: A meta-analysis. *Journal of Marriage and the Family, 53*, 43–58.

Amato, P. R., & Keith, B. (1991b). Parental divorce and the well-being of children: A meta-analysis. *Psychological Bulletin, 110*, 26–46.

Barker, J., Brinkman, L., & Deardorff, M. (1995). Computer interventions for adolescent children of divorce. *Journal of Divorce and Remarriage, 23*, 197–213.

Booth, A., & Edwards, J. N. (1990). The transmission of marital and family quality over the generations: The effects of parental divorce and unhappiness. *Journal of Divorce, 13*, 41–58.

Clarke, S. C. (1995). Advance report of final divorce statistics, 1989 and 1990. *Monthly Vital Statistics Report, 43*(8, Suppl.). Hyattsville, MD: National Center for Health Statistics.

Eitzen, D. S., & Baca Zinn, M. (1997). *Social Problems* (7th ed.). Boston: Allyn & Bacon.

Ford, G., & Ward-Wimmer, D. (2001). Playback theatre. In H. Kaduson & C. Schaefer (Eds.), *101 more favorite play therapy techniques* (pp. 390–394). North Bergen, NJ: Aronson.

Guldner, C. A., & O'Connor, T. (1991). The ALF group: A model of group therapy with children. *Journal of Group Psychotherapy, 43*, 184–190.

Hetherington, E. M., Bridges, M., & InSabella, G. M. (1998). What matters? What does not? Five perspectives on the association between marital transitions and children's adjustment: *American Psychologist, 53*(2), 167–184.

Kaduson, H. (2001a). The anger box. In H. Kaduson & C. Schaefer (Eds.), *101 more favorite play therapy techniques* (pp. 375–378). North Bergen, NJ: Aronson.

Kaduson, H. (2001b). Broadcast news. In H. Kaduson & C. Schaefer (Eds.), *101 more favorite play therapy techniques* (pp. 397–400). North Bergen, NJ: Aronson.

Kalter, N. (1998). Group interventions for children of divorce. In K. C. Stoiber & T. R. Krattochwill (Eds.), *Handbook of group interventions for children and families* (pp. 120–140) Boston: Allyn & Bacon.

Kalter, N., Pickar, J., & Lesowitz, M. (1984). School based developmental facilitation groups for children of divorce: A preventive intervention. *American Journal of Orthopsychiatry, 54,* 613–623.

Kalter, N., & Shreier, S. (1993). School-based support groups for children of divorce. *Special Services in the Schools, 8,* 39–66.

Neuman, G. M., & Romanowski, P. (1998). *Helping your kids cope with divorce the sandcastles way.* New York: Times Books.

Northen, H., & Kurland, R. (2001). *Social work with groups* (3rd ed.). New York: Columbia University Press.

Pedro-Carroll, J. L. (2005). Fostering resilience in the aftermath of divorce: The role of evidence based programs for children. *Family Court Review, 43,* 52–64.

Pedro-Carroll, J. L., & Cowen, E. L. (1985). The children of divorce intervention program: An investigation of the efficacy of a school-based prevention program. *Journal of Consulting and Clinical Psychology, 53,* 603–611.

Shapiro, L. (1994). *Tricks of the trade: 101 psychological techniques to help children grow and change.* King of Prussia, PA: Center for Applied Psychology.

Stolberg, A. L., & Garrison, K. M. (1985). Evaluating a primary prevention program for children of divorce: The divorce adjustment project. *American Journal of Community Psychology, 13,* 111–124.

Stolberg, A. L., & Mahler, J. (1994). Enhancing treatment gains in a school-based intervention for children of divorce through skill training, parental involvement and transfer procedures. *Journal of Consulting and Clinical Psychology, 62,* 147–156.

VanFleet, R. (2001a). Dynamic dinosaurs. In H. Kaduson & C. Schaefer (Eds.), *101 more favorite play therapy techniques* (pp. 359–361). North Bergen, NJ: Aronson.

VanFleet, R. (2001b). The gallery of goofy art. In H. Kaduson & C. Schaefer (Eds.), *101 more favorite play therapy techniques* (pp. 359–361). North Bergen, NJ: Aronson.

Young, D. M. (1989). Group intervention for children of divorced families. In M. R. Textor (Ed.), *The divorce and divorce therapy handbook* (pp. 267–284). Northvale, NJ: Aronson.

CHAPTER 13

The Use of Group Play Therapy for Children with Social Skills Deficits

JULIE A. BLUNDON
CHARLES E. SCHAEFER

Social skills are essential for the development and maintenance of positive peer relations, not only throughout childhood but in adulthood as well. Hay, Payne, and Chadwick (2004) describe how social competence begins as early as during the hospital stay immediately after birth and continues to develop throughout childhood and adolescence. As the infant develops, he or she begins to interact with peers and adults through smiling, touching, and reaching behaviors, though topic-related interaction does not fully develop until the second year. By 6 months of age, infants can be showing turn-taking behaviors, which is also known as contingency in terms of responsiveness. This turn-taking behavior by infants is present with both peers and adults. Mutual engagement, alternating turns, and other prosocial behaviors such as sharing, helping, and giving comfort develop around 1 year of age, when the child also begins to show interest in cooperative games. Children begin to have conflicts with others regarding both possessions and personal space by age 1, and how they deal with such conflicts can be predictive of how they deal with future conflicts and interactions. For example, if children deal with early conflicts with physical force, aggression is likely in the future as well. Likewise, children who develop more socially appropriate methods of dealing with conflicts tend to continue these patterns throughout their developmental stages.

SOCIAL SKILLS AND SOCIAL COMPETENCE

"Social skills" differs from "social competence" in that the skills are needed to develop and maintain competence. Gresham (1997) reviewed the literature from the 1970s to 1997 and found that three definitions of social skills were used most frequently: a peer acceptance definition, a competence-correlates definition, and a behavioral definition. The peer acceptance definition relies on peer acceptance or the popularity of the child to determine whether or not the child is socially skilled. The rationale is that a child who is more popular or well accepted will have more positive social skills. The competence-correlates definition focuses on the correlation between behaviors and peer acceptance, popularity, or some other measure of social competence. This means that children with higher levels of peer acceptance or popularity are likely to have higher levels of positive social skills than children with lower levels of acceptance. The behavioral definition states that social skills include behaviors that increase socially appropriate responses as well as extinguish socially inappropriate responses. For the purposes of this chapter, the behavioral definition is used. Thus, social skills are defined here as behaviors that increase positive social interactions (e.g., cooperation, starting conversations) and decrease negative interactions (e.g., conflict resolution).

Children exhibit a number of social skills that form the basis for social competence with others. These skills include conversation (both initiating and sustaining), cooperation, helpfulness, sympathy, kindness, conflict resolution, and many more. Spence's (2003) review of social skills training outlines a number of cognitive and emotional social skills that have been targeted for intervention. These include the development of interpersonal problem-solving skills, accurate processing of social information, social perception and perspective taking, cognitive distortion and maladaptive thinking styles, social knowledge, affect regulation and emotional skills, and self-regulation and self-monitoring skills. Training has been focused on both deficiencies in existing skills, and acquisition of new skills.

A review of the literature indicates that four general types of social skills are usually included in training programs: communication, interaction, self-control, and feelings/emotions. Within communication skills are conversation skills (both initiating and maintaining), recognizing and understanding interpersonal cues, eye contact, listening, and staying on topic. Interaction skills include taking turns, sharing, assertiveness versus aggression, making positive statements, cooperation, and empathy. Self-control primarily includes impulsivity control and problem solving. Finally, the feelings/emotions area includes the identification of emotions in the self and others, externalizing emotions, and regulation of emotions.

Differences have been noted between performance and acquisition deficits in regard to social skills (Bandura, 1969). Acquisition deficits are seen when a child does not have a certain skill in his or her repertoire, whereas a perfor-mance deficit is seen when a child has developed the skill but fails to appropri-ately perform the skill. This chapter focuses primarily on perceived acquisition deficits, although performance deficits are also targeted through coaching and modeling of appropriate social interactions.

TRAINING MODEL

Oden and Asher (1977), Ladd and Mize (1983), and Choi and Kim (2003) present a coaching model of social skills training that contains three steps: (1) encouraging skill acquisition through education, (2) increasing individual skill performance through practice, and (3) generalizing the new skills to daily life situations. The model is psychoeducational in nature, involving teaching a group of children basic information about a variety of social skills, practic-ing these skills in a group session with prompting, modeling, and reinforce-ment by therapists, and promoting generalization by outside practice of each skill.

The fun and enjoyment the children derive from playing in group games is another important aspect of the teaching program because such positive emo-tions make learning and practicing the skills a positive experience. Learning strategies presented in a game-like context have been found to be particularly effective with elementary school age children. The game-like atmosphere en-hances and maintains the children's interest and motivation to engage in the activities. Because the skills are associated with pleasant experiences, the children are able to remember more easily what they have learned in the sessions.

GENERALIZATION OF SKILLS

The generalization of social skills training to daily life is a problem that has challenged researchers for a number of years (Gresham, 1997). The teaching of social behaviors is typically done in the context of a group, held in a clinic or a school. As Gresham (1997) points out, researchers often give children set examples of when to use which behaviors and do not allow them an opportu-nity to learn how to generalize these skills on their own. Very rarely are chil-dren in daily life going to encounter the neatly designed "conflicts" presented to them in a training session. Children need to learn of a variety of situations in which they can best utilize their newly learned skills. One way of encourag-ing this is to keep parents informed of the skills that are being taught and ask-ing them to support their children with these skills daily. Informing parents of the skills that are taught and encouraging them to remind or reinforce their children to use the new skills encourages generalization of the skills. This active reinforcement of the skills by parents can also result in less deterioration over time (Gresham, 1997).

SOCIAL SKILLS OUTCOMES

To provide the most comprehensive social skills training, variables that increase effectiveness must be examined. A meta-analysis of 35 social skills training programs for children with emotional and behavioral disorders showed a pooled mean effect size of 0.20 (Quinn, Kavale, Mathur, Rutherford, & Forness, 1999). This indicates a small positive gain in increasing prosocial behaviors and decreasing negative behaviors. This meta-analysis included programs that were designed for research purposes as well as commercially available programs, and no differences were seen between the two.

SOCIAL SKILLS TRAINING PROGRAM

Social Skills Curriculum

A 10-session social skills curriculum for children and a corresponding curriculum for parents are presented in this chapter. The curricula focus on teaching social skills specific to common problems seen in children and engaging parents as coaches to the children's learning process. The 10 targeted skills were selected on the basis of their relevance to social relationships of this age group and were derived from the literature regarding social skills deficits. The instruction, reinforcement, and practice of these skills can benefit both older and younger children, and the activities can be modified to fit the developmental and cognitive levels of many children. The purpose of these curricula is to provide children with base skills that can help increase positive peer contacts, increase a child's appeal with peers, and decrease socially unpleasant and inappropriate behaviors.

While the children are in sessions, as described presently, the parents meet in their own group in a separate room. In the parent session, the goal is to enhance parents' ability to support their children's skill acquisition. Because much learning takes place outside the classroom, parents are trained in enhancing the children's skill development in the home and other settings. The support and encouragement of a parent are essential in facilitating generalization and maintaining treatment effects. When parents are taught the same skills that the children are learning, they are aware of what and how to reinforce and arrange social behaviors outside the group setting.

The leader of the parent group also explains what is known about children's social development and the importance of social skills and status as related to the various topics. Parents are consistently encouraged to take on a coaching role with their children and provide them with opportunities to practice their skills through play dates and other social gatherings. To help facilitate this process, parents are introduced to the same vocabulary and activities that their children are learning. Parents are also made aware of the children's homework assignments and, at times, given activities of their own for the week. Throughout the 10 sessions, parents are taught how to prompt and reward children's positive social behaviors and encouraged to seek new ways to introduce the skills during the week.

Parents are encouraged to role-play some of the skills, especially in assertion training, and discussions of how best to implement the skills in the home environment are expected. At the start of each session, parents are asked to relate any problems found with the previous week's skill and are encouraged to keep practicing the skills with their children to promote generalization. They are also encouraged to arrange play dates with the children in the groups, as these children have not previously interacted and are starting off with clean slates, which can provide good opportunities for positive social interactions.

Screening

Children and their parents attend a 1½-hour screening session conducted by a group leader prior to acceptance to the program. This session is used to determine the appropriateness of the child for the group, or the group for the child. The parents are interviewed to collect a variety of information about the child (including developmental history, family history and stressors, social history, school adaptation, special interests and talents, physical problems, medications, food restrictions, and goals for group participation).

While the leader meets with the child, the parents complete the Social Skills Rating Scale (Gresham & Elliot, 1990) and a measure of social skills related to the curriculum. The leader also meets with the parents and child together to discuss the purpose of the social skills group and the benefits of attending. When speaking with the child, it is useful to refer to the group as a "Friendship Group" to more clearly explain the purpose of the sessions.

Leaders must closely review the information obtained in the interviews to be sure that the children are appropriate for this group and the development of a safe and positive learning environment. There are a number of criteria for excluding a child from the group, including the following:

- Severely disruptive, aggressive, or oppositional behaviors
- Bizarre or psychotic behaviors
- Extreme social withdrawal (e.g., no eye contact, lack of verbal responsiveness, no social interest)
- Intense separation anxiety, inability to separate from parents
- Major depression or suicidal tendencies

If it is determined that a child is not appropriate for the group, other options are given to the parents, such as individual psychotherapy or other groups.

Group Composition

Each group consists of five to ten children of both genders. The children in the groups are no more than 4 years apart in age, such as 4–7 years old or 8–12 years old. It is optimal to mix children with internalizing and externalizing problems, such as social inhibition and aggressive tendencies. The size of the group should depend on the number of leaders available.

Group Leaders

Within each group, there should be leaders of both genders, preferably at a ratio of one leader for every two children. The same leaders meet with the same children for the 10 weeks. Another group leader meets separately with the parents. Leaders are typically graduate students or therapists within a mental health profession (e.g., psychology, social work, and counseling).

A leaders has several roles to fill, in addition to being a teacher; a major role of a group leader is to be a cheerleader, becoming excited about the group activities and reacting as if a child's response should be a headline of a newspaper. By being enthusiastic, energetic, and excited, leaders help the children to become more interested and involved in the group activities. Enthusiasm is contagious in group sessions.

Leaders should also be playful and fun loving (even a bit wacky at times) in order to capture and sustain children's interest and attention. In showing strong positive affect, such as by smiling and being cheerful, leaders make the gratifying fun elements of the group activities more obvious. In addition, group leaders need to have or to develop good "child-handling" skills. They must clearly be in charge of the group sessions and comfortable in enforcing group rules without becoming harsh or autocratic. Prior experience as a camp counselor, classroom teacher, coach, or youth club leader can help prepare a person to be a children's group therapist.

Group Sessions

The first 10 minutes of each 60-minute session are devoted to a group discussion in which the leaders review the previous week's homework and describe the target social skill to be practiced in the current session. The leaders explain in simple, concrete terms what the skill is and why it is important, give examples of the skill in action, and answer any questions. This instruction time is followed by 40 minutes of structured activities, such as games or art projects, that give the children an opportunity to practice the new social skill and receive feedback about their performances. The final 10 minutes of each session is reserved for snack time (which is used to promote a feeling of being nurtured), summaries by the leaders of the group members' performances on the target skill, rewarding the work done during the session, and presenting homework for the coming week.

Teaching Methods

A basic assumption of this training program is that children learn social behaviors best when group leaders use a very active instructional approach that includes multiple cognitive-behavioral strategies, such as direct instruction, role plays, supervised practice activity, prompting, corrective feedback, monitoring, and providing opportunities for independent practice in the natural environment. Specific teaching strategies used in this curriculum are as follows:

Modeling

This method is based on the principle of imitative learning. Appropriate social skills are modeled by group leaders, peers, and by the use of puppets, dolls, or story characters. Following a demonstration by a model, children are given an opportunity to practice the skill.

Operant Conditioning

Positive and negative reinforcement are used to gradually strengthen appropriate behaviors, such as cooperation, and weaken inappropriate ones, such as aggressiveness.

Social Cognition

The emphasis in this approach is not on external behaviors, but on the thoughts and feelings that underlie such behaviors. The social-cognitive approach is concerned with verbal and cognitive mediators such as thinking of alternative ways to solve a social problem, changing irrational beliefs, or thinking of the consequences to self and others of one's actions.

Coaching

Oden and Asher (1977) were among the first to use a coaching method to teach social skills to isolated children. This coaching process includes three components:

1. Children are verbally instructed in social skills (what they are, why they are important).
2. Children are provided with an opportunity to practice their social skills by playing with their peers.
3. Children have a postplay performance review with the group leader (coach).

In coaching, the goal is behavior change based on the child's knowledge of specific interpersonal behaviors, ability to convert social knowledge into skillful social behavior in interactive contexts, and ability to accurately evaluate his or her skill performance (Ladd & Mize, 1983).

Finally, the therapeutic factors in the group process such as universalization, cohesion, altruism, and vicarious learning are present to enhance the power of this intervention (Yalom, 1985). A major advantage of group play therapy over individual play therapy is the provision of a safe social setting for discovering and experimenting with new and more satisfying ways to relate to peers. The best way for children to learn social skills is to learn them in a real-life group situation with their peers, not in individual psychotherapy with an adult therapist.

Group Management Strategies

Perhaps the most challenging aspect of group work with children is finding ways to manage the broad range of inappropriate behaviors that may emerge in group sessions, such as name calling, play fighting, shouting, and not listening or participating. The goals of group discipline are twofold: to ensure the safety of the children and leaders and to create an environment conducive to learning new social skills. Group leaders use the a number of strategies, discussed in the following paragraph, to prevent or reduce behavioral disturbances during group sessions.

Rules

Rules provide children with concrete guidelines regarding appropriate behavior in sessions and send a clear message that the children will be safe in the group. Rules should be formulated during the first session with input from the children. A list of the rules should be displayed in a conspicuous location in the room. Go over the rules several times, and explain the reasons for constructing group rules.

GUIDELINES

1. Rules should be limited to four to six, because children will not remember more than this number. Give specific directives regarding other behaviors as the need arises.

2. Phrase the rules in a positive ("to do") manner rather than a negative ("don't do") manner. Examples include "Stay in your seat" rather than "Don't walk around."

3. Rules should refer to specific observable behaviors, such as "Keep your hands to yourself" rather than "Be nice to everyone."

4. Throughout the group, children should be reinforced for following the rules, and negative consequences attached for not following the rules. Examples of positive reinforcement include praising a child individually, as well as in front of the group, and negative reinforcement may include private reprimands or time-outs.

5. Review the rules at the start of each session by asking one child to select a rule and explain it to the group members.

6. The rules should be short and to the point so that they can be easily remembered. Examples include:
   • Wait your turn.
   • Hands to yourself.
   • Raise your hand.
   • Listen and pay attention.
   • Do your homework.

Social Reinforcement

Social reinforcement (such as smiling, saying "thank you," praising, patting on the arm, nearness, giving attention) should be given for appropriate social behaviors by the children (Madsen, Becker, & Thomas, 1968). Research has shown that social reinforcement is very effective in increasing children's positive social behaviors. Group leaders, like classroom teachers and parents, are inclined to take good behaviors for granted and to pay attention only when a child acts up or misbehaves. Give praise and appreciation freely when children follow the rules and show prosocial behaviors. It is very important to notice as many good behaviors as possible during a group session.

When praising children, labeled praise is much more beneficial than unlabeled praise. Labeled praise differs from unlabeled praise in that it clearly specifies the behavior that is being commended. A labeled praise for sharing is, "Eric, nice job sharing your markers with Bill." An unlabeled praise is, "Good work, Eric." The second comment fails to inform the child of the particular behavior that pleases the group leader. Leaders should remind children throughout the session when they are following a rule ("Great job raising your hand!") or still need to work on a rule ("I want you to earn your smiley face—remember to wait your turn!").

GUIDELINES

1. Be sure every group member is singled out for praise and attention.
2. Vary your expressions of praise rather than continually saying "Good."

3. Attempt to become spontaneous in your approval, and smile while giving it.
4. At first you will probably feel that you are expressing approval a great deal and that it sounds a bit phony. This is a typical reaction, but it will become more natural with the passage of time.
5. After a session, tell the parents about something their child did well in the session.

Ratio of Positive to Negative Responses

Leaders should positively reinforce desired behaviors much more frequently (about a 5:1 ratio) than they apply negative consequences for inappropriate behaviors. This may seem daunting, but as with praising, it becomes routine quickly.

Reward System

For appropriate social behavior in the group, each child can earn a happy (smiley) face on a reward chart. For noncompliant and disruptive behaviors, children receive sad (frowny) faces. These notations relate directly to the rules posted. At the end of each session, leaders should ask each child individually if he or she followed each of the rules. If the child did, a happy face is earned, and if there was trouble regarding a rule, a sad face is drawn by the leader. This discussion is best held in front of the entire group, as children should be expected to clap for their peers. This encourages cooperation and social approval. Children are encouraged to work on the rules they had trouble with during the next session. If the group receives more happy than sad faces, they each earn a reward of a small toy. This practice can be modified so that no prizes are given in individual sessions, but cumulative totals of more happy faces than sad can earn a full-group pizza party or another fun activity. Children should be reminded of this reward system throughout the group sessions.

Studies indicate that positive reinforcement is most powerful when it includes a combination of social approval and tangible rewards (Pfiffner, Rosen, & O'Leary, 1985). Moreover, children often give their best performances when their individual efforts contribute to a group reward (Slavin, 1983). This method of reward also encourages the idea of cooperation with the group members.

Negative Consequences

For minor or infrequent rule infractions (e.g., occasionally interrupting others), group leaders should try ignoring, reprimanding in private, prompting or reminding about the rule, or leading a group problem-solving effort. However, for more serious or frequent rule violations (e.g., physical or verbal hostility, frequent sex talk), group leaders are likely to use time-out or suspension for a session. Children who argue, fight, or act out when they are together need to be physically separated from each other. For example, a leader may sit between them during the session.

Time-out simply means time away from the group and group leaders. One group leader implements the time-out while the other group leaders continue to direct the group activity. The following guidelines can make time-out more effective:

1. A chair in the hallway outside the group room often works well, or a separate room can be used to isolate the child. Sitting in the corner of the group room (partial separation) can work for preschoolers or for short periods of time. This can also be called the "Focus Chair" to remove common negative stereotypes.

2. Short durations of time-out (5 to 10 minutes) are preferable. Longer durations have not been found to be more effective and are more difficult to enforce. The child must be quiet at the end of the time-out before he or she can return to the group. If a child resists or attempts to leave time-out, enforce this measure by physically holding the child with just enough force to contain him or her (basket hold) or by ending the session for that child.

3. Children should receive one warning before time-out is enforced. The frequency of time-outs tends to decrease when a warning is given. Keep warnings short and unemotional (e.g., "If you can't stop your shouting, you'll need to take time in the Focus Chair").

4. The group leader, not the child, should always control when a child is released from time-out.

5. Time-out works only if the environment the child is leaving (often termed the "time-in" environment) is more reinforcing than the time-out area. The relative difference is obtained reinforcement between the time-in and the time-out environments, and the main reason that time-out is effective (Christophersen, 1987).

6. During time-out, the group leader does not touch or talk with the child except as needed for physical restraint.

Prompting

Remind children of appropriate behavior by saying such things as:

- "Remember your inside voice."
- "Eyes on me."
- "I need your listening ears."
- "Freeze your body."
- "Right now it's my turn."

Prompts involving the rules of the group are also beneficial.

Reprimand

In reprimanding, you express your disapproval of a child's behavior. Use "I" statements to state how the behavior adversely affects you, your feelings about it, and to suggest an alternative behavior that is acceptable to you. Remember to disapprove of the specific behavior, not the child. Reprimand privately and quietly.

Programming

If a session is dull or boring, the children will likely be disruptive. It is important to make group activities fun, enjoyable, and interesting for both you and the children.

SOCIAL SKILLS MODULES

Session 1 (Children's Group): Conversation

After introductions, group leaders explain the purpose of the group, that is, to learn and practice some new friendly behaviors. When group members get really good at their friendship skills, they will enjoy themselves more with their friends and classmates and be more popular with their friends. Ask the children to think about and select a name for their friendship group. Encourage the quieter children to volunteer names as well.

With the children's input, generate a list of four to five group rules that can help make the group sessions an enjoyable and safe experience for everyone. Post the rules conspicuously on a wall and refer to them throughout the session. For younger children, you may have the rules developed before the session (Raise your hand, Wait your turn, Listen/Pay attention, Hands to yourself, Do your homework).

Learning Goals

- To enhance children's listening skills, including nonverbal behaviors (eye contact, close interpersonal distance such as 3 feet, forward body lean, pleasant facial expression and tone of voice) and verbal behaviors that indicate that one is attending and trying to understand (such as questioning, noncommittal acknowledgments such as "Mm-hmm," "OK," paraphrasing, and empathy).

- To increase children's ability to talk and hold up their end of a conversation (such as answering questions, engaging in small talk, and self-disclose).

Instruction

Introduce this session to the children by explaining that they will be learning some new conversation skills that will help them to better initiate conversations with each other, as well as with other children and adults. Then describe and ask for examples of specific behaviors that can enhance conversation such as:

- *Eye contact:* Show your interest in the other person by looking at him or her when you are talking and by saying the person's name when talking to him or her.
- *Asking questions:* When you ask someone a question, you show that you are interested in that person and want to learn more about him or her. Showing interest makes it more likely that the other person will like you and want to get to know you better.
- *Talking:* Answer questions that are asked of you with more than a one-word response. Tell about something interesting that happened to you. Wait for the other person to pause before you start talking. Don't do all the talking—others enjoy talking, too.

While you are giving examples of these behaviors to the children, invite them to come to the front of the group to help you demonstrate the skills. Encourage the children to think of different types of conversation starters and ways to show they are interested in what the other person is saying. When discussing this segment, encourage the children to stay on topic.

Activities

INTERVIEWING

In dyads, children take turns interviewing each other. Group leaders prompt and model the types of questions they might ask each other: personal inquiries such as age, where they live; inquiries about family, hobbies, vacations, school, TV/movies, pets After the interview, each child introduces the other and tells the group what he or she learned about the person interviewed.

CONVERSATIONS

While the group is sitting in a circle, one child starts a conversation by asking another child a question about one of the following topics: favorite movie, favorite food, place you would like to visit, person you would like to meet, pet you would like to own. The two children have a brief conversation, then one turns to the child on the right and includes him or her in the conversation.

TELEPHONE GAME

Begin by giving one child a message to whisper to the next child. The message should be only one to two sentences long, such as, "Tell your mother that a big, black, angry creature is hanging from the ceiling over her head." The message is whispered from child to child around the room. When it returns to first child, it is spoken aloud and examined for accuracy. The first message should be relatively simple to model the game ("Jen's hair looks nice today"). The goal of this game is to practice listening skills and to demonstrate how even simple repetition can be distorted.

Once these skills have been taught and practiced, gather the children into a group and ask them to go over the group rules once again individually. Have each child come to the front of the room, and for each rule that he or she has successfully followed, draw a smiley face next to the childs name on the chart. If the child still needs to work on following the rule, draw a frowning face next to his or her name. Add up the smiling and frowning faces on the chart, and if the number of smiling faces is greater, give each child a chance to select a toy to take home. Each child can choose a sticker to take home regardless of the number of smiling faces. Homework should be given and explained at this point. Give the children a snack and prepare for parents to pick them up.

Homework

Give each child a sheet with the following homework assignment:

Start a conversation with another child this week. Remember:

1. Make eye contact.
2. Ask good questions.
3. Don't forget to talk!

Name of child:_____

Where was the conversation? _____

How did the conversation start? _____

What did the other child say? _____

Were there any problems with the conversation? _____

Session 1 (Parents' Group): Conversation

Learning Goal

To inform parents about how they can help their children develop better conversation skills.

Introduction

Start by describing the children's group, what will be expected of the children, and what will be expected of the parents. In the children's group, they are told, "We are here to learn and practice some new friendly behaviors. When you get really good at your friendship skills, you will enjoy yourselves more with your friends and classmates and be more popular with your friends." Parents should be informed of the home practice assignments that correspond with the day's goals. Children are asked to practice the skills at home, and parents are encouraged to ask their children what they covered in the session, what they need to practice, and how they used the skills in school. Parents will be learning more about the skills their children are learning to aid in this process. Remind parents that only so much can be done in the group sessions—if they want to see generalization, their help is needed! It does not have to take a lot of effort, but there should some recognition of the group goals outside the sessions.

Instruction

Children need to speak with others and communicate effectively if they are to interact successfully with their peers. Popular children tend to engage in more verbal discourse with their peers than others do. Training conversation skills can lead to improvements in peer acceptance. Researchers have found that popular children ask questions and offer personal information more readily than unpopular children. Conversation skills that contribute to the formation of friendship include listening skills (in conjunction with asking questions, particularly open-ended questions that need more than a one-word response), talking skills (such as answering another's question, elaborating on responses, talking about interests or school activities, sticking to the topic of conversation), and nonverbally attending to the other person while conversing, (making eye contact, minimizing distracting gestures, etc.).

Activity

Discuss with the parents the ways in which they can instruct, prompt, reinforce, and model conversation skills with their children at home. List all of the ideas and ask the parents to select a few ideas to implement at home that week. Talk about such things as holding conversations over dinner (if they are getting one-word answers from their children, suggest writing questions that require more lengthy answers, such as "What celebrity do you most admire and why?" or "What is your favorite place in the world?" on cards and putting them in a box. Each night, someone chooses a card and the question on it becomes the topic for discussion).

Practice

To practice their own conversation skills (which is good for modeling to their children), parents split into groups of three. One parent is designated the "talker," who shares a personal experience; another is the "listener," who responds to the "talker" with good verbal and nonverbal listening skills; and the third parent is the "observer," who gives feedback at the end of the 5-minute exercise to the talker and the listener" about ways to improve their conversation skills. Be sure to alternate roles among the three parents. Leaders should watch and listen to these groups to see where improvements can be made.

Homework

Explain to the parents their child's homework assignment and the need for a parent to monitor the homework, show interest in it, and make sure that it is handed in. The homework is intended to help children practice the new skills outside of session. The child's homework for this week is to start a conversation with another child during the week and indicate what the topic was.

Parents should also play the Twenty Questions game with their child. Each person chooses a person, place, or thing that the other person must figure out by using only 20 yes/no questions. Parents may give suggestions of how to ask better questions. The purpose of this activity is to encourage their child to ask more thoughtful and informative questions with other children, which is an important conversation skill.

Session 2 (Children's Group): Peer Group Entry

Review the previous week's homework and ask if there are any related questions.

Learning Goal

To improve children's ability to join an ongoing activity or conversation with their peers.

Instruction

Studies show that children with high social competence often attempt to enter an ongoing game by following a three- or four-step procedure. First they stand nearby and watch their peers interacting. Then they make a positive comment about the game or the group playing (e.g., "Good shot!" or "That looks like fun!"). They may then engage in a similar activity on their own (e.g., bouncing a basketball). Finally, they ask the group members if they may join in the activity.

Similarly, for children to join an ongoing conversation between two or more of their peers, the following strategy may be offered:

1. Look at your peers with an interested, pleasant expression on your face. Try to make eye contact.
2. Wait for a pause.
3. Say something on the topic.
4. If your initiative is ignored, walk away with a good attitude and find someone else to talk with. If your initiative is accepted, try to use all of the skills taught in the previous session

Activities

ENTERING PLAY

Have the children practice how to enter the ongoing play activity of two or three other people. Use the principles of modeling to practice the skill between leaders and children. When modeling, present the children with examples of poor ways to enter groups and ask them to correct you. Ask them to show you how it should be done. Leaders should prompt, model, and reinforce effective entry strategies.

ROLE PLAYS

Ask the group to role-play ineffective strategies for joining a play activity of their peers, such as:

1. Claiming superiority over the other children (e.g., "I can do that better than you can.").
2. Criticizing th other children.
3. Barging right in without asking permission to play.
4. Protracted hovering about without any attempt to enter.

INVITATION ROLE PLAYS

To teach children how to invite a peer to join an activity in which they are involved, discuss the following strategies:

1. Ask the other child if he or she would like to join in the group activity.
2. If necessary, introduce the child to others in your group
3. Explain the activity and any rules to the new child.

Role-play scenarios in which a child invites a peer to join in a conversation he or she is having with two other friends.

HOMEWORK

Practice joining a conversation or a group at home or in school three times this week. Remember:

1. Use a pleasant face and voice.
2. Look at others.
3. Wait for a pause.
4. Say something on the topic.

Explain how you joined a conversation or a group.

First time:_____

Second time:_____

Third time:_____

Session 2 (Parents' Group): Peer Group Entry

Learning Goal

To coach parents on how to help their children enter ongoing activities of others.

Instruction

Children's entry behavior refers to how they approach and attempt to enter the ongoing activity of others, particularly their peers. The study of children's entry behavior has received more research attention than any other social skill. Because successful entry in a peer play group is a prerequisite for further social interaction, it is clearly an important task for children to master.

One of the most effective strategies for joining a peer group activity is to follow a three- or four-step behavioral sequence:

1. *Spectator behavior:* Quietly stand close by and watch the group activity. This initial spectator behavior allows the child to learn behaviors acceptable to the group and the group's frame of reference so he or she can engage in an entry behavior most likely to lead to the child's success in joining the group.
2. *Positive comments:* Make a positive statement about the group or the activity.
3. *Mimicking:* Engage in an activity similar to the group's behavior to show that you are interested in the activity and have the needed skills.
4. *Direct request:* Ask the group members if you can join their activity.

Remember that even when children master effective entry skills, they must learn that their peers will probably not accept them immediately into the group.

Often a child must convince others of his or her merits as a playmate. Parents are told that to inoculate their child against the stress of having his or her initiations ignored or rejected, they might role-play with their child how to handle this situation by calmly walking away and seeking another activity or playmate.

Activity

Ask the parents to discuss ways they used as children to join an ongoing peer activity and what types of activities they were most often asked to join. Ask what types of methods their children use, and how they can best encourage their children to join more positively.

Homework

Review with your child the steps to take to join an ongoing conversation of family members without interrupting the discussion. Encourage your child to use this skill at home this week.

Session 3 (Children's Group): Rejection

Review the previous week's homework and ask if there are any related questions.

Learning Goal

To help children deal appropriately with rejection by peers and determine alternate activities.

Instruction

Sometimes children do everything "by the book" for joining groups, but their peers still reject them. This may be because the children are not liked, or because there isn't enough room for them to play with that particular group, or for any number of other reasons. Children have already been exposed to spectator behavior, positive comments, and mimicking to make entry into groups. In this session the children continue to practice these behaviors, but all of the outcomes are going to be negative (i.e., the children will be rejected by the groups they are trying to enter) and the children will discover other activities to deal with the situation.

First, ask the children what it feels like to be rejected. Create a master list of all of the emotions they mention, and add some of your own that you deem appropriate to create a comprehensive list. Once the list is complete, ask children if they would like to figure out some ways to avoid these feelings when they are rejected.

Discuss the benefits of positive self-talk when rejected. Children are not always rejected because there is something wrong with what they did or with them personally. Helping them practice such statements as "That was a good try," or "Maybe they're just busy or don't have enough room for another player" can help them see that rejection is not always their fault.

Activities

LISTING ALTERNATIVES

Ask the children to create a list of things they could do instead of joining a group when they are rejected. Examples include trying a different group, creating your own group, doing a different activity, reading a book, riding your bike, and the like. Encourage a variety of activities so that many different types of rejection are covered.

ROLE PLAYS

Once the list is created, have the children role-play being rejected and figuring out something else to do. Just walking away is not always a good option, because it can lead to many of the feelings they listed previously. Remind them of this when they suggest just walking away. Ask the participants how they think they would feel after trying a different activity. Would they feel the same way as when they were rejected in the first place?

GAME

In this game, all of the children line up against a far wall and leaders stand at an opposite location. The leaders call the children to their side by specifying attributes. For example, leaders ask for all of the children with brown hair to come over and play a game with them (e.g., Hangman, hula hoops, etc.). The other children remain against the wall and watch the activities. After a few minutes, the leaders call over children with a different attribute and the process is repeated. After a few rounds, gather all of the children together and ask them how they felt about not being called—that is, rejection—and how they dealt with it in their heads. What were they thinking? Did they try positive self-talk or other methods? This is a situation in which children cannot just leave the uncomfortable place, but must come up with other ideas to deal with the rejection.

Homework

Tell about a time you were rejected this week. How did you feel, and what did you do to deal with the situation? Did you talk positively to yourself, find something else to do, or come up with a new strategy by yourself?

Session 3 (Parents' Group): Rejection

Learning Goal

To coach parents on how to help their children deal appropriately with rejection by peers and determine alternate activities.

Instruction

Sometimes children do everything appropriately for joining groups, but their peers still reject them. This may be because the children are not liked for some reason, or because there isn't enough room for them to play with that particular group. Children have already been exposed to spectator behavior, positive comments, and mimicking to make entry into groups. In this session they continue to practice these behaviors, but all of the outcomes are going to be negative (i.e., the children will be rejected from the groups they are trying to enter).

The children then learn about different things they can do when rejected from groups and shown that the reasons they are rejected may not have anything to do with them personally. Ask parents to develop a list of alternative activities their children can do when rejected from a group.

Discuss the benefits of positive self-talk when rejected. Children are not always rejected because there is something wrong with what they did or with them personally. Let the parents know that helping their children practice such statements as "That was a good try," or "Maybe they're just busy or don't have enough room for another player" can help them see that rejection is not always their fault.

Activity

Ask the parents to discuss how they handle peer rejection now, and what methods their children use. Suggest alternatives to the methods that have not been working.

Homework

Discuss different ways to deal with rejection, and talk with your child about how you felt when you were rejected as a child. When you see yourself as an example, the child sees that rejection happens to everyone and does not make him or her a bad person. What is another thing the child can do? What can the child change about how he or she handled the situation?

Session 4 (Children's Group): Assertiveness

Review the previous week's homework and ask if there are any related questions.

Learning Goal

To teach children how to stand up for themselves without being aggressive or passive.

Instruction

Assertiveness can be defined as the thoughts, feelings, and behaviors that can help a child obtain personal goals or defend his or her rights in a socially acceptable manner. Teach the children to use "I statements" to assert themselves in situations of conflict. The basic components of an "I" message are:

1. Briefly describe the behavior of concern.
2. State the reason that this is a problem for you.
3. Request an alternate behavior that is acceptable to you.
4. Show understanding of the other person's good intentions, or extenuating circumstances.
5. Share your negative feelings.

Activities

MODELING

First, the leaders should model using "I messages" to handle common conflicts they encounter in daily living. Examples of an "I" statement include "When put-downs are used, I am disappointed because you're hurting each other. We can't enjoy ourselves in group when we worry about bad names being called." "Tapping your pencil is distracting to me. Thanks for stopping."

Model all three common conflict resolution styles: aggressive (verbal and physical), assertive, and passive/avoidant. Aggressive reactions include those in which a person behaves as though he or she is better than or more important than another person. A passive reaction is one in which a person behaves as though another person's feelings or rights are more important than his or her own. An assertive reaction is one in which both people are respected. Ask group members for suggestions of "I" statements as well as examples of the conflict resolution styles to be sure they understand.

Next, ask the group members to role-play being assertive in response to common conflicts with their peers, siblings, or parents. The role plays can be done as a whole group or in smaller groups. Ask the children to generate some examples similar to the following:

1. A friend won't play by the rules of a game.
2. A friend never wants to play anything you want to play.
3. A classmate cuts in front of you in line.

4. A sibling takes your possession without permission.

5. A parent forgets to wake you up on time in the morning.

DETECTIVE GAME

Have one child volunteer to play the part of the detective, and one to be the person being watched. The person being watched has to interact with a leader in either a passive, assertive, or aggressive manner. The detective must watch eye contact, listen to tone of voice, and listen to the reactions of the person being watched to determine which type of response is being used. If the reaction is decided to be aggressive or passive, group members work together to determine what an assertive response should have been. This activity should first be modeled, with three leaders participating.

Homework

Practice being assertive during the next week and tell the group about that time. Remember:

1. Say what bothered you.
2. Tell why this is a problem to you.
3. Request an alternate behavior that would work.
4. Show understanding of other person.
5. Share your negative feelings.

When:_____

With whom:_____

What was the situation?_____

How were you assertive?_____

Session 4 (Parents' Group): Assertiveness

Learning Goal

To teach parents the difference between assertiveness, aggression, and passive/avoidant responses.

Instruction

Explain that the best way to teach assertiveness to children is by parental example. If a child tracks mud all over the kitchen floor, parents tend to respond in one of three ways:

1. *Aggressive:* "How could you be so dumb!? You made a mess of the floor. You never think about what you're doing!"
2. *Assertive:* "I'm really upset. I worked so hard to clean this floor, and now it's dirty again."

3. *Passive/avoidant:* Parent mutters to him- or herself but says nothing directly to the child.

Describe the components of an assertive "I" message (the problem behavior, concrete effect on you, your feelings about it) and point out how an "I" message differs from a blaming "you" message that attacks a child's personality and is likely to make the child defensive.

Activity

Parents role-play giving aggressive, assertive, and avoidant responses to problem behaviors of children, such as a child's making a peanut butter sandwich and leaving the kitchen table a mess. For a physical altercation between siblings, an "I" statement can be, "When fights occur, I'm concerned about your safety, and in this house we solve our differences peacefully without fights." Encourage volunteers to role-play for the group, then have a leader demonstrate with one of the volunteers a more assertive way to handle the conflict.

Homework

In addition to monitoring their child's homework (being assertive three times during the week), parents practice giving "I" messages to other family members at home. Ask them to think about when it is most difficult to remember to give these messages and how conflicts are typically solved in their homes.

Session 5 (Children's Group): Social Problem Solving

Review the previous week's homework and ask if there are any related questions.

Learning Goal

To assist children in solving social conflicts by learning the five steps of effective problem solving:

1. Identify the problem.
2. Generate alternate solutions.
3. Choose the best solution.
4. Implement the solution.
5. Review solution effectiveness and revise as needed.

Instruction

Explain to the children what a social conflict is, and ask them to give examples. Explain that they will be learning better ways to deal with such conflicts.

STEP 1

A social problem exists when there is a conflict between the needs or desires of two or more persons. If two children are fighting over possession of the same toy, the basic problem is not the fighting but the fact that two children want the same toy at the same time. To determine the source of the conflict (i.e., why they are upset), each child must take responsibility for his or her own actions and use his or her assertiveness and active listening skills. Children need to learn to attack the basic problem or conflict, not the other person by blaming or name calling.

STEP 2

The focus shifts from the problem to solutions. Leaders engage the children in brainstorming possible solutions. Each child thinks of a variety of solutions to the problem by following the basic rules of brainstorming:

- No criticism of other people's ideas during brainstorming.
- Quantity is wanted (at least five possible solutions).
- Piggybacking, modifying another's idea to improve it, is encouraged.
- Wild, creative ideas are welcome.

In addition to recording their ideas, the leaders suggest some possible solutions when the children are having difficulty doing so.

STEP 3

Discuss the pros and cons of each solution (for example, the consequences of each solution) so as to decide on a solution everyone can live with. Seek a "win–win" solution whereby each child has at least part of his or her desires met (compromise).

STEP 4

Decide who does what, when, and where in order to implement the agreed-upon solution.

STEP 5

At the end of a preestablished interval (a day, a week, a month) all parties to the dispute meet to discuss how well the solution is working, and revise the solution as necessary. If the solution is inappropriate, try another.

Activities

BRAINSTORMING "WHAT IF?" SITUATIONS

Group leaders describe a series of common social conflict situations in childhood, such as peers provoking you by cheating on board games, taking something without permission, losing something you have borrowed from a friend, or wanting something that isn't yours. The group brainstorms as many solutions to each problem situation as possible. Explain that having a large number of ideas increases chances that a successful solution will be found. List the ideas on an easel or blackboard and add a few ideas that the group members have not mentioned. To loosen up their thinking, suggest a crazy idea.

GAME

All group members line up against a far wall, and two leaders model an activity with some kind of conflict (someone steals a ball, cheats on a test, etc.). Each child is asked to give a solution, and a leader writes it on the board. For every different solution given, the child can move forward one step. The winner has the greatest number of unique solutions and reaches the finish line first.

Homework

Describe how you applied the problem-solving method to a conflict you had at school or home this week. Remember:

1. Figure out the problem.
2. What else can you do?
3. Choose the best solution.
4. Carry out the solution.
5. How did it work? Do you need to change your solution?

When:_____

With whom:_____

What was the conflict?_____

How did you solve it?_____

Session 5 (Parents' Group): Social Problem Solving

Learning Goal

To review the five-step problem-solving process.

Instruction

Explain that when parents articulate the problems they face and discuss solutions with their children, the children become more aware of the significance of the problem-solving process. When effective problem-solving behaviors are modeled by parents, children emulate these behaviors.

Problem solving is a skill that can be learned and must be practiced. Outline the five steps in effective problem solving (writing them on a board or easel may be useful):

- Identify the problem.
- Brainstorm a wide range of possible solutions.
- Consider the pros and cons, and choose a good solution.
- Plan how to carry out the solution, and then implement it.
- Review the success of the solution and modify as necessary.

Often the most difficult of these steps is identifying the problem. If a child complains, "Alice is hitting me," the basic problem to be solved is not the hitting, but rather the reason that Alice is hitting. Therefore, the investigation of solutions must relate to the cause of the problem instead of its effect.

The process of problem solving—making choices and learning from them —is facilitated by parents who observe, listen, and ask open-ended questions that further the process. Useful questions are:

- What's the problem?
- What will happen if . . . ?
- What other ways can you think of to . . . ?
- How would you feel if someone did that to you?

Remember that when parents invite "give and take" in a conflict with their child through the use of listening, reasoning, empathy, and compromise, the child tends to employ similar conflict resolution strategies with his or her peers (Crockenberg & Lourie, 1996). Researchers have found that it is the ability to resolve conflicts quickly and amicably, not the ability to avoid conflict altogether, that distinguishes close peer relationships from other peer relationships in childhood (Carlson-Jones, 1985).

Activity

Ask parents to role-play, using the five-step problem-solving process, a common parent–child conflict at home. This can be done in front of the group, and leaders can give suggestions and ask the parents to make comments.

Homework

Apply the problem-solving process with your child at home this week. (The children must use this process in school or at home).

Session 6 (Children's Group): Cooperation

Review the previous week's homework and ask if there are any related questions.

Learning Goal

To teach the children to share, to work together toward a common goal, to take turns, and to do their share of the group work.

Instruction

Explain to the group what "cooperation" means. In a cooperative situation, the combined behavior of two or more individuals is needed to reach a goal. The goal can be attained by an individual only if all the individuals involved can also attain the goal. In a competitive situation, goal attainment by one or a number of individuals precludes attainment by the remaining individuals. Many believe that our culture suffers from a "cooperation deficiency." It tends to be a highly individualistic, competitive society.

Activities

CREATE A MONSTER

Each child in the group draws part of a monster. One child draws the head, one the upper body, another the lower body, another the tail, and so forth. For an older group, have children work in pairs to draw sections. The drawings are then taped together to form the monster and the group names the creature.

LINE BY LINE STORYTELLING (FOR YOUNGER CHILDREN)

A leader starts the story by saying, "Once upon a time, long, long ago, there lived a monster named _____." Then each child in turn contributes the next line to the composite story. Each child should contribute at least two lines until the last child in the sequence gives the last line and says, "The end."

BLINDFOLDED OBSTACLE COURSE

While the children have their eyes closed, leaders place chairs around the room to create an easy obstacle course. Two children are blindfolded, and two others serve as their guides. Attempting to get across the room to a designated point, the guides must verbally lead their partners around the obstacles.

CREATE A GAME (FOR OLDER CHILDREN)

Split the group into two smaller groups. Give each group some crayons, paper, cards with the numbers 1–10 written on them, and any other materials that are available. Tell them that they need to work together to create a game they can teach to the other team. Encourage quieter children to participate, and help restrain the more assertive children if necessary.

Homework

Offer to help someone at home three different times this week. Remember: you have to offer, the other person can't ask you!

Session 6 (Parents' Group): Cooperation

Learning Goal

To teach the parents how to coach their children in sharing, working together toward a common goal, taking turns, and doing their share of group work.

Instruction

Cooperation is defined as each person in a group doing his or her share, plus aiding or giving assistance to the others, and all working together without conflict. This behavior is especially relevant for maintenance tasks around the house. Children occasionally disagree as to whose job it is to empty the trash or put away the dishes. They try to avoid the task, wait until others do it, or come to parents to settle the disagreement. These behaviors take time and effort and can be avoided if children learn to help around the house at an early age. Young children (ages 3–4) can help to clean and set the table, put toys away, and help to make their beds. Discuss specific chores that each child in the group can do at home.

Some children have difficulty in cooperating with their peers because they are too bossy and used to having everything their own way. Explain that if parents observe their child being too bossy with a playmate, their should talk with their child in private at a later time. They might say, "I don't think Sarah likes it when you insist that she follow your rules every time you play together."

After citing some specific examples of bossy or self-centered behaviors, parents should ask their child, "How would you feel if someone spoke to you that way?" Then they should ask their child to think of another way to say what he or she wants without sounding quite so bossy.

Also explain the need for parents to pay attention to and praise cooperative behaviors by their children. Have the group discuss examples of various cooperative behaviors around the house. What do the children currently do, and how can they, as parents, encourage more cooperation?

Homework

Complete a jigsaw puzzle by working together with your child.

Session 7 (Children's Group): Complimenting

Review the previous week's homework and ask if there are any related questions.

Learning Goal

To teach children the importance and "how-to's" of giving positive feedback to others ("warm fuzzies") as opposed to negative comments ("cold prickles.")

Instruction

Positive reactions (warm fuzzies) make other people feel good and include such behaviors as:

- *Appreciation:* Telling another person what you like about his or her behavior or appearance.
- *Praise:* Telling someone that you think he or she did something well.
- *Polite comments:* Saying, "Thank you," "Please," "I'm sorry."
- *Agreeableness:* Finding something about another's remarks that you agree with.
- *Encouragement:* Offering encouragement such as "You can do it."
- *Affection:* Hugs, pats on the back, saying, "I love you."

Activities

SPECIAL PEOPLE

Throughout the session, leaders stop the session and call out the name of one child. The rest of the group gives compliments to that person and/or asks questions to get to know him or her better. Each child should be called on throughout the session. Leaders should help the children to give compliments that go further than physical characteristics; for example, "You are really great at problem solving!"

ACCEPTING VERSUS REJECTING

Each child gives a partner a compliment, which the other rejects. For example, "That shirt looks really good on you." "I hate this shirt—I had nothing else to wear today." The children then give each other a compliment, which they accept with a "thank you" and a smile. The children then discuss how it feels to have a compliment accepted versus rejected. What could they say when a compliment is rejected?

OPINIONS

In a circle, one child states an opinion about something, such as a favorite base-ball team, type of animal, or favorite TV show, and rolls a ball to another child. The second child finds something about the first child's comments to agree with, and this continues around the circle until everyone has participated.

ROLE PLAYS

Children and leaders role-play different situations in which compliments, agreeable comments, praise, or encouragement can be given. The group re-sponds by suggesting other appropriate compliments for the actors.

Homework

Tell members of your family what you like about them or their behavior three different times.

Session 7 (Parents' Group): Complimenting

Learning Goal

To explain the importance of giving positive feedback to children.

Instruction

Describe the concept and importance of being a positive person and how this increases one's attractiveness to others. Ask the parents to consider how often they give "warm fuzzies" versus "cold prickles" to their children. Ideally, par-ents should give five positives to every one negative comment. This is a very dif-ficult skill to learn. It is also the guideline that the children's group leaders use.

Discuss the main types of positive feedback (praise and appreciation), rewards (token and concrete), and negative feedback (criticism, put-downs, sarcasm, commands, threats, etc.). Notice that there are many more types of negative feedback than positive—our society focuses much more often on the negatives than on the positives.

There are three main reasons to give a child positive feedback:

1. It bolsters the child's self-esteem. Children, like adults, like to be noticed. This kind of recognition increases their good feelings about themselves.
2. It builds a close, warm relationship. This is good for both the parent and the child.
3. It is a method of positive discipline. It gets children to do more of what parents want.

Explain to the parents that there are three kinds of things they should notice in their child: behaviors, ideas, and personal characteristics. For example, parents can notice and express approval when their daughter helps to clean off the kitchen table. They can notice that she thinks recycling is a great way to care for the environment.

What parents notice can be big or little. They should try to look for a lot of little things to notice, as often these little things grow into bigger things. For example, parents' recognizing their son for clearing his plate from the table can lead to his clearing a few serving dishes as well.

Giving positive feedback should not be an isolated occurrence. Rather, parents should be constantly looking for chances to "catch him (or her) being good" whenever they are with their child. At a minimum, they should recognze the child for positive behavior several times a day. Eventually, this will become a style of relating to the child (looking for positive behaviors, ideas, and characteristics).

Homework

List the positive qualities you noticed in your child this week and what your child did to make you notice him or her. Some qualities other parents have noticed in their children are: generosity, being proud, caring, helpfulness, being clever, being creative, and standing up for their beliefs. Also note your responses (positive, it is hoped) to these qualities.

Session 8 (Children's Group): Awareness of Feelings

Review the previous week's homework and ask if there are any related questions. Children who have difficulty in managing their emotions tend to have few friends. Emotional regulation refers to the ability to modulate one's emotions in response to situational demands. Difficulty in regulating emotions is evident in hot-tempered, deliberately annoying, irritable, easily frustrated, hostile, moody, and fearful behaviors. The first step in emotional regulation is the awareness of one's emotional states and the ability to label them and express them to others.

Learning Goals

- To help children identify the wide variety of feelings that a person can experience.
- To assist children to identify situations that lead to different feelings and to discuss what happens when feelings are kept inside for a long time.

Instruction

Ask the children to name a variety of emotions and write the responses on an easel or blackboard. Suggest variations of emotions to supplement their list.

Activities

FEELINGS WALL

Ask each child to choose one feeling from the list generated previously and tell the group about a time he or she felt that way and why. Continue until each child has chosen two feelings. Then select a feeling, and have each child tell what makes him or her feel that way.

FEELINGS CHARADES

Ask each child to select, without looking, from a pile of notes that have various feelings written on them (created from the list developed earlier). Without showing the note to anyone, each should then act out the feeling, using body language but no sounds. The other group members then try to identify the feelings.

GOOD FEELINGS/BAD FEELINGS

One child sits in the center of a circle while the other group members ask him or her what happened during the week that made the child feel good. When the child has given a description of his or her good feelings, the others ask what made the child feel bad and what the child did to make him- or herself feel better. Let each child have a turn until everyone has had a chance to talk. The purpose of this game is to help children identify their feelings and link them to events in their lives.

Homework

Write down every time this week when you felt scared. Describe what happened just before you got scared and what you did about it.

Session 8 (Parents' Group): Awareness of Feelings/Emotional Intelligence

Learning Goal

To increase parents' awareness of their role in developing their child's "emotional intelligence."

Instruction

The children's session focuses on awareness of feelings. "Emotional intelligence" (EI) refers to the ability to recognize feeling states in oneself and others, and to control the expression of one's emotions. This ability plays a major role in determining a person's success and happiness in all aspects of life. The components of EI are (writing these out for parents will be useful):

- *Awareness of feeling states in self and others.* This means tuning into the bodily sensations of various feelings in yourself, and empathically putting yourself in another's shoes to imagine what that person is feeling at the moment.
- *Emotional understanding:* This refers to the ability to connect feelings to antecedent events (the triggers that produce an emotional reaction, like feeling sad after losing a ball game) and to the ability to anticipate how your emotional reactions will affect future behaviors toward yourself and others.
- *Emotional control:* This is the ability to moderate and control the intensity of your emotional reactions (feelings and behaviors) by the use of self-control coping strategies such as the following:
  - Catharsis: emotional release of psychological and physical tension by pounding a pillow, crying, tearing up a newspaper, and the like.
  - Relaxation: deep breathing, tensing and relaxing muscle groups.
  - Imagery: picturing a calm and comforting place.
  - Positive self-talk: calming self-statements ("I'm OK," "It's fine").
  - Physical activity: going for a walk, shooting hoops.

Researchers have discovered that parents fall into one of two categories in terms of coaching about emotions. Parents in the first group give their children guidance about emotions. They reflect and validate their children's emotions and are empathic to their children's emotional reactions. Those in the second group do not give any substantial guidance in this area. Research has indicated that children whose parents coach them on emotions are better in academics, social competence, emotional well-being, and physical health.

There are five main components of "emotions coaching":

1. Be aware of your child's emotions.
2. Tune into both the verbal and nonverbal ways children express their emotions.
3. Recognize that negative emotions (anger, fearfulness, jealousy, anxiety) are opportunities for teaching.
4. Help your child express and control his or her feelings before they escalate and explode.
5. Try not to ignore, trivialize, criticize, or punish the expression of negative emotions.

Parents should help their child verbally label his or her emotions ("You seem a little bored today," "You're feeling proud because you worked hard and got a lot done today"). Labeling feelings gives children a sense of being able to cope with them. Studies show that the act of labeling emotions can have a calming effect on the nervous system and help children recover more quickly from upsets.

Parents are told to listen empathically and validate their child's feelings. For instance, if a child is upset about being teased at school, the parent might say, "I can understand why that would make you feel sad. That's how I feel when people are mean to me." Invalidating the feeling ("That's nothing to be upset about. Don't let it bother you") will not help the child learn about the appropriate way to express and understand emotions. In regard to ambivalent feelings, at about age 7, children can recognize conflicting emotions, so parents can help them understand that it is OK to feel two ways at once ("I imagine you're excited about sleeping over at Marie's house, but a little scared too?").

Parents should set limits on emotional expression while helping their child problem-solve. They help their child problem-solve to find more constructive ways of handling emotionally charged situations ("Your brother is not there for you to hit! What can you do instead when you are angry with him?"). Problem solving before the situation occurs helps the child realize that there is a range of solutions to a problem to choose from.

Activity

The ability to describe personal emotional experiences (recalling and describing emotional situations) is central to controlling emotional reactions. Knowledge here can lead to better control. For example, self-awareness of sadness can lead to changes in a person's thoughts or situations.

Ask the following questions to start a group discussion of emotional awareness:

- How do you know when your children are angry/sad/happy?
- How do you help your children tune into their emotional states?

Homework

Talk with your child about how you are feeling at different times throughout the day. Ask him or her to do the same and discuss how you dealt with the various feelings.

Session 9 (Children's Group): Awareness of Feelings in Others

Review the previous week's homework and ask if there are any related questions.

Learning Goal

To help children recognize emotions in other people and learn about empathy.

Instruction

Remind the children that last week they learned about feelings and how they can feel differently in different situations. This week, they are going to talk about recognizing these same emotions in other people.

Ask the children how they can tell when their parents are feeling angry (they may yell, wrinkle up their faces, etc.). How about when they are feeling happy? Sad? Talk about how each emotion has distinct effects on a person's face and body, and that some emotions can also have the same effects of others; for example, sad and angry, confused and sad, among others. How can they tell the difference between the emotions? They may need to think about the what has been happening in the other person's life, and how they might feel in that situation. This is empathy—the experiencing of the same emotions as another person.

Activities

ROLE PLAY

Have one leader and one child demonstrate a situation that would make one of them feel sad or angry. Ask the children to guess what emotion the person is probably feeling, and how they can tell. What could they say to the person to improve the situation?

FEELINGS MATCH

Cut out pictures from magazines of people experiencing various emotions and use them to make a collages on pieces of paper. Create a list of various emotions and have the children work in groups to match the appropriate feelings to the faces.

Homework

Tell about a time this week when your parent or teacher was feeling happy or mad. How could you tell what he or she was feeling? How did you respond?

Session 9 (Parents' Group): Awareness of Feelings in Others

Learning Goal

To help parents help their children recognize feelings in other people and learn about empathy.

Instruction

First, go over anything from last week that was missed or needs further discussion. This is an important topic and needs sufficient discussion.

Empathy is the ability to experience the same emotions as another person. The children are learning how to visually recognize the emotions of others (i.e., people who are sad may pout, angry people may screw up their faces). They are also learning how to read a situation and use the context of a conversation to figure out what emotions might be involved.

Activity

Have another discussion about emotional awareness and emotions the parents noticed in their children during the week. Ask how they know when their children are feeling happy, sad, angry, scared, or jealous. For example, do the parents notice their children's body language (facial expressions, sagging shoulders, etc.) or do they use empathy to identify with their children? Ask the parents how they can discuss their own feelings more openly with their children. Be sure to explain that certain boundaries should be in place when discussing emotions, as children do not need to know that their parents are worried because of financial concerns or about some sensitive topics.

Homework

Discuss various emotions with your child. Ask your child during a movie or television show what he or she thinks the characters are feeling, and what makes the child think of those emotions.

Session 10 (Children's Group): Good Sportsmanship

Review the previous week's homework and ask if there are any related questions.

Learning Goal

To help children understand the concept of good sportsmanship.

Instruction

A good sport is a person who accepts victory or defeat graciously and who does not cheat at games. To become a good sport, you must handle the stresses of competitive play, such as losing a game, making mistakes and bad choices when playing, waiting your turn, and accepting constructive criticism to improve your competence at play.

Effective ways to handle frustration and stress without losing your temper or becoming upset are:

- Relaxation reponses
  - Take a deep breath, hold to the count of three, release slowly. Repeat two or three times.
  - Count to 10 before responding.
- Self-talk: Ask the group to generate and practice saying some comforting self-statements, such as:
  - "Stay cool."
  - "I can handle this."
  - "It's OK to lose."
  - "This is helpful advice."
- Identifying irrational beliefs
  - Help the group examine common irrational beliefs: "I have to be perfect at everything," "Things must go my way," "It's awful to lose or fail!"
  - Suggest more rational thoughts: "It doesn't matter if I win or lose as long as I try my best," "If I make a mistake people won't think I'm a failure," "Having a good time with friends is more important than winning a game."

Activities

TWENTY QUESTIONS

The group must work together to figure out a person, place, or thing, asking only yes/no questions. Group members should be encouraged to compliment good questions and give suggestions for altering questions when necessary.

ROLE PLAYS

In small groups or in the whole group, children and leaders develop role plays that show people being both good and bad sports. If a role play demonstrates bad sportsmanship, the children must decide how the players could have shown good sportsmanship. If a role play demonstrates good sportsmanship, the children must compliment those performing the role play.

Session 10 (Parents' Group): Good Sportsmanship

Learning Goal

To help parents understand the importance of developing good sportsmanship in their children.

Instruction

Children like to play with other children who are good sports (who keep a good attitude even though losing a game, making a poor move while playing, or during other frustrating events).

Children who can cope well with stress and frustration tend to be better sports. Three ways in which children can cope with frustration without becoming unduly upset are:

1. Relaxation responses.
2. Positive self-talk.
3. Changing irrational beliefs ("I'm OK," "This isn't a big deal," etc.)

Explain and practice these techniques.

Activity

Ask the parents to discuss how they teach children to be good sports when playing games with them (e.g. modeling, prompting, coaching, reinforcing good sportsmanship, and ending the game if a child continues to act like a poor sport after one warning by the parent).

CONCLUSION

The primary objectives of this short-term social skills program are to enhance children's social knowledge, help children translate their concepts into skillful interpersonal behaviors, and foster skill maintenance and generalization of the children's social competence.

Using an active and direct teaching approach, group leaders coach children in social skills within a group play format of fun and games. Generalization of the social skills is promoted by the use of homework assignments and by training the children's parents to be social skill coaches in the home environment.

REFERENCES

Bandura, A. (1969). *Principles of behavior modification*. New York: Holt, Rinehart & Winston.

Carlson-Jones, D. (1985). Persuasive appeals and responses to appeals among friends and acquaintances. *Child Development, 56,* 757–763.

Choi, D. H., & Kim, J. (2003). Practicing social skills training for young children with low peer acceptance: A cognitive-social learning model. *Early Childhood Education Journal, 31*(1), 41–46.

Christophersen, E. R. (1987). *Little people: A common-sense guide to child rearing* (3rd ed.). Kansas City, MO: Westport Publishers.

Crockenberg, S., & Lourie, A. (1996). Parents' conflict strategies with children and children's conflict strategies with peers. *Merrill-Palmer Quarterly, 42,* 495–518.

Gresham, F. M. (1997). Social competence and students with behavior disorders: Where we've been, where we are, and where we should go. *Education and Treatment of Children, 20*(3), 233–249.

Gresham, F. M., & Elliot, S. N. (1990). *Social Skills Rating System Manual.* Circle Pines, MN: American Guidance Service.

Hay, D. F., Payne, A., & Chadwick, A. (2004). Peer relations in childhood. *Journal of Child Psychology and Psychiatry, 45*(1), 84–108.

Ladd, G. W., & Mize, J. (1983). A cognitive-social learning model of social-skill training. *Psychological Review, 90*(2), 127–157.

Madsen, C. H., Becker, W. C., & Thomas, D. R. (1968). Rules, praise, and ignoring: Elements of elementary classroom control. *Journal of Applied Behavior Analysis, 1*(2), 139–150.

Oden, S., & Asher, S. R. (1977). Coaching children in social skills for friendship making. *Child Development, 48*(2), 495–506.

Pfiffner, L. J., Rosen, L. A., & O'Leary, S. G. (1985). The efficacy of an all-positive approach to classroom management. *Journal of Applied Behavior Analysis, 18*(3), 257–261.

Quinn, M. M., Kavale, K. A., Mathur, S. R., Rutherford, R. B., Jr., & Forness, S. R. (1999). A meta-analysis of social skill interventions for students with emotional or behavioral disorders. *Journal of Emotional and Behavioral Disorders, 7*(1), 54–64.

Slavin, R. E. (1983). When does cooperative learning increase student achievement? *Psychological Bulletin, 94*(3), 429–445.

Spence, S. H. (2003). Social skills training with children and young people: Theory, evidence, and practice. *Child and Adolescent Mental Health, 8*(2), 84–96.

Yalom, I. D. (1985). *The theory and practice of group psychotherapy* (3rd ed.). New York: Basic Books.

Index